Cariology

FOURTH EDITION

Other Related Titles in Medical and Dental Sciences

Cariology

FOURTH EDITION

E. Newbrun, DMD, PhD
Professor of Oral Biology and Periodonotology
Department of Stomatology
School of Dentistry

MEDTECH
A Division of Scientific International
Engaging Sciences—Developing Minds!

Cariology

MEDTECH
A Division of
Scientific International Pvt. Ltd.

Fourth Edition: 2018

ISBN: 978-93-87210-32-5

Published by: Vinod Kumar Jain, Scientific International (Pvt.) Ltd.

Registered Office: • **New Delhi:** 4850/24, Ansari Road, Daryaganj, New Delhi-110002

Branch Offices:
• **Bengaluru:** House No. 1665, Ground Floor, 18th Main, BSK 2nd Stage, Bengaluru-560070
• **Guwahati:** House No. 31, 1st Floor, KKB Road, Chenikuthi, Opp. Sirdi Sai Bidya Mandir High School, PO-Silpukhuri, District-Kamrup, Guwahati-781003
• **Kerala:** Ponary House, Paudua Raod, Konthuruthy - 682013 Thevara P.O Ernakulam district, Kerala, India
• **Kolkata:** 127/G, Manicktala Main Road, Kankurgachi, Near Yogodyan, Kolkata-700054

Laser typeset by SIPL

Printed in India

Contents

Chapter 1	**History and Early Theories of the Etiology of Caries**	**13**
	Early theories of caries etiology	13
	Evaluation of the various theories of caries	19
Chapter 2	**Current Concepts of Caries Etiology**	**29**
	Host factors: saliva	30
	Host factors: immunization	44
	Host factors: tooth	52
Chapter 3	**Microflora**	**63**
	Evidence of bacterial role in caries etiology	63
	Localization of the oral flora related to caries	64
	Flora of pits and fissures	66
	Root caries	67
	Transmissibility of the cariogenic flora	70
	Bacterial interactions	71
	Bacteriology of smooth surface dental plaque	73
	Oral streptococci	75
	Oral lactobacilli	86
	Oral *Actinomyces*	87
Chapter 4	**Substrate: Diet and Caries**	**99**
	Influence of diet on the caries process	99
	Epidemiological observations of caries and diet	100
	Interventional human studies	102
	Special population groups	104
	Noninterventional human studies	107
	Assessment of cariogenic potential of foodstuffs	107
	Experimental caries of animals	112
	Cariogenicity of sucrose and other carbohydrates	115
	Other dietary components and dental caries	121
	Frequency of eating and caries formation	124
Chapter 5	**Sugar, Sugar Substitutes, and Noncaloric Sweetening Agents**	**135**

	Taste and sweetening agents	136
	Sucrose	140
	Sugar substitutes	145
	Noncaloric sweetening agents	159
	Discussion	166
Chapter 6	**Dental Deposits**	**177**
	Terminology	178
	Acquired pellicle	181
	Morphology of dental plaque	189
	Microbiology of dental plaque	200
	Chemical composition of plaque	214
	Pathogenic potential of plaque	217
	Control of dental plaque	219
Chapter 7	**Histopathology of Dental Caries**	**245**
	Time factors in caries development	246
	Caries of enamel	248
	Caries of coronal dentin	258
	Root caries	265
Chapter 8	**Caries Activity Tests**	**273**
	Lactobacillus colony count	274
	Snyder test	276
	Reductase test	277
	Buffer capacity test	278
	Fosdick calcium dissolution test	278
	Dewar test	279
	Mutans group of streptococci screening tests	279
	Prediction of future caries activity based on previous caries experience	283
	Relationship between tests and cariogenic factors	285
	Relationship between tests and cariogenic substrate	287
	Relationship between tests and resistance of the host: tooth and saliva	288
	Value of laboratory tests for control of dental disease	289
Chapter 9	**Dentifrices**	**295**
	Functions of a dentifrice	295
	Composition	296
	Packaging	302
	Ingestion	303
	Contact sensitivity and irritation due to dentifrice ingredients	304
	Therapeutic dentifrices	304
	Cost of dentifrices	309
Chapter 10	**Occlusal Sealants**	**315**
	Susceptibility of occlusal surfaces	315
	Historical efforts at prevention of occlusal caries	315

	Development of occlusal sealants	317
	Materials assessed for use as sealants	320
	Technique for the use of sealants	323
	Factors affecting clinical use of available sealants	324
Chapter 11	**The Uses of Fluorides in Preventive Dentistry**	**331**
	Fluorides	331
	Systemic fluoride	332
	Topical fluoride	340
	Agents and systems used for topical fluoride therapy	347
	Fluoride toxicology	348
	Guide to the use of fluoride agents	349
Chapter 12	**Control and Prevention of Dental Caries**	**357**
	Extent of the problem	358
	Approaches to prevention of caries	359
	Preventive programs for the individual at home	359
	Preventive programs for the dental office	362
	Preventive programs for the community	367
Index		**377**

Foreword

There is an increasing tendency to equate the marked reduction in caries in children in many countries with the demise of the disease and to view caries as a vestigal remnant of a bygone time. Neither position is valid. Epidemiologically, caries has become a dichotomous disease in children in most developed countries; 50% of the children are caries-free whereas 20% of them account for 75% of the lesions. In the older, post-fluoride generations, teeth are being retained much longer than in the past, and they are subject to recurrent enamel caries and an increasing occurrence of root caries. In developing countries, where 50% of the people are under 15 years of age, changing life-styles and dietary patterns are markedly increasing caries incidence. This picture is hardly reflective of a dying disease. What we are really seeing is a dramatic change in the patterns of disease. Development of an appropriate response to these changes by academic and public health institutions requires students and practitioners to have available a continued updating on the etiologic and preventive aspects of caries.

Cariology continues to be a major area of research by investigators around the world. Dr Newbrun is an active participant in this community, both as a researcher and as a scholar reviewing and integrating new findings. *Cariology, Third Edition* reflects this dual role, exhibiting insight into the research and placing it into the appropriate perspective. This new third edition continues the superb comprehension, organization, and clarity that have been the hallmarks of its predecessors. It is as up to date as a textbook is possible to be because it reflects Dr Newbrun's participation in the conferences at which new information is presented. His personal mental computer is always at the ready, and the new is being constantly integrated into the established framework.

In this age of subspecialization it is becoming rare to find a single-authored textbook. Dr Newbrun is a unique multidisciplinarian who continues to keep abreast of all aspects of cariology and has provided students, teachers, and academically oriented practitioners with a very valuable guide to a rapidly changing field.

Irwin D. Mandel
Professor of Dentistry
Director of the Center For Clinical Research In Dentistry
School of Dental and Oral Surgery
Columbia University

Preface

Dental caries is a multifactorial disease. Consequently, in many dental schools the teaching of cariology has been hopelessly fragmented, with a little information included in each of the basic science courses—biochemistry, microbiology, oral pathology, and nutrition—and with further amplification in clinical or applied courses such as operative, public health, community, preventive, or pediatric dentistry. Yet the patient with dental caries is not a set of separate disciplines. An integrated approach to the teaching of cariology makes good sense but has been hampered for several reasons. There is the practical difficulty of a joint course crossing traditional departmental boundaries. An adequate text in this field suitable for undergraduate dental and dental hygiene students as well as for students in specialty or graduate programs is also required.

Cariology, Third Edition is a sophisticated and comprehensive text. It is intended for students who have already completed courses in general biochemistry, histology, microbiology, nutrition, and pharmacology. Preferably a course using this text should be taught before students start clinical dentistry. It can serve to bridge the gap between the basic science and clinical courses. Each chapter concludes with a series of questions (objectives) intended to help students test their understanding of the subject. A list of selected readings suggests major reviews or books for further study. In addition, there is a comprehensive bibliography based on original research relevant to each section. Thus, each chapter provides information at several levels. For the beginning student the contents of each chapter should suffice, while for the advanced or graduate student there are abundant references for more detailed study.

During the past decade, dental research has undergone unprecedented growth, as reflected by the large number of abstracts (now exceeding 2,000) presented annually at the meetings of the International Association for Dental Research. Accordingly, any textbook in dentistry requires periodic updating in order to remain current. In this new edition, every chapter has undergone some degree of revision. Not only the text, but also many tables and figures have been updated.

A better understanding of salivary components, xerostomia, and saliva substitutes is reflected in chapter 2. Acceptance of a new nomenclature for the mutans group of streptococci necessitated changes in chapter 3. Some of the recommendations of a recent consensus conference on the assessment of the cariogenic potential of foods are included in chapter 4. New developments on the use of sweeteners such as acesulfame-K, aspartame, high-fructose corn syrup, and xylitol are included in chapter 5. Continuing interest in antiplaque agents prompted revisions in chapter 6. Simplified screening tests for mutans group streptococci and the concept of using computer technology to predict caries risk by mathematically combining results of several measurements are described in chapter 8. Dentifrices have undergone important changes in formulation during the last decade, requiring a major rewriting of chapter 9. Occlusal sealants have now been available for about 17 years, so that assessment of their longevity is possible; new sealants and their applications are discussed in chapter 10. A totally new chapter (11), briefly reviewing the systemic and topical uses of fluorides in caries prevention, has been included in response to the desire of some teachers and students to have a single textbook dealing with caries. Those who require a broader understanding of the biological, toxicological, social, political, and legal aspects of fluorides and fluoridation, as well as the clinical application, are referred to other sources (eg, *Fluorides and Dental Caries, 3rd ed,* Charles C Thomas Publishers, 1986; *Fluoride in Preventive Dentistry,* Quintessence Publ Co, 1983; and *Fluorides and Caries Prevention, 2nd ed,* John Wright & Sons, Ltd, 1982).

Finally, because the prevalence of caries among children in several developed countries has declined, some administrators and dental educators have prematurely pronounced the topic of prevention of dental caries to be irrelevant in a modern dental curriculum. Nevertheless, as discussed in chapter 12, caries continues to be the major cause of loss of teeth in both children and adults. Clearly, control and prevention of dental caries are integral parts of every dentist's and dental hygienist's responsibility to his or her patients.

As an oral biologist, I have attempted a multidisciplinary presentation of the available knowledge of cariology, crossing the borders of biochemistry, epidemiology, histopathology, immunology, microbiology, nutrition, and physiology. In these days of scientific specialization, conventional wisdom would suggest that such a text be written by a group of expert contributors from various fields. There is a danger that such a multiauthor text may lack a unified concept, may have considerable overlap, and may often experience inordinate delays because all chapters are not ready at the same time. In writing a single-author text I have tried to compensate for my own limitations by having experts in different fields read and comment on relevant chapters or sections.

I am indebted to many colleagues for valuable suggestions during the long gestation and revisions of *Cariology.* These include Drs G. Armitage, W. Bowen, D. Bratthall, J. Bulkacz, B. Burt, N. Chilton, T. Christie, T. Daniels, J. Felton, P.O. Glantz, J.M. Goodson, J.S. Greenspan, B. Guggenheim, S. Heifetz, C. Hoover, A. Horowitz, H. Horowitz, R. Isman, K. Konig, W. Loesche, I. Mandel, F. McIntire, R. Micik, K. Miyasaki, I.

Mjör, M. Newman, A. Nizel, R. Page, C. Schachtele, H. Schroeder, D. Scott, G. Stookey, and A. Tatevossian. Photographs, photomicrographs, radiographs, and line drawings were generously made available by Drs J. Arends, G. Armitage, J. Carlos, N. Chilton, A.D. Eastcott, S. Edwardsson, J. Egelberg, T. Fusayama, B. Guggenheim, B. Gustafsson, P. Keyes, M. Listgarten, T. Marthaler, J.R. McGhee, S. Micik, K. Miyasaki, C.A. Saxton, H. Schroeder, P. Schüpbach, D. Scott, S. Silverman, and A. Thylstrup. The sterling editorial assistance of Ms E. Leash is much appreciated.

Chapter 1

History and Early Theories of the Etiology of Caries

The evil that men do lives after them,
The good is oft interred with their bones.

Julius Caesar, Act 3

Dental caries, or tooth decay, is a pathological process of localized destruction of tooth tissues by microorganisms (Latin: *caries* = rottenness). It is something of a paradox that teeth can be destroyed relatively rapidly in vivo and yet are almost indestructible post mortem. A few cases of caries have been found in fossil teeth of prehistoric dinosaurs, reptiles, and early mammals. Caries appears to have been evident in *Homo sapiens* since Paleolithic times, but the incidence of caries increased during the Neolithic Period.[3,40] Records have been found concerning dental problems in ancient Asia, Africa, and America; the earliest were the wall paintings of the Cro-Magnon Period (22,000 years ago). In ancient humans caries was usually located at the cementoenamel junction or in the cementum, whereas in modern man grooves and fissures are the most common sites of decay. To better understand current concepts of the etiology of caries, earlier theories will be discussed briefly.

Early theories of caries etiology

Worms

According to an ancient Sumerian text, toothache was caused by a worm that drank the blood of the teeth and fed on the roots of the jaws. This legend of the worm was discovered on one of many clay tablets excavated near Niffer, Ur, and other cities within the Euphrates Valley of the lower Mesopotamian area and estimated to date from about 5000 BC.[31] Oracle bones from the Shang dynasty, dating before 1000 BC, bear the Chinese character for caries. The character combines the ideas for "mouth" and "worm" and shows the worm invading the mouth.

The idea that caries is caused by a worm was almost universal at one time, as evidenced by the writings of Homer and popular lore of China, India, Finland, and Scotland. Guy de Cahuliac (1300–1368), the greatest surgeon of the Middle Ages, believed that worms caused dental decay. As a cure he advocated fumigation with seeds of leek, onion, and hyoscyamus. Note that hyoscyamine is an alkaloid obtained from henbane and is used as a hypnotic, sedative, and smooth muscle relaxant. Fumigation was used by Chinese and Egyptians in earlier times, and fumigation devices continued to be used in England as late as the nineteenth century. Antony van Leeuwenhoek (1700), the father of modern microscopy, wrote a letter to the Royal Society of London describing little worms "taken out of a corrupt tooth" and said that they caused the pain in toothache.[32]

Shakespeare alludes to worms in *Much Ado about Nothing* (Act III, Scene 2, Line 20). Benedick, complaining of a toothache, is rebuked by his friends:

> What! Sigh for the tooth-ache?
> Where is but a humour or a worm?

At least at the subconscious level this theory survives to our day when we refer to a toothache as a "gnawing pain."

Humors

The ancient Greeks considered that a person's physical and mental constitution was determined by the relative proportions of the four elemental fluids of the body—blood, phlegm, black bile, and yellow bile—which correspond to the four humors—sanguine, phlegmatic, melancholic, and choleric. All diseases, including caries, could be explained by an imbalance of these humors. Hippocrates, while accepting the prevailing Greek philosophy, drew attention to the stagnation of food and suggested that both local and systemic factors were related to the cause of caries. Aristotle, an astute observer, noticed that soft, sweet figs adhered to the teeth, putrified, and produced damage.[1]

Vital theory

The vital theory regarded dental caries as originating within the tooth itself, analogous to bone gangrene. This theory, proposed at the end of the eighteenth century, remained dominant until the middle of the nineteenth century. A clinically well-known type of caries is characterized by extensive penetration into the dentin, and even into the pulp, but with a barely detectable catch in the fissure. It is not so surprising, therefore, that the vital theory attracted many supporters.

Chemical theory

Parmly (1819) rebelled against the vital theory and proposed that an unidentified "chymical agent" was responsible for caries. He stated that caries began on the enamel surface in locations where food putrified and acquired sufficient dissolving power to produce the disease chemically. Support for the chemical theory came from Robertson (1835) and Regnart (1938), who actually carried out experiments with different dilutions of inorganic acids (such as sulfuric and nitric) and found that they corroded enamel and dentin.

Parasitic or septic theory

In 1843, Erdl described filamentous parasites in the "surface membrane" (plaque?) of teeth. Shortly thereafter, Ficinus, a Dresden physician, observed filamentous microorganisms, which he called *denticolae,* in material taken from carious cavities. He implied that these bacteria caused decomposition of the enamel and then the dentin. Neither Erdl nor Ficinus explained how these organisms destroyed tooth structure.

Chemo-parasitic theory

The chemo-parasitic theory is a blend of the above two theories because it states that caries is caused by acids produced by microorganisms of the mouth. It has been customary to credit this theory to W.D. Miller (1890), whose writings and experiments helped to establish this concept on a firm basis. However, Miller owes much to the observations of his predecessors and contemporaries. Pasteur had discovered that microorganisms transform sugars to lactic acid in the process of fermentation. Another Frenchman, Emil Magitot (1867), demonstrated that fermentation of sugars caused dissolution of tooth mineral in vitro. Artificial lesions similar to caries were produced when sound adult teeth, covered by wax except for a small opening, were exposed to dilute acids or fermenting mixtures for an extended period of time. Magitot also opposed the vital theory on the basis that caries occurred in natural teeth when used in artificial dentures.

In Berlin, Leber and Rottenstein (1867) presented additional experimental evidence implicating acids (which made enamel porous) and bacteria as the causative agents of caries. They described a specific microorganism, *Leptothrix buccalis,* in tubules of carious dentin and thought that it was responsible for enlarging the tubules and facilitating the rapid penetration of acids. Micrococci, oval, and round bacteria were found in histological sections of carious dentin by Underwood and Miles (1881). They considered caries to be absolutely dependent on the presence of organisms that "create an acid which removes the lime salt."

The work of an American, Willoughby D. Miller (1853–1907), at the

University of Berlin had a most profound effect on the understanding of caries etiology and subsequent caries research. Miller learned the methods of isolating, staining, and identifying bacteria in the laboratories of Koch. In a series of experiments Miller demonstrated the following facts:

1. Acid was present within the deeper carious lesion, as shown by reaction on litmus paper.
2. Different kinds of foods (bread, sugar, but not meat) mixed with saliva and incubated at 37°C could decalcify the entire crown of a tooth.
3. Several types of mouth bacteria (at least 30 species were isolated) could produce enough acid to cause dental caries.
4. Lactic acid was an identifiable product in carbohydrate-saliva incubation mixtures.
5. Different microorganisms (filamentous, long and short bacilli, and micrococci) invade carious dentin.

Miller concluded that no single species of microorganism caused caries, but rather that the process was mediated by an oral microorganism capable of producing acid and digesting protein[26]:

> Dental decay is a chemo-parasitic process consisting of two stages: *decalcification* or softening of the tissues and *dissolution* of the softened residue. In the case of enamel, however, the second stage is practically wanting, the decalcification of enamel signifying its total destruction.

Further weight was added to the chemo-parasitic theory by Williams (1897), who observed dental plaque on the enamel surface. Plaque was considered to be a means of localizing organic acids formed by microorganisms in contact with the tooth surface. The plaque partially prevented dilution and neutralization of the organic acids by the saliva.

Proteolytic theory

The classical chemo-parasitic theory has not been universally accepted. Instead, it has been proposed that the organic or protein elements are the initial pathway of invasion by microorganisms. Mature enamel is more highly mineralized than any other vertebrate tissue. The human tooth contains only about 1.5% to 2% organic material, of which 0.3% to 0.4% is protein. According to the proteolytic theory, the organic component is most vulnerable and is attacked by hydrolytic enzymes of microorganisms. This precedes the loss of the inorganic phase.

Gottlieb (1944) maintained that the initial action was due to proteolytic enzymes attacking the lamellae, rod sheaths, tufts, and walls of the dentinal tubules. He suggested that a coccus, probably *Staphylococcus aureus*, was involved because of the yellow pigmentation that he considered pathognomonic of dental caries. According to Gottlieb, acid alone produces chalky enamel but not true caries. Gottlieb's ideas were based on the observations of histological specimens and on the similarity between carious enamel and enamel whose organic components were stained with silver nitrate. There has been no bacteriological confirmation of his proposed link between *Staphylococcus pyogenes* and caries.

Frisbie (1944) also described caries as a proteolytic process involving depolymerization and liquefaction of the organic matrix of enamel. The less soluble inorganic salts could then be freed from their "organic bond," favoring their solution by acidogenic bacteria that secondarily penetrate along widening paths of ingress.

Pincus (1949) contended that proteolytic organisms first attacked the protein elements, such as the dental cuticle, and then destroyed the prism sheaths. The loosened prisms would then fall out mechanically. He also suggested that sulfatases of gram-negative bacilli hydrolyzed "mucoitin sulfate" of enamel or chondroitin sulfate of dentin and produced sulfuric acid. The released sulfuric acid could combine with the calcium of the mineral phase. It should be noted that the composition of the organic components of enamel does not resemble that of connective tissue, and an abundance of sulfated polysaccharides has not been demonstrated. Pincus' theory remains, therefore, without experimental support.

Proteolysis-chelation theory

A chelate results from combining an inorganic metal ion with at least two electron-rich functional groups in a single organic molecule. The chelating agent is a molecule capable of seizing and holding a metal ion in a claw-like grip (Greek: *chele* = claw) and forming a heterocyclic ring. The atoms holding the metal ion are called *ligands* and are usually oxygen, nitrogen, or sulfur. In biology there are many well-known chelates, including hemoglobin (containing iron), chlorophyll (containing magnesium), vitamin B-12 (containing cobalt), and the enzymes cytochrome oxidase (containing both iron and copper) and carboxypeptidase A (containing zinc).

Examples of chelate structures involving lactate or citrate and calcium are shown in Fig 1-1. The calcium is held covalently by two oxygens of the carboxyl groups and in a coordinate covalent bond involving the unshared electrons of the alcohol groups. Citrate can effectively form chelates of calcium and may be important for the physiological mobilization of calcium from the skeleton and transport of complexed calcium to the serum. By comparison, lactate is of negligible importance as an organic chelator of calcium.[28] Of course, this does not rule out the role of lactate in acid decalcification.

Chelation has been proposed as an explanation for tooth decay whereby the inorganic components of enamel can be removed at neutral or alkaline pH.[24] The proteolysis-chelation theory considers dental caries to be a bacterial destruction of teeth where the initial attack is essentially on organic components of enamel. The breakdown products of this

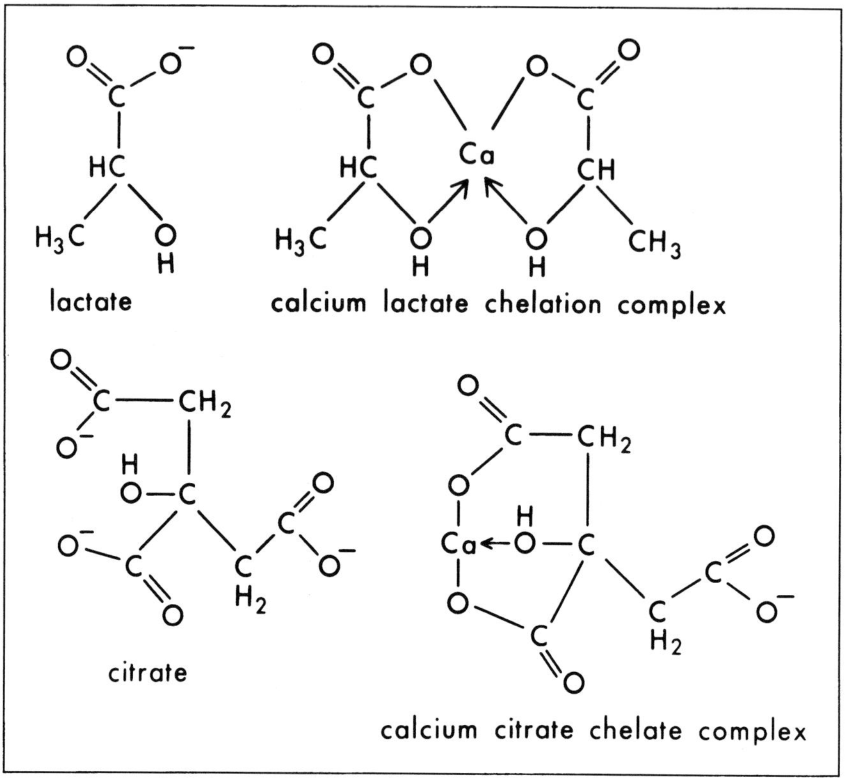

Fig 1-1 The formulas of lactate and citrate and of the calcium chelate compounds that they form. Note the difference between the covalent bonds from the carboxyl groups and the coordinate covalent bonds involving the unshared electrons of the alcohol groups *(arrows).*

organic matter have chelating properties and thereby dissolve the minerals in the enamel. Thus, both the organic and inorganic constituents of enamel are simultaneously demolished.

According to this theory, decalcification is mediated by a variety of complexing agents, such as acid anions, amines, amino acids, peptides, polyphosphates, and carbohydrate derivatives. These substances are microbial breakdown products of either the organic components of enamel or dentin, or of food that is ingested and diffuses through the plaque. Oral keratinolytic bacteria are thought to be involved in the process. Differences in keratin content of the enamel in children with high caries and low caries experience are considered important. It should be noted that only a small fraction of the protein of enamel bears any resemblance to the keratin of hair.

Schatz and Martin[33] challenged the chemo-parasitic theory, advocated the proteolysis-chelation theory, and stated that acid may prevent tooth decay by interfering with growth and activity of proteolytic bacteria. They suggested that acid protects the enamel organic matter.

The validity of the proteolysis-chelation theory has been seriously questioned[4,19] primarily because of the lack of supporting data.

Solutions of the sodium salts of various amino acids (alanine, aspartate, glutamate) and lactate at or near neutral pH can increase the uptake of radioactive phosphorus by enamel[27] or loss of calcium from enamel.[29] This has been interpreted as evidence of demineralization occurring at neutral pH. Mörch et al[27] proposed the hypothesis that demineralization is initiated by acid dissolution when the pH of plaque is low and is continued by complex-forming agents when the pH of plaque is neutral.

Other theories of caries

Numerous experiments on rodents have demonstrated that phosphate salts have the potential to retard dental caries. It is not surprising, therefore, that several theories have been proposed dealing with the role of phosphate in the process of caries formation. Using radioactive phosphorus, Luoma[22] showed that inorganic phosphate was taken up by plaque bacteria during metabolism of carbohydrates, the phosphate being required for phosphorylation of sugars and for polyphosphates that store energy. It has been postulated that a steady-state equilibrium exists between the inorganic phosphate of saliva and the mineral phase of enamel. According to the phosphate sequestration theory,[12] as bacteria take up phosphate, inorganic phosphate must be removed from enamel. However, in vivo, there is a continual flow of saliva containing soluble inorganic phosphates that are more readily available to bacteria than the insoluble mineral phase of enamel, provided the saliva can diffuse through the plaque to the bacteria.

Alternative explanations consider caries as a nutritional deficiency caused either by insufficient phosphate intake[2] or by an improper dietary calcium-to-phosphate ratio.[33] Neither of these latter explanations has adequate statistical or experimental support, and both remain primarily conjectural.

Bacterial alkaline phosphatase was found to release phosphate from enamel in vitro. It was speculated that this enzyme could participate in caries destruction[21] by acting on phosphoproteins of enamel. A commercial enzyme preparation obtained by sulfate precipitation was utilized, but it was subsequently observed that ammonium sulfate itself can release phosphate from teeth.[23] Another difficulty with this theory is that the alkaline phosphatase of the bacteria is an intracellular enzyme. Therefore, lysis of cells would have to occur to free the enzyme.

Evaluation of the various theories of caries

Chemo-parasitic theory

There is no doubt that acids are involved in the formation of caries.

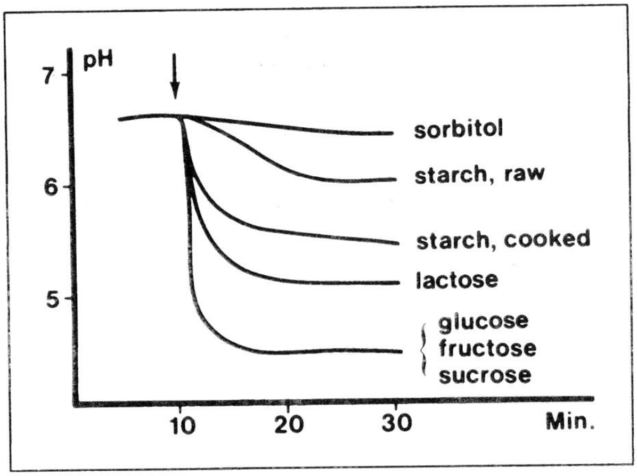

Fig 1-2 pH changes in plaque following application of different carbohydrate solutions. Time of application is indicated by *arrow* (Stephan curve). (Adapted from Neff, D. Acid production from different carbohydrate sources in human plaque in situ. *Caries Res* 1:78-87, 1967.)

Within carious lesions and in plaque, the pH decreases following a rinse with a suitable substrate for bacterial fermentation. By inserting fine antimony electrodes into plaque on the smooth surface of anterior teeth, Stephan[35] showed that within 2 to 4 minutes of rinsing with glucose or sucrose solution, the pH fell from about 6.5 to about 5 and gradually returned to the original pH within 40 minutes. More recently, by using telemetry and a miniature glass electrode pH sensor built into a removable appliance, it has been possible to obtain continuous and direct measurements of the pH of interproximal plaque in situ at the tooth/plaque interface.[5,6,16] These studies indicate that the presence of acid at the tooth/plaque interface may last longer (up to 2 hours) and the pH may drop lower than was observed by Stephan (Fig 1-2). The amount and duration of the drop in pH are influenced by *(1)* the amount of interdental plaque, *(2)* the predominant flora, *(3)* the rate of salivary flow, *(4)* the type and concentration of substrate, and *(5)* the location of the plaque (ie, buccal or lingual as compared with interproximal surfaces).

A variety of organic acids have been identified by specific chromatographic techniques in dental plaque, in bacterial cultures isolated from plaque, and in carious lesions. These include lactic, acetic, propionic, formic, and butyric acids. However, the relative concentrations of these acids may vary. This is to be expected, because plaque harbors a mixed bacterial population of homo- and heterolactic fermentative microorganisms, as well as mixed acid fermentative microorganisms, which differ in their fermentative capabilities. Not only are the proportions of these organisms in a dynamic state of flux, but the relative proportions of their end products are not constant and are influenced by such variables as pH, type and concentration of substrate, and oxygen tension.

The pathways by which bacteria form different acid end products from hexose sugars are shown in Fig 1-3. Intermediate steps and other end products have been omitted for simplification. Glycolysis of one 6-carbon sugar (C_6) yields two molecules of pyruvate (C_3). In homofermentative lactic acid formers, about 90% of the pyruvic acid is converted

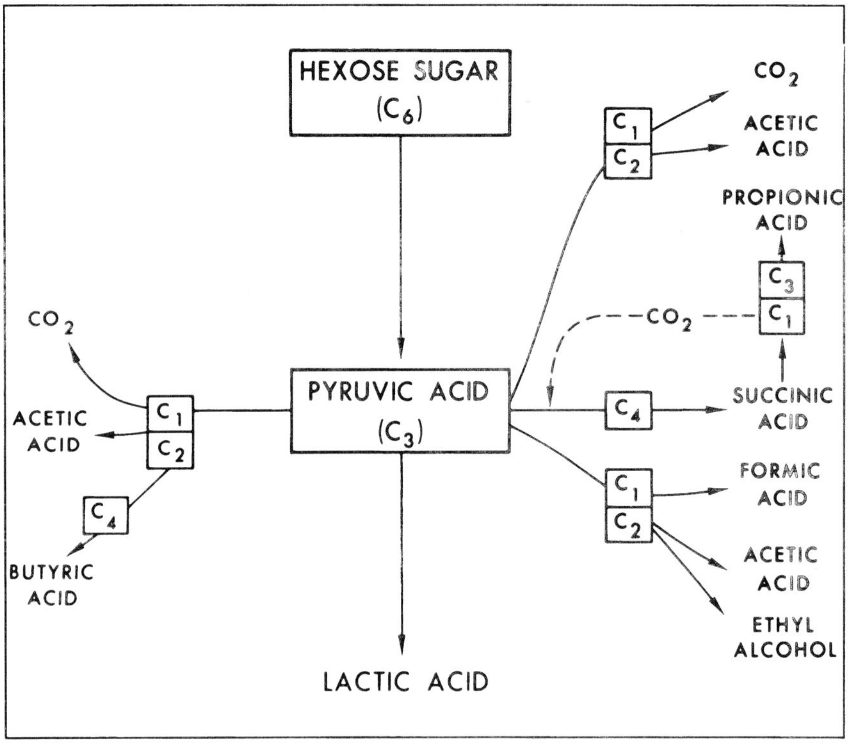

Fig 1-3 Simplified pathway showing how various end products are derived from hexose sugars in different glycolytic bacterial fermentations.

to lactic acid, while the remainder is converted to other acids, carbon dioxide, and ethyl alcohol. The caries-inducing *Streptococcus mutans* falls into this category.[36] Glucose is metabolized mainly to lactate by the Embden-Meyerhof pathway.[39] Some of the noncariogenic oral streptococci do not differ in their fermentation end products or in the amounts of acids produced when grown in liquid culture[11,20] (Table 1-1). However, on solid media (which more closely resemble growth in plaque) the acid accumulation by *S mutans* is substantially greater than by *Streptococcus sanguis* or *Streptococcus mitis*.[29] The high acid-accumulating capacity of *S mutans* may be an important factor in its cariogenicity.

Actinomyces are gram-positive rods or filaments consistently found in plaque. Under anaerobic conditions without CO_2 they are homolactic fermenters, but in the presence of CO_2 the fermentation is heterolactic with formate, acetate, lactate, and succinate as products. In air, acetate and carbon dioxide are the main products of glucose metabolism.

Lactobacilli, numerically relatively minor components of plaque, are either homofermentative or heterofermentative; the latter form less than 90% lactic acid and more acetic and other acids. Veillonellae (gram-negative anaerobic cocci), peptostreptococci (gram-positive anaerobic cocci), *Arachnia* (gram-positive facultative rods or filaments), and pro-

Table 1-1 End products of glucose metabolism by rat streptococci

	mM/100 mM glucose used	
End product	Strain FA1*	Strain JR8LG†
Lactate	181.09	184.54
Acetate	9.18	9.52
CO_2	8.31	10.96
Ethanol	2.77	5.75
Formate	3.42	4.52
Acetoin	0.60	0.20
Diacetyl	0.01	0.01
Glycerol	0	0
% glucose utilized	44.17	52.63
% carbon recovered	96.98	100.08

*Caries active.
†Caries inactive.

pionibacteria (gram-positive anaerobic rods) found in plaque form propionic acid on fermentation. Neisseriae (gram-negative cocci) degrade glucose, pyruvate, and lactate to acetate. Due to the various types of organisms present, plaques differ inherently in their content of fermentation products.

Most studies have used pure strains of organisms, so that very little is known about the biochemical capabilities of dental plaque per se. According to one report on plaque incubated in vitro for 5 hours, the concentration of lactic acid was similar to or less than that of either acetic or propionic acids.[15] Immediately after sucrose is ingested, total lactic acid production by plaque exceeds total volatile acids; acetic is greater than propionic, and only traces of *n*-butyric acid can be detected.[13] Several hours later volatile acids (especially acetic) account for most of the total acid in plaque.[14] *S mutans* and *S sanguis* grown in pure culture under conditions of nitrogen limitation or glucose limitation produced volatile end products.[7] When glucose was available, and the nitrogen source limited growth, lactate was the main fermentation product. However, when glucose was limited (as might occur in starved plaque) the main fermentation products were ethanol, acetate, and formate. *S mutans* grown by continuous culture forms various fermentation products in addition to lactate. During rapid growth of *S mutans* lactate is the major end product, whereas the volatile fatty acids predominate during slow growth rate.[25]

A proposed scheme for the regulation of glucose metabolism of *S mutans* during continuous growth under glucose limitation and nitrogen limitation in the presence of excess glucose is shown in Fig 1-4. When *S mutans* is growing under glucose limitation (Fig 1-4, *a*) the low intracellular concentration of glucose 6-phosphate restricts the activity of pyruvate kinase, and the increased level of phosphoenolpyruvate is used for effective transport of glucose into the cell. In addition, the pyruvate formate-lyase activity responsible for the formation of formate, acetate,

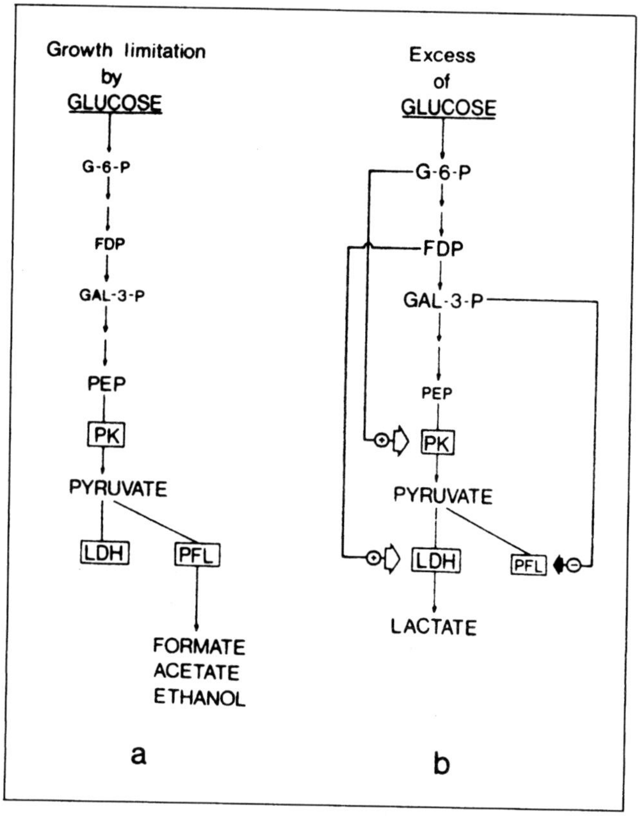

Fig 1-4 Scheme for the regulation of glucose metabolism of *S mutans* during continuous growth under glucose limitation *(a)* and nitrogen limitation in the presence of excess glucose *(b)*. *G-6-P,* glucose 6-phosphate; *FDP,* fructose 1,6-diphosphate; *GAL-3-P,* glyceraldehyde 3-phosphate; *PEP,* phosphoenolpyruvate; *PK,* pyruvate kinase; *LDH,* lactate dehydrogenase; *PFL,* pyruvate formate-lyase. +, activation; −, inhibition. *Large capital letters,* high concentration of intracellular intermediates in the cell; *small capital letters,* low concentration of intracellular intermediates in the cell. (Courtesy of Yamada and Carlsson.[38])

and ethanol is greatly increased; presumably it is an inducible enzyme.[38] On the other hand, when *S mutans* is growing in the presence of excess glucose (Fig 1-4, *b*) this enzyme is inhibited by d-glyceraldehyde 3-phosphate. Furthermore, fructose 1,6-diphosphate levels are raised, favoring lactate dehydrogenase activity and, therefore, lactate formation.[37]

Nonvolatile lactate can be converted by *Veillonella* species to propionate, acetate, and CO_2.[10,25] Under aerobic conditions oral isolates of *Neisseria* degrade lactate to acetate and CO_2, mostly via pyruvate but in part directly by lactate oxidase.[18] All of these findings can explain the presence of various volatile end products as well as lactate in dental plaque.

Interest in the qualitative and quantitative production of acids is more than academic. Table 1-2 shows the dissociation constants of some of these acid end products, and it can be readily seen that there are significant differences in the amount of available hydrogen ions (ie, resulting pH). Lactic acid is a much stronger acid than acetic or propionic acid at the same concentration. Accordingly, one would predict that it would be clinically more effective in enamel demineralization.

Formation of propionic acid can occur by a complex pathway involving carbon dioxide fixation to form oxaloacetate (C_4), and succinate intermediates (see Fig 1-3). Lactic acid formed by homofermenters can be

Table 1-2 Dissociation constants of organic acids found in plaque*

Acid	Constant for the first hydrogen	pK_1
Lactic	74.1×10^{-5}	3.13
Formic	17.6×10^{-5}	3.75
Succinic	6.9×10^{-5}	4.16
Butyric	2.0×10^{-5}	4.70
Acetic	1.8×10^{-5}	4.75
Propionic	1.3×10^{-5}	4.87

*Acids are arranged in decreasing order of available hydrogen ions, at 25°C in aqueous solution.

broken down to the weaker acetic and propionic acids. To what extent this plays a role in altering the pH of plaque is not known. Modern sophisticated methods have confirmed the formation of acid by microorganisms in plaque. They support the conclusions of the early investigators who first enunciated the chemo-parasitic theory.

However, the pH of plaque is not always acidic and may rise after the initial drop caused by fermentable substrate. This is partly due to salivary buffering but may also be explained by other metabolic processes within plaque. The mixed flora of dental plaque can decarboxylate certain amino acids (arginine, aspartic and glutamic acids, histidine, lysine, and ornithine) and form carbon dioxide and the respective amine.[17]

$$\text{L-Amino acid} \xrightarrow{\text{decarboxylase}} \text{amine} + \text{carbon dioxide}$$

Certain plaque organisms such as *Fusobacterium nucleatum, Bacteroides melaninogenicus, Treponema* species, peptostreptococci, and others will ferment and release ammonia as well as volatile end products. Ammonia is formed either directly by oxidative deamination:

$$\underset{\text{L-Amino acid}}{RCHNH_2COOH} + 0.5\ O_2 \longrightarrow \underset{\alpha\text{-keto acid}}{RCOCOOH} + NH_3$$

or indirectly by transamination forming glutamate, followed by oxidative deamination:

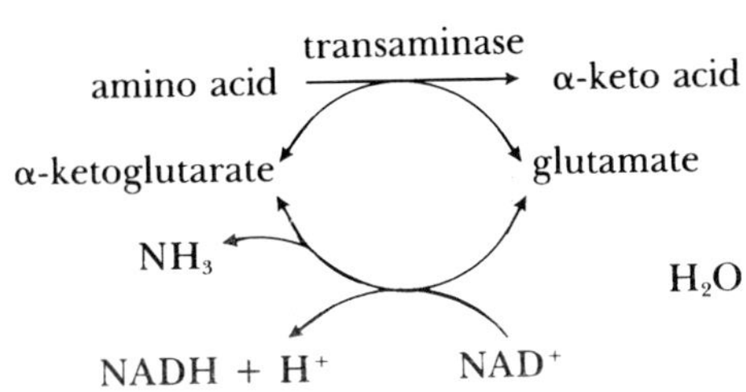

In anaerobic bacteria the Strickland reaction—the coupled oxidation-reduction of pairs of amino acids (eg, glycine-alanine; proline-alanine)—forms ammonia:

$$RCHNH_2COOH + 2R'CHNH_2COOH + H_2O \rightarrow RCOOH + CO_2 + 2R'CH_2COOH + 3NH_3$$

The process may be divided into three steps: *(1)* the NAD^+-linked deamination of the oxidizable component of the pair to its corresponding α-keto acid and ammonia; *(2)* oxidative decarboxylation, again NAD^+-linked, of the keto acid to an acyl coenzyme A and CO_2; *(3)* the oxidation of the NADH from the first two reactions by amino acid reductase system. This third reaction is not deaminative in the case of proline, forming δ-NH_2 valeric acid that is found in high levels in dental plaque.[8,9] Proline is a major amino acid constituent of salivary proteins. Though proline is the foremost hydrogen acceptor in these reactions, other equally abundant amino acids in plaque may function in a similar capacity.

The formation of amines or ammonia, as well as removal of lactate by oxidation to weaker acids, will help to restore the pH to neutrality following carbohydrate metabolism.

Proteolytic theory

The proponents of this idea were primarily histologists who based their case on the observation of microorganisms within the lamellae or prism sheaths of enamel. However, it is a dangerous trap to interpret biochemical events on the basis of histopathological specimens. There is no doubt that organisms do invade the enamel and can be found in structures of relatively higher organic content, but this explains neither their metabolism nor how they got there. It has been found that gnotobiotic rats inoculated with a single strain of a nonproteolytic *Streptococcus* developed extensive cavitation. The infecting streptococcus could not hydrolyze gelatin, casein, collagen, or chondroitin. Although proteolysis of the organic matrix of dentin may indeed occur after demineralization, there is no satisfactory evidence to support the claim that the *initial attack* on enamel is proteolytic. In fact, gnotobiotic studies show that caries can occur in the absence of proteolytic organisms. Furthermore, chemical analyses of early carious enamel lesions show a rise in nitrogen content and a fall in specific gravity that indicate a persistence or increase in organic matter (probably bacterial enzymes or cells).

Proteolysis-chelation theory

The weaknesses and strengths of this theory are as follows. Proteolysis is not an important step in the carious process. Carious lesions and plaque are acid in the presence of suitable substrate. Chelation, on the other hand, is a widespread biological process, and amino acids, citrate, and lactate, which are capable of chelate formation, are present in the saliva and plaque. It is not clear whether these chelators are present in sufficient quantities. What proportion of calcium is removed as an ionic salt versus a calcium chelate complex is also not clear.

Chapter review

- Name the structures of enamel attacked in caries according to the proteolytic theory.
- Define chelation. Give some examples of biological chelates.
- State the "vital" theory of caries and say how it was derived.
- State the proteolysis-chelation theory of caries.
- State the chemo-parasitic theory of caries. List some early investigators who contributed to this theory.
- List the organic acids that have been identified in dental plaque or carious lesions.
- State which is the main organic acid formed immediately after ingestion of a fermentable substrate. Describe what happens several hours later. Explain.
- Indicate which of these acids is the strongest and which is the weakest.
- Explain how different acids can be formed in dental plaque.
- List the factors that influence *(1)* the pH fall, and *(2)* the pH rise of dental plaque.
- Draw a Stephan curve, indicating the coordinates representative of the pH of plaque following the ingestion of equal amounts of *(1)* glucose, *(2)* sucrose, and *(3)* sorbitol.
- List the four general factors that influence the etiology of caries.

Selected readings

Ellen, T.K. 1961. Some notes on dental caries and the chemo-parasitic theory. *Ala Dent Rev* 8:11–14.

Harris, R.S. (ed) 1968. *Art and Science of Dental Caries Research.* New York: Academic Press.

Levine, R.S. 1977. The aetiology of dental caries—an outline of current thought. *Int Dent J* 27:341–348.

Mandel, I. 1983. Caries through the ages: A worm's eye view. *J Dent Res* 62:926–929.

Miller, W.D. 1890. *The Micro-organisms of the Human Mouth.* K. König (ed), Basel: S. Karger, 1973.

Sanders, H.J. 1980. Tooth decay. *Chem Eng News* 58:30–42.

References

1. Aristotle. *Opera omnia.* Paris: I. Billaine, Simon Piget, Frederic Leonard, 1654. 4 vols. Vol. 4, p 182. Problemata. Section 22, Eorum ad fructus arborum, question 14.
2. Aslander, A. 1961. Lifetime teeth, *NYJ Dent* 31:346–348.
3. Auernhammer, S., and Mayer, R. 1984. Milchzahnkaries in laufe der jahrtausende. *Dtsch Zahnarztl Z* 39:324–327.
4. Bibby, B.G., Gustafson, G., and Davies, G.N. 1958. A critique of three theories of caries attack. *Int Dent J* 8:685–695.
5. De Boever, J., and Mühlemann, H.R. 1969. pH of interproximal plaque with regard to continuous sucrose application. *Helv Odontol Acta* 13:97–99.
6. De Boever, J., Hirzel, H.C., and Mühlemann, H.R. 1969. The effect of concentrated sucrose solutions on pH of interproximal plaque. *Helv Odontol Acta* 13:27–28.
7. Carlsson, J., and Griffith, C.J. 1974. Fermentation products and bacterial yields in glucose-limited and nitrogen-limited cultures of streptococci. *Arch Oral Biol* 19:1105–1109.
8. Curtis, M.A., and Kemp, C.S. 1984. Nitrogen metabolism in dental plaque. In *Cariology Today Int Cong,* B. Guggenheim (ed), Basel: S. Karger, pp. 212–222.
9. Curtis, M.A., Kemp, C.W., Robrish, S.A., and Bowen, W.H. 1983. Strickland reactions of dental plaque. *Infect Immun* 42:431–433.
10. Distler, W., and Kröncke, A. 1980. Acid formation by mixed cultures of cariogenic strains of *Streptococcus mutans* and *Veillonella alcalescens. Arch Oral Biol* 25:655–658.
11. Drucker, D.B., and Melville, T.H. 1968. Fermentation end-products of cariogenic and non-cariogenic streptococci. *Arch Oral Biol* 13:563–570.
12. Eggers Lura, H. 1967. *The Non-acid Complexing and Phosphorylating Theory of Dental Caries.* Holbaek: Ator Tryk, Denmark.
13. Geddes, D.A.M. 1972. The production of L(+) and D(−) lactic acid and volatile acids by human dental plaque and the effect of plaque buffering and acid strength on pH. *Arch Oral Biol* 17:537–545.
14. Geddes, D.A.M. 1973. Acids produced by human dental plaque metabolism in situ. *Helv Odont Acta* 17:45.
15. Gilmour, M.N., and Poole, A.E. 1967. The fermentative capabilities of dental plaque. *Caries Res* 1:247–260.
16. Graf, H., and Mühlemann, H.R. 1966. Telemetry of plaque from interdental area. *Helv Odontol Acta* 10:94–101.
17. Hayes, M.L., and Hyatt, A.T. 1974. Decarboxylation of amino acids by bacteria derived from human dental plaque. *Arch Oral Biol* 19:361–369.
18. Hoshino, E., Yamada, T., and Araya, S. 1976. Lactate degradation by a strain of *Neisseira* isolated from human dental plaque. *Arch Oral Biol* 21:677–683.
19. Jenkins, G.N. 1961. A critique of the proteolysis-chelation theory of caries. *Br Dent J* 11:311–330.
20. Jordan, H.V. 1965. Bacteriological aspects of experimental dental caries. *Ann NY Acad Sci* 131:905–912.
21. Kreitzman, S.N., Irving, S., Navia, J.M., and Harris, R.S. 1969. Enzymatic release of phosphate from rat molar enamel by phosphoprotein phosphatase. *Nature* 223:520–521.
22. Luoma, H. 1964. Lability of inorganic phosphate in dental plaque and saliva. *Acta Odontol Scand* 22:Suppl. 41.
23. Mäkinen, K.K., and Paunio, I.K. 1970. The pH-dependent liberation of phosphate from human dental enamel and dentine by ammonium sulphate. *Acta Chem Scand* 24:1541–1550.
24. Martin, J.J., Isenberg, H.D., Schatz, V., Trelawny, B.S., and Schatz, A. 1954. Chelation, or metal-binding, as a new approach to the problem of dental caries. *Revista Mensual de Ciencias Exactas (Madrid)* 14:311–317.
25. Mikx, F.H.M., and van der Hoeven, J.S. 1975. Symbiosis of *Streptococcus mutans* and *Veillonella alcalescens* in mixed continuous culture. *Arch Oral Biol* 20:407–410.
26. Miller, W.D. 1890. *The Micro-organisms of the Human Mouth.* K. König (ed), Basel: S. Karger, 1973, p. 205.
27. Mörch, T., Punwani, I., and Greve, E. 1971. The possible role of complex forming substances in the decalcification of the caries process. *Caries Res* 5:135–143.
28. Neuman, W.F., and Neuman, M.W. 1958. *The Chemical Dynamics of Bone Mineral.* Chicago: University of Chicago Press, pp. 142–143.
29. Onose, H., and Sandham, H.J. 1976. pH changes during culture of human dental plaque streptococci on mitis-salivarius agar. *Arch Oral Biol* 21:291–296.

30. Plasschaert, A.J.M., Mörch, T., and König, K.G. 1972. Effect of sodium lactate under conditions of neutral pH on the release of calcium from the enamel surface. *Caries Res* 6:334–345.
31. Prinz, H. 1909. *A History of Dentistry*. Philadelphia: Lea & Febiger, pp. 15–16.
32. Ring, M.E. 1971. Anton van Leeuwenhoek and the tooth worm. *J Am Dent Assoc* 83:999–1001.
33. Schatz, A., and Martin, J.J. 1955. Speculation on lactobacilli and acids as possible anticaries factors. *NY State Dent J* 21:367–379.
34. Stanton, G. 1969. Diet and dental caries. The phosphate sequestration hypothesis. *NY State Dent J* 35:399–407.
35. Stephan, R.M. 1940. Changes in the hydrogen ion concentration on tooth surfaces and in carious lesions. *J Am Dent Assoc* 27:718.
36. Tanzer, J.M., Krichesvsky, M.I., and Keyes, P.H. 1969. The metabolic fate of glucose catabolized by a washed stationary phase caries-conductive streptococcus. *Caries Res* 3:167–177.
37. Yamada, T., and Carlsson, J. 1975. Regulation of lactate dehydrogenase and change of fermentation products in streptococci. *J Bacteriol* 124:55–61.
38. Yamada, T., and Carlsson, J. 1976. The role of pyruvate formate-lyase in glucose metabolism of *Streptococcus mutans*. In *Microbiol Aspects of Dental Caries,* H.M. Stiles, W.J. Loesche, and T.C. O'Brien (eds), Sp. Suppl. Microbiol. Abstr. 3:809–819.
39. Yamada, T., Hojo, S., Kobayashi, K., Asano, Y., and Araya, S. 1970. Studies on the carbohydrate metabolism of cariogenic *Streptococcus mutans* strain PK-1. *Arch Oral Biol* 15:1205–1217.
40. Zhang, Y-Z. 1982. Dental disease of Neolithic age skulls excavated in Shaanxi Province. *Chinese Med J* 95:391–396.

Chapter 2

Current Concepts of Caries Etiology

Saliva is one of our natural resources. As with most resources, it is unappreciated until there is a shortage. It is not only the patients who seem ungrateful, however; the profession treats saliva as an enemy to be expunged, aspirated and dammed.

Irwin Mandel in *Cariology Today*, S. Karger, pp 332–339, 1984

Dental caries is a multifactorial disease in which there is an interplay of three principal factors: the host (primarily the saliva and teeth), the microflora, and the substrate, or diet. In addition, a fourth factor—time—must be considered in any discussion of the etiology of caries. Diagrammatically, these factors can be portrayed as four overlapping circles (Fig 2-1). For caries to occur, conditions within each of these factors must be favorable. In other words, caries requires a susceptible host, a cariogenic oral flora, and a suitable substrate that must be present for a sufficient length of time. Conversely, caries prevention is based upon attempts to *(1)* increase the resistance of the host (fluoride therapy, occlusal sealants, immunization), *(2)* lower the numbers of microorganisms in contact with the tooth (plaque control), *(3)* modify the substrate by selecting noncariogenic foodstuffs, and *(4)* reduce the time that the substrate is in the mouth by limiting the frequency of intake.

The next three chapters will examine these factors for the role each plays in the carious process.

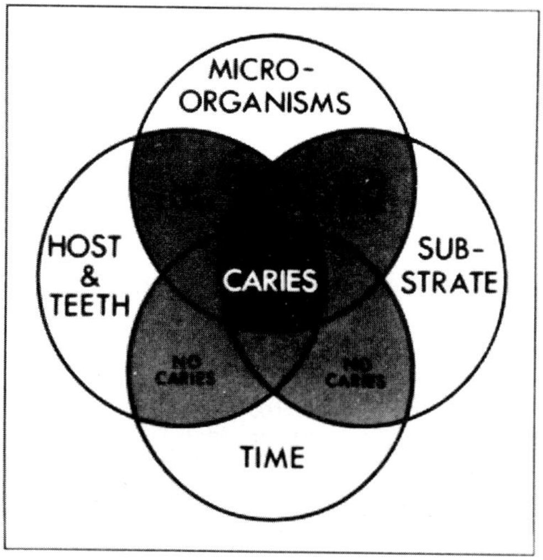

Fig 2-1 The four circles diagrammatically represent the factors involved in the carious process. All four factors must act concurrently (overlapping of the circles) for caries to occur.

Host factors: saliva

Terminology

In the following discussion, the term *saliva* refers to the mixture of secretions in the oral cavity. This mixture consists of fluids derived from the major salivary glands (parotid, submandibular, sublingual), from the minor glands of the oral mucosa, and traces from the gingival exudate. The latter is not a glandular secretion. Accordingly, it has been proposed that the term *oral fluid,* which is more encompassing, be substituted for saliva. In this text, unless stated otherwise, saliva is used synonymously with oral fluid.

Effect of desalivation on incidence and extent of caries in animals

There is no doubt that saliva significantly influences the carious process as evidenced by animal experiments in which the salivary glands are surgically extirpated.[44] When fed a diet containing 66% sucrose, uninfected hamsters with intact salivary glands developed relatively few carious lesions, whereas desalivated hamsters on the same diet developed more than five times as many carious teeth and much more extensive lesions (Table 2-1).

Table 2-1 Effect of desalivation on caries in hamsters[44]

Group	No. hamsters	Avg. no. carious teeth	Avg. caries score
Intact salivary glands	20	2.3	4.0
Desalivated*	10	10.5	39.0

*Parotid, submandibular, and sublingual glands.

These experiments have been reproduced in several laboratories. It is only fair to point out that removal of salivary glands is a drastic procedure affecting, in addition to saliva, other factors which in themselves influence caries development. These factors include:

1. Differences in food and water consumption
2. Longer eating time (animals modify their eating habits to compensate for the lack of saliva)
3. Greater food retention
4. Possible alterations in the bacterial flora of the mouth
5. Maturation of the enamel

It should be noted that in desalivated animals a cariogenic substrate is still required for caries to occur. Low-carbohydrate or carbohydrate-free diets will not cause caries in these animals, which again indicates the multifactorial nature of the carious process.

Decreased salivary flow and caries in humans

Xerostomia (Greek: *xeros* = dry; *stoma* = mouth) was first described by Bartley in 1868, and a detailed historical review is available.[9] Synonyms for xerostomia include oligosialia, asialia, and stomatitis sicca. Humans suffering from decreased or lack of salivary secretion often experience an increased rate of dental caries and rapid tooth destruction. Xerostomia may be the consequence of a variety of different human pathological conditions, as listed below.

1. Sarcoidosis may involve reduced salivary gland functions.[3]
2. Sjögren's syndrome consists of xerostomia, xerophthalmia, and a connective tissue disease. This syndrome includes what is sometimes called Mikulicz's disease.
3. Therapeutic radiation of the head and neck leads to xerostomia if glands are within the primary beam. Such glands undergo progressive atrophy, fibrosis, and severe reduction in output.
4. Surgical removal of salivary glands for neoplasms may cause localized xerostomia.
5. Chronic administration of anticholinergic or parasympatholytic drugs can produce clinical manifestation of xerostomia.
6. In diabetes mellitus, a frequent complaint is dryness of the mouth.
7. Patients with Parkinson's disease have decreased salivary flow. Drooling is sometimes seen in these patients, probably due to defective swallowing.[7]
8. Rarely, xerostomia may be due to congenital absence or malformation of salivary glands.
9. Acute virus infection involving salivary glands results in temporary xerostomia.
10. Anxiety, mental stress, and depression may temporarily decrease salivary flow.[6]

In some of these conditions decreased salivary flow has been quantitatively demonstrated[35]; in others it is only a clinical impression. Increased caries associated with xerostomia in cases of Sjögren's syndrome, or following prolonged medication with salivary depressant drugs, has been reported.[106] Because of the insidious onset of Sjögren's syndrome, it is difficult to design well-controlled clinical trials comparing caries increments of affected and normal subjects. Accordingly, much of the evidence is anecdotal. Nevertheless, these patients regularly develop cervical caries and incisal edge lesions, the severity of which depends on the duration and intensity of the syndrome.[30] Rampant caries has been well documented in numerous patients following radiation therapy of the mouth,[36,45,64] regardless of whether the teeth were inside or outside the field of radiation. In all patients having such lesions, the salivary glands had been irradiated and the quantity of saliva was greatly reduced. The caries is atypical: decay often attacks the cervical area, involves cementum and dentin, and progresses inwardly until the crown is amputated (Fig 2-2). Occasionally, a rapid wearing-away of the incisal and occlusal surfaces occurs with or without cervical lesions. Heavy brownish black discoloration of the whole tooth may be seen. In some patients the clinical pattern of tooth loss is characterized by rapid demineralization over broad surfaces with little, if any, cavitation. Rampant dental caries develops in monkeys whose salivary glands have been deliberately irradiated.[37] This is attributable not to a specific change in the quality of the saliva produced by the residual gland tissue after irradiation, since no such change could be identified, but rather to the great reduction in the quantity of saliva and thus in its protective constituents.

Under conditions of xerostomia, alterations in both the amount and bacteriological composition of the plaque occur. Following irradiation of the main salivary glands, *Streptococcus mutans, Lactobacillus* species, yeasts (especially *Candida albicans*), *Actinomyces,* and *Staphylococcus* increase in plaque.[18,74] Decreases in *Veillonella, Streptococcus sanguis, Neisseria, Bacteroides,* and *Fusobacterium* have been observed. The most marked changes usually occur during the first 3 months postradiotherapy. These alterations in plaque flora may be responsible for the increased incidence of caries. In patients with Sjögren's syndrome, there is also a significant increase in the proportion of *C albicans.*[75] This alteration in oral flora may be a reflection of a lower environmental pH due to decreased salivary buffering, and it would favor the growth of the more aciduric yeasts.

An interesting case of rampant caries has been reported following partial surgical desalivation of a 12-year-old girl who had been treated for a mucoepidermoid carcinoma of the right parotid gland.[56] The patient's right parotid and submandibular glands and left submandibular gland had been removed 2 years previously. Widespread caries affecting maxillary and mandibular quadrants on the right but not the left side were described. Severe carious destruction of the lingual surfaces of the mandibular incisors had occurred. These surfaces are usually the least susceptible to decay. A diet history did not reveal any unusual eating habits to account for the caries pattern.

Many drugs have a side effect of dry mouth, and it has been pointed out that prolonged medication with these drugs may result in rampant caries.[2,4,49,50,95,97,106] Drugs with either major or minor xerostomic potential include antispasmodics, antidepressants, antipsychotics, skeletal muscle relaxants, antiarrhythmics, antihistaminics, appetite depressants, anticonvulsants, anxiolytics, antihypertensives, diuretics, and anti-Parkinsonism agents, as well as miscellaneous drugs.[105a] Some of these are listed in Table 2-2. Tranquilizers are widely used for long periods of time in some psychic disorders to relieve anxiety, tension, and agitation. Nearly half of the drugs used by psychiatrists are tranquilizers.

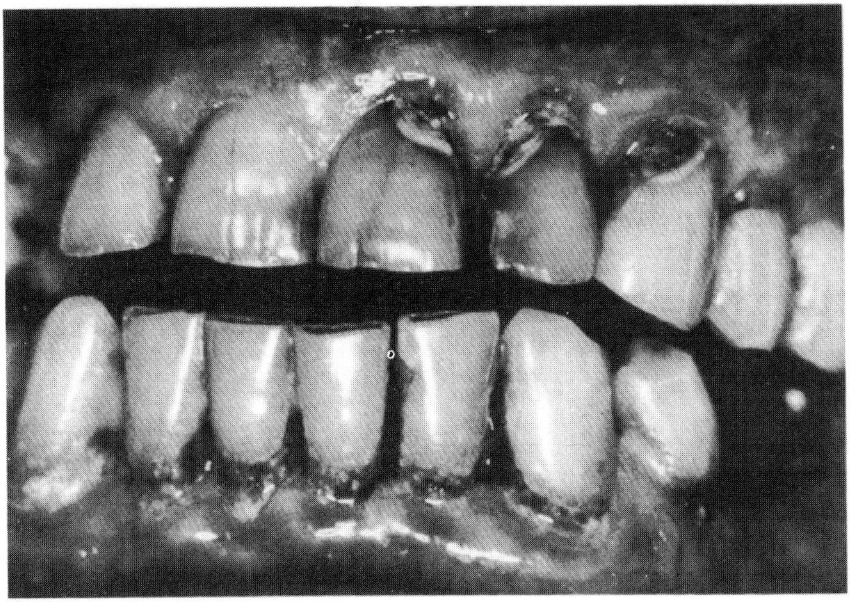

Fig 2-2 Dental caries 10 months following irradiation of the parotid glands. Prior to radiation therapy there was no evidence of decay. (Courtesy of S. Silverman, Jr.)

Diazepam is the drug most frequently used by psychiatrists, followed by chlorpromazine, thioridazine, and trifluoperazine HCl.[87] Long-term use of lithium carbonate, to prevent the manic episodes of manic-depressive illness, causes decreased salivary function and has been associated with cervical caries. In general practice, nonbarbiturate sedative-hypnotics and tranquilizers are also among the most frequently used drugs next to antibiotics and analgesics. Amphetamines, and similar sympathomimetic amines are taken as anorectics in attempting to control obesity. Prolonged use of these drugs may cause dry mouth and extensive caries.

Quantitative estimations of antisialagogue effects of several anticholinergic and sedative-antihistaminic-antiemetic drugs have been reported.[33,34] In order to standardize conditions, salivary flow was stimulated by a mixture of carbachol and adrenaline. Most of the anticholinergic drugs tested reduced salivary secretion 90% to 100%. Salivary flow was decreased 93% with promethazine and 33% with chlorpromazine. Antihistamines are frequently used for long periods of time to relieve the distress of allergies.

Considering the widespread use of many drugs with xerostomic side effects, and their cariogenic potential, it is surprising that there are very few well-documented cases of iatrogenic caries. Winer and Bahn[127] described a patient with severe depression and Parkinsonism. He was treated simultaneously with imipramine (a tricyclic antidepressant), trihexyphenidyl (a parasympathetic blocking agent), and diphenhydra-

Table 2-2 Drugs causing xerostomia*

Classification	Major effect	Minor effect
Antispasmodic	Belladonna alkaloids (Belladenal, Bellergal) Glycopyrrolate (Robinul) Hyoscine (Buscopan) l-hyoscamine (Levsin) Isopropamide (Darbid) Oxybutynin (Ditropan) Pirenzipine (Gastrozepin) Propantheline (Pro-Banthine)	Anisotropine (Valpin); dicyclomine (Bentylol); orphenadrine (Diminul); pinaverium (Dicetel)
Antidepressant	Amitriptyline (Elavil) Amoxapine (Asendin) Doxepin (Sinequan) Protriptyline (Triptil) Trimipramine (Surmontil)	Clomipramine (Anafranil); desipramine (Norpramin, Pertofrane); imipramine (Tofranil); isocarboxazide (Marplan); nomifensine (Merital); nortriptyline (Aventyl); phenelzine (Nardil); trancylpromine (Parnate); trazodone (Desyrel)
Antipsychotic	Chlorpromazine (Largactil) Chlorprothixene (Tarasan) Promazine (Sparine) Thioridazine (Mellaril)	Haloperidol (Haldol); fluphenazine (Permitil); lithium carbonate (Carbolith); loxapine (Loxapac); mesoridazine (Serentil); methotrimeprazine (Nozinan); perphenazine (Trilafon); piperacetazine (Quide); thiopropazate (Dartal); thiothixene (Navane); trifluoperazine (Stelazine)
Skeletal muscle relaxant	Clyclobenzaprine (Flexeril)	Baclofen (Lioresal); diazepam (Valium); orphenadrine (Norflex)
Parkinsonism therapy	Benztropine (Cogentin) Biperiden (Akineton) Trihexyphenidyl (Artane)	Amantadine (Symmetrel); benserazide (Prolopa); carbidopa (Sinemet); dextroamphetamine (Dexedrine); levodopa (Larodopa); orphenadrine (Disipal); procyclidine (Kemadrin)
Antiarrythmic	Disopyramide (Norpace)	

*From Grad, H., Grushka, M., and Yanover, L. 1985. Drug induced xerostomia. *J Can Dent Assoc* 51:296–299. Reprinted with permission.

Table 2-2 Drugs causing xerostomia—cont'd

Classification	Major effect	Minor effect
Antihistamine		Antazoline (Antistine); astemizole (Hismanal); azatadine (Optimine); brompheniramine (Dimetane); chlorpheniramine (Chlortripolon); clemastine (Tavist); cyproheptadine (Periactin); dexchlorpheniramine (Polaramine); diphenhydramine (Benadryl); hydroxyzine (Atarax); promethazine (Phenergan); trimeprazine (Panectyl); tripelennamine (Pyribenzamine)
Appetite depressant		Chlorphentermine (Pre-Sate); diethylpropion (Tenuate); fenfluramine (Ponderal); mazindol (Sanorex); phenteramine (lonamin)
Anticonvulsant		Carbamazepine (Tegretol); clonazepam (Rivotril); nitrazepam (Mogadon)
Anxiolytic		Alprazolam (Xanax); bromazepam (Lectopam); chlorazepate (Tranxene); chlordiazepoxide (Librium); chlormezanone (Trancopal); lorazepam (Ativan); oxazepam (Serax); temazepam (Restoril); triazolam (Halcion)
Antihypertensive	Clonidine (Catapres)	Atenolol (Tenormin); catopril (Capoten); debrisoquine (Declinax); guanethidine (Ismelin); labetolol (Trandate); methyldopa (Aldomet); metoprolol (Lopressor); nadolol (Corgard); oxyprenolol (Trasicor); pindolol (Visken); propranolol (Inderal); timolol (Blocadren)
Diuretic (dry mouth may be a symptom of a serious potassium loss)		Amiloride (Midamor); chlorothiazide (Diuril); chlorthalidone (Hygroton); furosemide (Lasix); hydrochlorthiazide (Hydro Diuril); indapamide (Lozide); metolazone (Zaroxolyn); methychlothiazide (Diuretic); polythiazide (Renese); spiranolactone (Aldactone)
Miscellaneous	Bleomycin (Blenoxane) Busulfan (Myleran) Doxorubicin (Adriamycin) Isotretonoin (Accutane)	Cimetidine (Tagamet); meclizine (Bonamine); procarbazine (Natulan); ranitidine (Zantac); sucralfate (Sulcrate)

Table 2-3 Sucrose content of antacid tablets or gums*

Product	Manufacturer	Sucrose (%)
Bisodol	Whitehall Laboratories, Inc	12.9
Camalox	William H. Rorer, Inc	0.02
Chooz Gum	Plough, Inc	48.0
Di-Gel	Plough, Inc	6.5
Kolantyl	Merrell Dow Pharmaceuticals, Inc	0.23
Maalox #1	William H. Rorer, Inc	0.4
Milk of Magnesia	Roxane Laboratories, Inc	17.2
Mylanta	Stuart Pharmaceuticals	0.08
Pepto-Bismol	Procter & Gamble	0.03
Rolaids	Warner-Lambert Co	56.5
Titralac	3M Company	0.02
Tums	Norcliff Thayer, Inc	41.0
Walgreen Antacid	Walgreen Labs, Inc	31.8

*I. Shannon (personal communication).

mine (an antihistamine). On admission to a Veterans Administration Hospital he had 12 teeth, of which only one was carious (it was restored). During hospitalization the patient complained almost constantly of dry mouth and developed irritation and ulceration from a maxillary denture. Within 12 months all of the patient's remaining teeth developed deep carious lesions and had to be extracted. Another case[89] involved a 21-year-old man who had developed rampant decay, including multiple carious exposures of the pulps of the mandibular incisors, over the preceding 24 months. While in college the patient had had symptoms of duodenitis for which he took antacid tablets (aluminum magnesium silicate—Gelusil). Many of the antacid preparations available across the counter have a high sucrose content (Table 2-3). The patient drank large quantities of milk and avoided spicy foods. Nevertheless, the symptoms did not abate so he sought medical attention. Propantheline bromide (Pro-Banthine), 15 mg four times a day before meals and before retiring, was prescribed. The patient's condition improved with only occasional stomach pain. However, he did complain of dry mouth. After a year the patient suffered a relapse and was given Combid Spansules (prochlorperazine maleate and isopropamide). The symptoms of dry mouth continued throughout this period. Clinical and roentgenographic examination revealed multiple restorations of many teeth and active carious lesions (Figs 2-3 and 2-4). The patient had a decayed, missing, filled teeth (DMFT) score of 27 and decayed, missing, filled surfaces (DMFS) score of 63. Information obtained from the patient's earlier treatment charts and radiographs revealed that at age 18 he had what would be considered average caries prevalence with a DMFT score of 15, with lesions restricted to occlusal pits and fissures (Fig 2-5). Examination of this patient's medical history revealed prolonged use of propantheline bromide and isopropamide. Both drugs have anticholinergic action. The coincidence of this therapy, the patient's symptoms of dry mouth, and

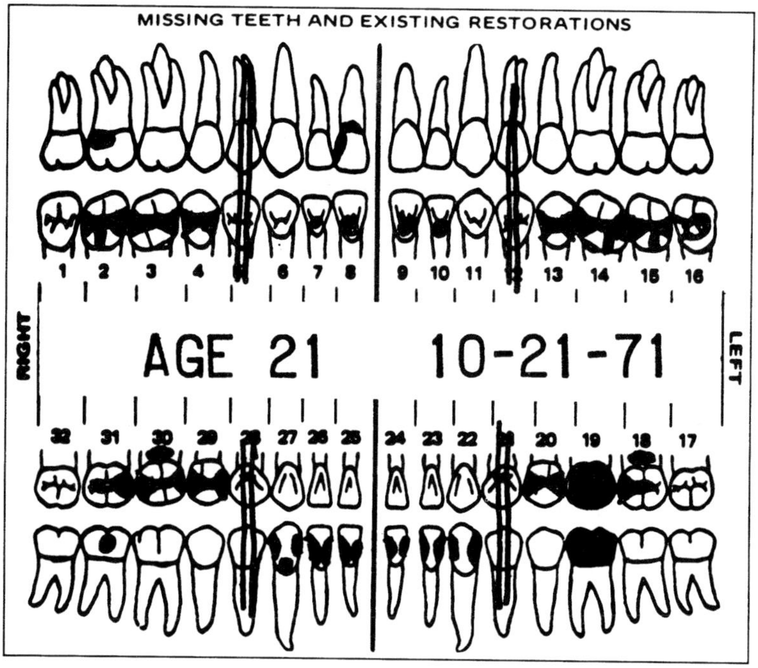

Fig 2-3 Decayed, missing, and filled teeth of a patient who received prolonged anticholinergic therapy for a duodenal ulcer. Note the steep caries increment (DMFT 27) that occurred during the time of xerostomia.

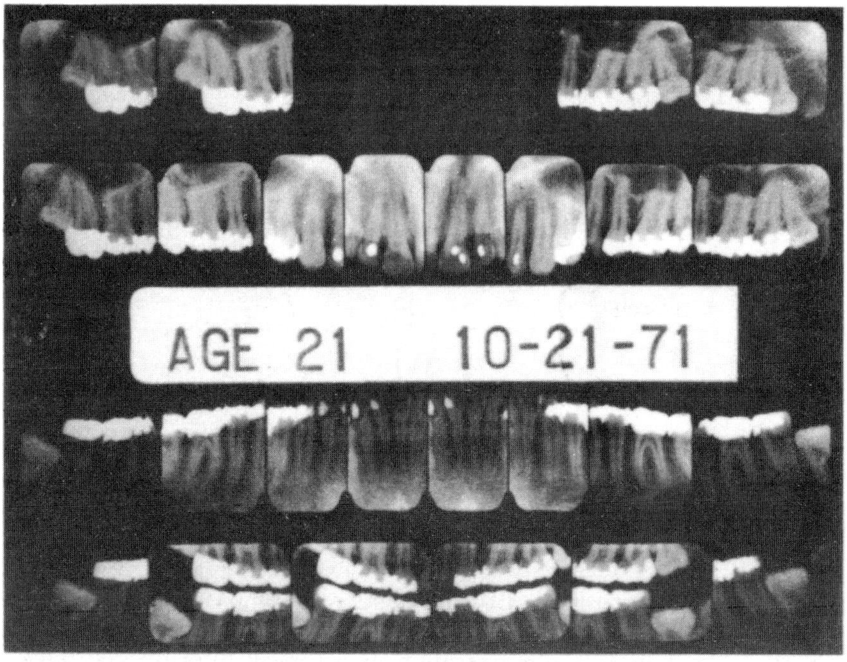

Fig 2-4 Full-mouth roentgenographs of patient showing rampant caries and pulpal involvement of mandibular anterior teeth.

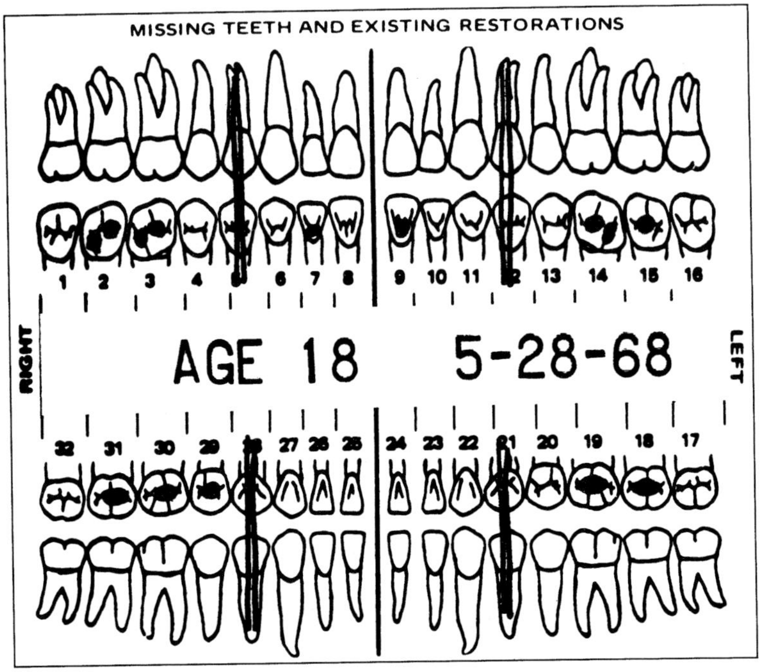

Fig 2-5 Decayed, missing, and filled teeth prior to the anticholinergic therapy obtained from the patient's dental records and roentgenographs.

Table 2-4 Components of various saliva substitutes

Category	Ingredients
Salt	NaCl, KCl, $CaCl_2$, $MgCl_2$, K_2HPO_4, KH_2PO_4
Lubricant	Carboxymethyl cellulose, animal mucins, glycerin
Sweetener	Sorbitol, xylitol
Flavor	Mint, wintergreen, coriander-spice, lemon
Preservative	Methyl p-hydroxybenzoate, paraben
Color	FD & C Red Dye No. 40
Therapeutic	NaF

the onset of rampant caries is strong circumstantial evidence of caries produced iatrogenically. It is also worth noting that Pro-Banthine tablets are sugar coated.

The management of patients with xerostomia includes the following: *(1)* fluoride therapy, *(2)* dietary control, *(3)* oral hygiene, *(4)* avoidance of xerostomic drugs, and *(5)* the use of artificial saliva.

The most effective caries-preventive regimen for these patients is the daily self-administration of a topical fluoride gel (0.5% fluoride) in a custom-made tray, because it provides the longest contact between agent and teeth—5 minutes or more. A daily fluoride rinse (0.05% sodium fluoride) for 1 minute is also effective. Details of caries prevention by dietary control and oral hygiene are discussed in chapter 12. Various formulations of artificial saliva have been proposed.[47,86,99] These usually contain anions and cations in approximately the proportions found in naturally secreted saliva. In addition, carboxymethyl cellulose or animal mucin is included to provide viscosity, and sodium fluoride may be included to promote remineralization (Table 2-4). Five preparations of artificial saliva that are commercially available (OTC) have been granted acceptance by the Council on Dental Therapeutics (Moi-Stir Artificial Saliva and Oral Swabs, Kingswood Laboratories, Inc; Orex Saliva Substitute, Young Dental Mfg Co, Inc; Salivart Synthetic Saliva, Westport Pharmaceuticals, Inc; Saliva Substitute, Roxane Laboratories, Inc; and Xero-Lube Artificial Saliva, Scherer Laboratories, Inc).[28] In Europe an artificial saliva containing mucin instead of carboxymethyl cellulose is marketed (Saliva Orthana, Orthana Ltd). This latter product may be preferable for xerostomic patients because its longer retention time means less is needed.[124] Most currently available products are less than ideal, since their effects are of limited duration, and some may have an unpleasant taste.[73]

Physiological xerostomia occurs in all humans during sleep because the salivary glands do not secrete spontaneously.[96] Since there is no saliva to buffer and wash away fermentation products of plaque during sleep, the most important time for plaque removal (tooth brushing, flossing, etc) is just before bedtime.

Salivary composition and caries

The aforementioned findings have led to the conclusion that saliva is in some way necessary to maintain the integrity of the teeth. Identification of the specific constituents of saliva that might be involved in protecting against or limiting the caries attack has remained frustratingly elusive. Many physical, chemical, and biological characteristics of saliva have, at one time or another, been implicated as important. To date the findings have been contradictory. Some investigators claim a relationship exists between caries prevalence and salivary amylase, urea, ammonia, calcium, phosphate, pH, etc; others find no such relationship.

A major problem in studying saliva is that its composition varies with flow rate, nature of stimulation, duration of stimulation, plasma composition, the time of day at which samples are collected, and the serial dependency of saliva samples, ie, the effect of previous stimulation on the composition of saliva collected subsequently.[31,72] Unfortunately, in many studies these variables have not been adequately controlled. In other instances, the assay methods were inadequate (eg, amylase measurements based on the time to reach the achromatic point) or the treatment of the data was inadmissible (eg, arithmetic averaging of pH, which is a logarithmic function). Another difficulty in interpreting results of

Table 2-5 Relationship between salivary characteristics and caries prevalence

Property	Relationship	Property	Relationship
Flow rate	±	pH	–
		Ca	–
Buffer capacity	+	PO_4	–
		NH_3	–
		Amylase	
		Viscosity	–
		Urea	–

+ positive relation; ± some relation; – no relation.

studies on salivary composition is that saliva is a mixture of the secretions from the three pairs of major salivary glands with contributions from numerous minor mucous glands. The secretion of each type of gland has a unique composition. For example, the secretion of the submandibular salivary glands contains about 50% more calcium (6.8 mg calcium/100 ml) than that of the parotid glands (4.1 mg calcium/100 ml).[88] Such regional differences may, in part, account for the observed relative immunity of the mandibular anterior teeth to caries and the higher frequency of supragingival calculus deposits.

Currently, no consistent relationship has been established between dental caries prevalence and salivary amylase, ammonia, urea, calcium, phosphate, pH, or viscosity (Table 2-5).

An inverse relationship between salivary flow rate and caries may exist, but the literature is in conflict on this point. The flow rate itself influences the salivary Na^+/HCO_3^- ratio; at higher flow rates there is an increased buffer capacity. Patients whose saliva has a higher buffer capacity tend to have less caries.[38,39]

Salivary buffers

A buffer is a solution that tends to maintain a constant pH. A graph of the pH versus the equivalent of acid or alkali added to a buffer is the titration curve. The pK marks the point on the curve at which the pH changes the least (when the concentration of conjugated base and conjugated acid are equal). In saliva, the chief buffer systems are bicarbonate-carbonic acid (HCO_3^-/H_2CO_3, $pK_1 = 6.1$) and phosphate ($HPO_4^{=}/H_2PO_4^-$, $pK_2 = 6.8$). Bicarbonate is by far the most important salivary buffer for several reasons.

1. It can buffer rapidly by losing carbon dioxide (compare with blood).
2. Its pK is close to that encountered in plaque, and, therefore, it is more effective in that range.
3. As the flow rate increases, the bicarbonate concentration increases

dramatically (as does Na^+), whereas phosphate falls slightly with increased flow rate.

4. After removal of bicarbonate by a current of CO_2-free air at pH 5, the buffering capacity of saliva is markedly reduced.

Dialysis of saliva, which removes both bicarbonate and phosphate but not protein, results in total loss of salivary buffering capacity. This indicates that salivary proteins can be disregarded as buffers in saliva.[55]

Urea is continuously secreted in saliva. Plaque microorganisms can convert urea to other nitrogenous products and ammonia. The ammonia thus formed can also serve as a buffer.

In a longitudinal study of caries incidence, a fall in buffer capacity preceded the highest peak in caries increment by about 9 months.[77]

Further evidence of the importance of saliva as a buffer was demonstrated when the pH of carious lesions and of dental plaque was studied. Within active carious lesions (dentin), a pH gradient exists. The deep advancing edges of such lesions are more acidic than the shallower layers, which have a pH similar to that of saliva. In enlarged and exposed cavities that are emptied of their contents, the carious layer is shallower and the pH closer to neutrality, probably because of the better access to saliva.[32]

It will be recalled that the pH of plaque falls to between 4 and 5 following a rinse with a suitable substrate and after a period of time returns to the original "resting" level in the pH range of 6 to 7 (see chapter 1, "Evaluation of the various theories of caries—Chemo-parasitic theory"). Studies on the pH of plaque in hamsters infected with *S mutans* have provided further insight as to why the pH of plaque returns to resting value.[24,25] When plaque was exposed to a low concentration of sucrose (2.5%), the pH dropped and then after a short time began to rise. However, if the plaque and tooth were isolated with a Parafilm cup, the pH of plaque decreased further and remained low. In view of the prolonged high levels of acid found when the plaque was isolated, it is presumed that normally pH reverts toward neutrality due to the gradual diffusion of saliva into plaque coupled with exhaustion of substrate and diffusion out of acid end products.

Concept of a "critical pH"

The pH at which any particular saliva ceases to be saturated with calcium and phosphate is referred to as the "critical pH"; below this value, the inorganic material of the tooth may dissolve. Critical pH varies according to the calcium and phosphate concentration, but it is usually about 5.5. With increasing concentration of hydrogen ions in the plaque, more phosphate ions will leave the solid apatite phase, according to the following equation:

$$PO_4^{3-} \underset{-H^+}{\overset{+H^+}{\rightleftharpoons}} HPO_4^{2-} \underset{-H^+}{\overset{+H^+}{\rightleftharpoons}} H_2PO_4^-$$

The concentration of calcium and phosphate influences the rate at which apatite dissolves by the law of mass action.

Antibacterial factors of glandular origin

Several salivary antimicrobial factors protect oral mucosal and hard surfaces by helping to regulate the quantity and species distribution of oral microbes. These factors are of both "ready-to-wear" nonimmunological and "made-to-order" immunological types. Nonimmunological factors include lysozyme and the salivary peroxidases.

Lysozyme

Lysozyme (*N*-acetylmuramide glycanohydrolase: EC 3.2.1.17), a hydrolytic enzyme, cleaves the β 1-4 linkage between *N*-acetylglucosamine and *N*-acetylmuramic acid, which constitute the repeating units of the cell wall peptidoglycans of bacteria. Certain organisms, such as *Micrococcus lysodeikticus,* are rapidly destroyed by this enzyme; others are destroyed more slowly, and some are resistant to lysozyme action. In 1922, Fleming discovered lysozyme in nasal secretion. This enzyme is also found in saliva, tears, egg white, most tissues, and body fluids. Sublingual and submandibular saliva contain higher levels of lysozyme than parotid saliva.[57] Lysozyme alone does not lyse or prevent growth of pure cultures of the predominant bacteria in the oral cavity of man.[48] In the presence of sodium lauryl sulfate, a detergent, lysozyme can lyse many cariogenic and noncariogenic streptococci. When lysozyme (from egg white) was added to a cariogenic diet, no cariostatic effect could be found in experimental rats.[66,85,107] Lysozyme activity in whole saliva has been found to be significantly greater in a group of caries-free preschool children than in a caries-susceptible group.[12] Although lysozyme may not be effective specifically against cariogenic microorganisms, it probably influences the ecological balance of the oral flora by discriminating against transient organisms introduced into the mouth.

Salivary peroxidase system

The salivary glands secrete salivary peroxidase and thiocyanate ion (SCN^-), which act on hydrogen peroxide generated by certain bacteria. This oxidoreductase system catalyzes the oxidation of the thiocyanate ion (SCN^-) to hypothiocyanate ion ($OSCN^-$). The net reaction is:

$$H_2O_2 + SCN^- \rightarrow OSCN^- + H_2O$$

The product $OSCN^-$ reacts rapidly with sulfhydryl compounds of low molecular weight and certain protein sulfhydryls. The oxidation reaction may inactivate various enzymes of the glycolytic pathway and thereby temporarily inhibit the growth, respiration, and metabolism of most species of oral bacteria.[116] The hypothiocyanate ion must reach a minimum threshold concentration before bacterial inhibition occurs, and this threshold concentration varies from species to species.

In addition, the products of the salivary peroxidase-thiocyanate system may be less deleterious to mammalian cells, and may serve to protect the mucous membranes of the mouth from the toxic effects of hydrogen peroxide produced by oral bacteria and activated phagocytes.[1,21] The precise role of the peroxidase system in oral biology remains unclear.[118]

In the absence of an extraneous source of peroxide, peroxidase is active against microorganisms that accumulate peroxide, such as *Lactobacillus acidophilus* and *Streptococcus cremoris*. The system appears to operate by preventing cells from accumulating lysine and glutamic acid, both of which are essential for growth.[26] Peroxidase activity has been demonstrated in human saliva by a number of workers. It is present in both submandibular and parotid secretions,[65,75a] and in the latter it has been separated into three fractions, each of which inhibits the growth of *Lactobacillus casei*. Pig peroxidase-thiocyanate, when added to pure cultures of different strains of *S mutans*, inhibits their growth.[84] Further investigation is necessary to determine whether this enzyme can control cariogenic bacteria in vivo. Substantial evidence suggests that peroxidase is involved in an antibacterial system in saliva.[101,116] However, no significant differences in peroxidase levels in parotid or submandibular secretions have been found between caries-resistant and caries-susceptible subjects.[128]

Immunoglobulins

The major immunoglobulin in saliva and other external secretions is secretory IgA, which differs from the serum IgA.[14] Whereas serum IgA exists as a 7S monomer, secretory IgA (sIgA) exists as an 11S dimer consisting of two IgA molecules joined by a J-chain, plus a secretory component (SC).[12,13] Secretory IgA is the product of two distinct cell types. Plasma cells synthesize polymeric IgA containing J-chain, a small peptide (15,000 daltons). Glandular cells synthesize a glycoprotein (60,000 to 70,000 daltons) secretory component. SC is a receptor for polymeric immunoglobulin A containing J-chain; the IgA binds to SC below the tight junction of glandular epithelial cells and is then transported across to the luminal surface. Besides facilitating transport, the presence of SC makes sIgA much more resistant than serum IgA to proteolytic enzymes, conferring on the sIgA molecule a remarkable stability in the hostile environment of external secretions.

Antibodies against specific bacteria have been reported in human saliva.[40-42,67,119] Purified salivary IgA and IgG fractions have been found with agglutinating activity against oral isolates of α-hemolytic streptococci.[100] IgA isolated from human parotid secretions specifically inhibits the adherence of certain strains of streptococci to human buccal epithelial cells,[126] facilitating their elimination from the oral cavity by swallowing. IgA antibodies that predominate in external secretions may represent a defense mechanism against superficial infections of mucous membranes; antibodies present in serum may play little role in such local infections.

Host factors: immunization

During the last three decades we have witnessed the worldwide eradication of smallpox as an infectious disease by means of vaccination. The development of the Salk and later the Sabin polio vaccines has also virtually eliminated poliomyelitis. Both depend on the host's immunological response to a vaccine against a specific virus. Since the recognition of *S mutans* as the most virulent cariogenic organism (see chapter 3), the possibility of developing a vaccine against dental caries has become increasingly attractive.

The mouth is provided with both humoral and cellular arms of the immune system, both of which could influence the composition of the microbial communities in the oral cavity (Fig 2-6). Humoral mechanisms could function through local immunoglobulins produced in the gingiva or salivary glands, and through systemic (serum) immunoglobulins entering via the gingival exudate (crevicular fluid). Cellular mechanisms would depend upon polymorphonuclear leukocytes, lymphocytes, and monocytes that presumably would also reach the plaque via the gingival exudate. These immune mechanisms, along with bacterial antagonism, appear to control or prevent colonization by *allochthonous* species (those found at other sites, such as Enterobacteriaceae and *Clostridium*) but do not seem to control *autochthonous* species (those normally found at the site), which may not be recognized. The fact that indigenous flora survives the immune system is of considerable importance to the design of immunological control of an oral population. We do not know if these immune mechanisms regulate the indigenous normal flora or understand how they prevent overt pathogens from initiating disease, partly because we do not know how well these mechanisms function in external fluids. Theoretically, antibodies could control populations of cariogenic streptococci in either of two ways: *(1)* they could inhibit colonization, by reacting with bacterial surface receptors or by inhibiting glucosyltransferase and thereby blocking glucan-induced irreversible adherence (see chapter 4 under the heading, "Cariogenicity of sucrose and other carbohydrates"), or *(2)* they could opsonize bacteria, permitting phagocytosis by polymorphonuclear leukocytes or possibly macrophages.

Animal studies

Active immunization with *S mutans* and certain antigens from this organism have been tested in rodents[114] and primates.[11] In these studies,

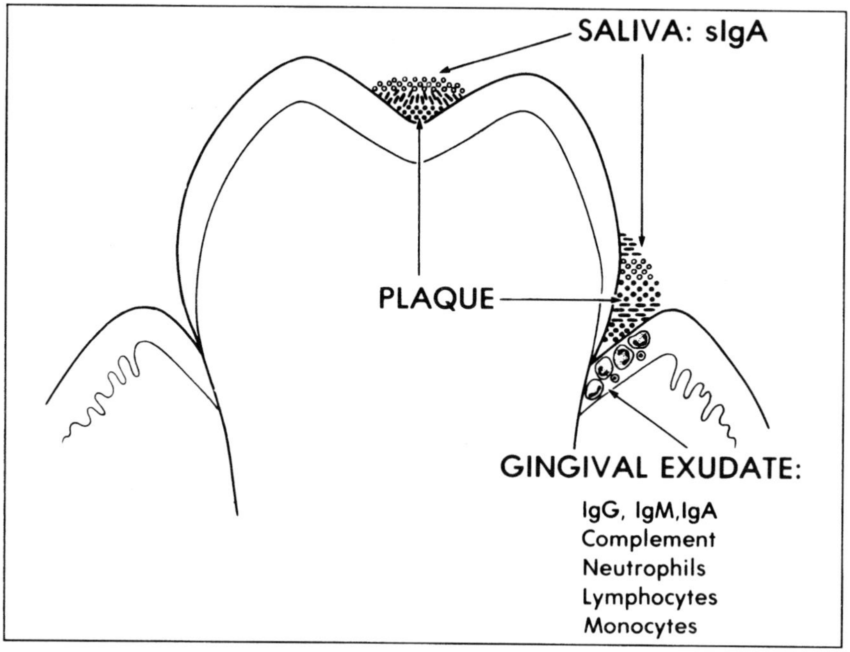

Fig 2-6 Humoral and cellular factors at the plaque/tooth interface. Saliva provides secretory IgA, which can reach plaque both at the gingiva and at occlusal fissures. Gingival exudate provides both humoral (IgG, IgM, and IgA) antibodies and cellular components (neutrophils, lymphocytes), but only to plaque in the gingival region.

animals fed a diet containing sucrose (to favor colonization by *S mutans*) were immunized and subsequently challenged with the virulent bacterium from which the vaccine was derived. Caries immunity was assessed by comparing the development of caries in animals that had been immunized with those that were sham-injected and similarly infected. Monoinfected rats offer the simplest model for evaluation of specific caries immunity, since noninfected animals remain caries free.

Various antigens have been used, including whole cells of killed *S mutans,* cell extracts, cell-free culture fluid, glucosyltransferase (GTF), and other purified antigens. Complete Freund's adjuvant (CFA) has also been used to augment the immune response. However, CFA is not acceptable for use in humans because of the resultant localized inflammation. A simpler synthetic muramyl dipeptide can augment salivary IgA and IgG response and holds considerable promise for future human as well as animal studies of caries prevention by immunization.[112]

These animal studies can be further divided into two groups:

1. Those involving stimulation of secretory IgA, either directly, locally, or indirectly via the gut
2. Those involving stimulation of serum antibodies, which reach the plaque via the gingival sulcus

Local immunity (direct stimulation of sIgA)

Rodents immunized by repeated injections in the vicinity of each parotid and submandibular gland with a vaccine prepared from *S mutans* (either killed cells or GTF) produced salivary IgA that agglutinated *S mutans* or inhibited glucan synthesis. These animals had fewer colonies of *S mutans* on their teeth[105] and significantly less caries than nonimmunized or sham-immunized animals.[79,101,113,115] The reductions in caries were greater on smooth surfaces than on occlusal surfaces (Table 2-6).[82,113,115] These and other studies have confirmed that the induction of salivary antibodies to *S mutans* correlates with protection against dental caries.

Oral immunization (indirect stimulation of sIgA)

The Peyer's patches (gut-associated lymphoid tissues, GALT) contain B cells that can populate the lamina propria of the gastrointestinal tract and become IgA-producing plasma cells, which subsequently migrate to local sites. Antigen-sensitized T and B cells leave GALT via efferent lymphatics, pass through the inductive environment of the mesenteric lymph nodes, and evidently reach the blood stream via the thoracic duct lymph. From the blood stream these cells selectively settle in the lamina propria of the gut, upper respiratory tract, and glandular tissues, including the mammary, lacrimal, and salivary glands (Fig 2-7).

Feeding whole cells of *S mutans* to gnotobiotic rats selectively induces sIgA antibodies in saliva but no serum response. The presence of sIgA to *S mutans* correlated with a reduced caries incidence in rats challenged with this organism.[81] The amount of antigen administered is important; a dose of approximately 10^8 colony-forming units per milliliter of drinking water yielded optimal responses. Hamsters orally immunized with the culture supernatant of *S mutans*, containing GTF, will develop salivary anti-GTF antibodies and fewer caries than controls.[103,104]

These studies suggest that salivary IgA responses can be induced by oral administration of *S mutans* antigens of various forms, and that the antibody-mediated protection may result from inhibition of GTF activity or from reaction with cell surface receptors important in adherence.

Stimulation of serum antibodies

There have been several attempts to prevent caries in experimental animals by repeatedly injecting killed cariogenic bacteria. The immunized animals developed high serum levels or specific antibodies (IgG) to these bacteria, but the effects on caries were not uniform. Rats monoinfected with *Streptococcus faecalis* had depressed cariogenic activity when thus immunized.[125] Monkeys immunized intravenously or submucosally against *S mutans* and fed a caries-promoting diet had variable susceptibility to caries, depending upon the immunogen used and the route of administration: whole cells or broken cells conferred some protection (although not statistically significant), whereas GTF preparations did not,

Table 2-6 Effect of immunization near the salivary glands with *S mutans* vaccine on salivary agglutinin titer and caries score of rats*

Group	Mean agglutinin titer†	Mean buccal	Caries score‡	
			Sulcal	Proximal
Noninfected	0.0	0.1	1.8	0.0
Infected	5.0	2.1	10.5	1.6
Infected and immunized	40.0	0.6	8.7	0.3

*Adapted from Michalek et al.[82]
†Expressed as reciprocal.
‡Lesions slightly penetrating into dentin.

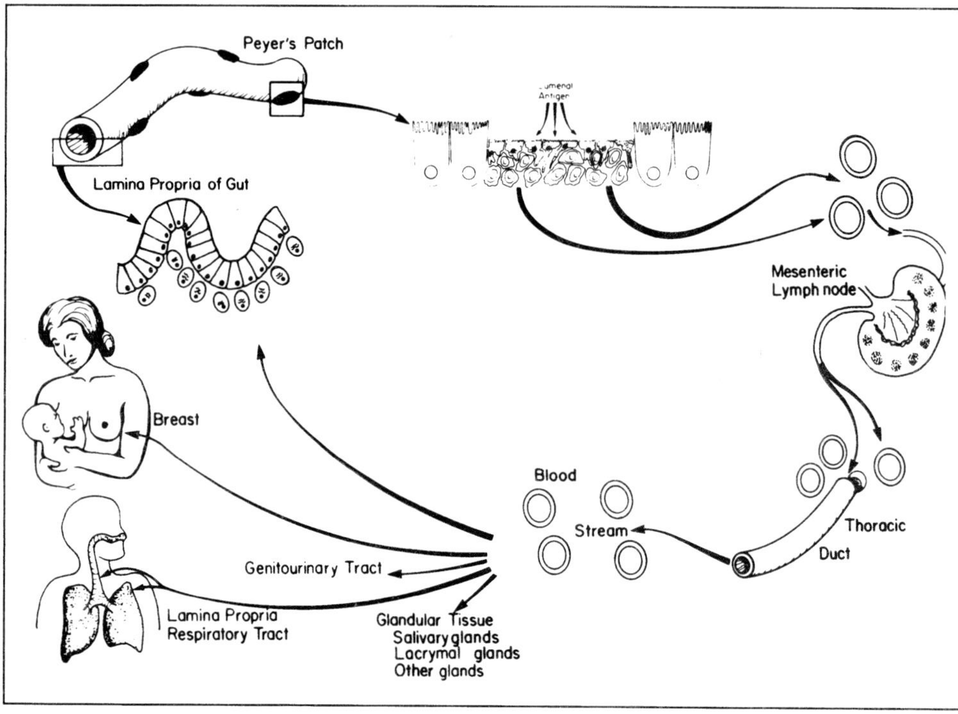

Fig 2-7 Illustration of the circular pathway for the induction of sIgA responses in distant mucosal tissues to antigens encountered in gut-associated lymphoid tissues (GALT). Antigen-sensitized cells leave GALT via efferent lymphatics, pass through the mesenteric lymph nodes, and eventually reach the blood stream. Eventually the cells settle in the gut, upper respiratory tract, and glandular tissues (eg, mammary, lacrimal, and salivary glands). (Courtesy of J.R. McGhee.)

and intraoral submucosal injection was apparently more effective than intravenous. Salivary antibody titers were not measured.[11] Specific pathogen-free rats immunized against *S mutans* developed high levels of antibody in the blood and saliva; these rats were partly protected against caries, but the protection was variable.[109] Rats immunized against crude GTF from *S mutans* developed less caries than sham-immunized animals, but the protection or lack of protection was not uniform.[54] In other studies using conventional rats, no protection against caries in immunized versus nonimmunized animals was observed.[53,108] In rhesus monkeys, subcutaneous injection of heat-killed whole cells of *S mutans* plus incomplete Freund's adjuvant in the upper arm, contralateral leg, and oral submucosa resulted in good serum antibody responses to the bacterium and partial caries protection. Although salivary antibodies were detected, the immunity to caries was correlated with complement-fixing serum antibodies.[69,70]

Whether to approach immunization through stimulation of serum or of salivary antibodies is currently the subject of some debate. Serum immunoglobulins (mainly IgG) enter the oral cavity via the gingival exudate,[23] especially when the gingiva are inflamed (pathotropic potentiation). IgG antibody and complement obtained from immunized rhesus monkeys result in increased phagocytosis and killing of *S mutans*.[98] Accordingly, Lehner and associates[23,69-71,98] have concluded that opsonization and phagocytosis of *S mutans* by leukocytes may occur in gingival exudate and plaque, and that this activity probably accounts for the observed caries reduction in immunized animals. The concentration of IgG in human dental plaque fluid is more than three times higher than that of IgA, indicating that the protein composition of plaque is greatly influenced by the gingival exudate.[110] The relative biological activity of IgA or IgG cannot be inferred, however, because of the proteolytic activity in plaque. On the other hand, McGhee and Michalek[78] consider that since sIgA is the principal immunoglobulin in external secretions, including saliva, local induction of antibodies of this type should be of greater importance in caries immunity.

Human studies

Secretory IgA

Studies on the relationship between caries and the total concentration of IgA in saliva of humans have given conflicting results. An inverse relationship between IgA concentration and caries prevalence has been reported,[128] but this negative correlation has not been confirmed by all investigators, some of whom employed stimulated and others unstimulated saliva. When the salivary flow rate is taken into consideration, a significant negative correlation has been found between DMF score and IgA secretion rate.[93] However, such studies take into consideration only the total IgA secreted, whereas specific anti-*S mutans* IgA may be more important. Significant antibody activity to five different serotypes of *S mutans* has been found in human parotid saliva.[3]

Such specific anti-*S mutans* antibodies in saliva can be induced by oral ingestion. In volunteers who swallowed capsules containing formalin-killed *S mutans* daily for several weeks, salivary and lacrimal antibodies of the IgA class were detected within 1 week, whereas no changes in serum antibody titers were noted during the immunization period.[78] Similarly, oral administration of glucosyltransferase (GTF) from *Streptococcus sobrinus* raised the level of anti-GTF salivary IgA and interfered with repopulation of the oral cavity by mutans-group streptococci, but the effects were relatively short-lived.[102]

Another approach to determining the relationship of immunoglobulins to caries protection or susceptibility has been to study the oral status of children with IgA deficiency.[68,94] These patients typically exhibit symptoms of chronic rhinitis, sinusitis, and recurrent nasopharyngeal infections. Oral manifestations included habitual mouth breathing, gingivitis, frequent labial caries, and tetracycline staining (caused by frequent administration of the drug during the mineralization period). Several adverse factors could be responsible for the poor oral health of these patients: oral hygiene is frequently neglected during periods of acute illness, and, in addition, these children often receive syrup-based oral medications and are bottle-fed in an effort to calm them at night during periods of upper respiratory distress. Most likely their caries and periodontal disease are also indirectly due to an increased susceptibility of the upper respiratory tract to infections.

Subsequent studies have compared salivary immunoglobulin levels, antibody titers to *S mutans*, and past caries experience of selective IgA-deficient patients with age- and sex-matched controls.[78] Immunodeficient subjects were divided into two groups: those without detectable salivary immunoglobulin, and those apparently compensating with sIgM. This latter group had significant titers of sIgM antibodies to six different *S mutans* serotypes. Control subjects had significant salivary antibody activity that could be associated with the IgA isotype. Only those patients who could not produce any salivary antibody had much higher levels of dental caries than matched controls, whereas those patients with compensating sIgM antibodies had less caries than those without any antibody. Patients with immune dysfunction (panhypogammaglobulinemia or agammaglobulinemia) tend to have more caries than normal, but statistical analyses are not possible because of the few patients involved.

Serum antibodies

The presence and the titer of serum antibodies to *S mutans* and *S sanguis* increase with age from early infancy to 16 years.[8] This might be expected from the observation that neither *S mutans* nor *S sanguis* becomes established in the mouth until the teeth have emerged into the oral cavity.[22] Surprisingly, in young children, serum antibodies against *S mutans* are found whether or not this organism is present in their plaque samples.[116] Presumably, these children swallowed *S mutans* cells via parental transmission, and because of their incomplete epithelial structure and immature mucosal secretory IgA system, the intestinal epithelial surface of these infants is more permeable to *S mutans* antigens.

In a study of young naval recruits, a caries-free group had significantly higher serum antibody levels to two strains of *S mutans* than did a caries-rampant group.[63] But in another study the opposite pattern was found: subjects with a low DMF score had lower serum antibody titers to two of seven types of cariogenic streptococci and one type of *Lactobacillus* than did subjects with a high DMF score.[71] In a third study, no correlation could be established between caries activity and levels of serum antibody against three strains of *S mutans* and one of *S sanguis*.[8]

There are several explanations for these anomalous results. First, *S mutans* has several different antigens,[15] one of which forms the specific antigen for identification (see chapter 3, "Serological classification of mutans group"). The other antigens of *S mutans* may also be found in other streptococci (eg, *S sanguis* and *S salivarius*) that do not induce caries. Antibodies against these antigens react both with *S mutans* and with other bacteria. Such "unwanted" reactions cannot be separated from specific reactions by the agglutination techniques commonly used. Second, many antibodies against lipoteichoic acids have been found in human serum.[76] Lipoteichoic acid occurs as a cell surface antigen in a number of gram-positive species such as streptococci, lactobacilli, and micrococci. The discrepancy of various studies relating serum antibody titer to caries prevalence may be because the antibodies are not specific toward *S mutans*. A third explanation may be the cross-sectional nature of antibody and caries analyses in such epidemiological studies. Caries is a chronic process, and caries scores (DMFT) are cumulative. At the time saliva or serum is tested for antibody titer, the lesion may have been restored or arrested. In this case the antibody titer may be low, although cumulative caries score could be high. Conversely, in adults who are no longer experiencing caries, it would not be surprising to find antibodies to cariogenic organisms in the serum and saliva, since these organisms could be introduced into the blood stream through the gingival crevice when hard foods are chewed. Furthermore, the organisms are also being swallowed, which means that humans could immunize themselves with their own oral microflora by stimulating antibody production via the intestinal route (see Fig 2-7).

S mutans possesses antigenic components that elicit antibodies that cross-react with human heart muscle (sarcolemmal sheaths).[43,61,122,123] As yet, postmortem examinations of monkeys immunized with *S mutans* have not revealed any indications of heart damage.[27] But since dental caries is not a life-threatening disease, advocates of a caries vaccine must show its safety as well as its efficacy. Any vaccine that may induce myocarditis represents an unacceptable risk; therefore, any vaccine intended for parenteral administration must be free of antigens that might stimulate antibody cross-reactions with human heart muscle.

Passive immunity

Although active immunization has received the most attention, studies on rats have shown that the offspring of vaccinated dams were protected from colonization by *S mutans* by the passive transfer of antibody via the colostrum and milk. Of course in humans, infection by *S mutans* does not occur until after the deciduous teeth have erupted, by which time infants are no longer nursing. However, these studies have prompted tests in which weanling rats were fed milk either from cows that had been previously immunized with *S mutans* vaccine or from nonimmunized cows. When the rats were subsequently challenged with an infecting dose of *S mutans,* those rats that had passively received the antibody in the cow's milk were protected against the infection.[80]

Caries immunization in perspective

The practicality of caries prevention by specific immunization has not yet been resolved from the point of view of safety. Induction of sIgA-mediated caries immunity offers the best prospects for a safe approach. However, antigenic shifts, whereby bacteria elude antibodies, are an important consideration. The agglutinating activity of standardized salivary IgA against strains of oral streptococci changes over time because of detectable alterations in bacterial antigens.[16,17] Immunological selection pressure mediated by these antibodies in the bathing secretion is responsible for those antigenic shifts. Serum antibodies may be an effective approach to vaccination, but the application of such a vaccine requires elimination of possible antibody cross-reactions with human heart muscle. Modern techniques of genetic bioengineering permit the cloning of genes that make cell wall antigen. Recently, such a gene has been isolated from *S mutans,* inserted in the DNA of *Escherichia coli,* and specific proteins synthesized.[5,29,58] Similarly, the gene responsible for glucosyltransferase activity has been isolated from *S mutans* and inserted into the DNA of *E coli.*[49] Another approach, based on the monoclonal antibody technique, has been to fuse spleen cells of mice immunized with purified cell wall antigen to myeloma cells, thereby generating a murine hybridoma cell line secreting antibodies against the cell wall antigens. These antibodies are further purified and immobilized for affinity chromatography. Culture fluid of *S mutans* is passed through the column and only the specific antigen is absorbed.[59,60] Thus protein antigens that are suitable as a vaccine but do not elicit antibodies cross-reacting with cardiac tissue can be prepared in unlimited quantities. We still need information on immunization routes and schedules and on forms of antigen that will stimulate optimal and persistent protective immunity to dental caries without causing adverse side effects. Much additional experimental work and human trials will be required before a caries vaccine can be applied to clinical practice. While a vaccine against caries is not imminent, the future partial prevention of caries by this means has been predicted.[20] In none of the experiments in which animals were immunized has there been an absolute protection against caries.

Immunization may supplement the established caries prevention obtained by fluoride (systemic and/or topical) but not replace it.

Summary

Saliva plays an extremely important role in attenuating caries. In part, this can be explained simply by the mechanical washing away of some of the food debris, bacteria, and their soluble products. Certainly the buffering action of saliva should not be overlooked. Although several different antibacterial factors have been isolated and identified in the individual secretions, the antibacterial activity of whole saliva gradually loses potency. To what extent the antibacterial action of saliva contributes to caries prevention is not clear.

Host factors: tooth

Tooth morphology and arch form

A susceptible host is one of the factors required for caries to occur (see Fig 2-1). Tooth morphology has long been recognized as an important determinant. For example, attempts to induce caries in dogs have been unsuccessful mainly because of the wide spacing and the conical shape of their teeth.

On the basis of clinical observations, it is known that the pit and fissure areas of the posterior teeth are highly susceptible to caries. Food debris and microorganisms readily impact in the fissures. Investigations have shown a relationship between caries susceptibility and the depth of the fissure.

Certain surfaces of a tooth are more prone to decay, whereas other surfaces rarely show decay. For example, in mandibular first molars the likelihood of decay in descending order is occlusal, buccal, mesial, distal, and lingual, whereas in maxillary first molars the order is occlusal, mesial, lingual (palatal), buccal, and distal. On maxillary lateral incisors, the lingual (palatal) surface is more susceptible to caries than the buccal surface. These differences in decay rates of various surfaces on the same tooth are in part due to morphology, for example, the buccal pit on mandibular molars, lingual groove of maxillary molars, and lingual cingulum of maxillary incisors. The distal surface of first permanent molars is freely accessible to saliva for about 4 to 5 years until the second molars erupt at age 10 or 11, whereas approximal plaque may form on the mesial surface shortly after eruption at age 6 or 7.

An intraoral variation exists in susceptibility to caries between different tooth types. The most susceptible permanent teeth are the mandibular first molars, closely followed by the maxillary first molars and the mandibular and maxillary second molars. The second premolars, maxillary incisors, and first premolars are the next in sequence, whereas the mandibular incisors and canines are the least likely to develop lesions (see Fig 7-2). A similarity of occurrence of caries in the corresponding tooth on the opposite quadrant has frequently been observed.

Irregularities in arch form, crowding, and overlapping of the teeth also favor the development of carious lesions. Experimentally this has been verified by the gold plate technique in which stagnation areas are deliberately created on selected tooth surfaces. These surfaces develop "white spot" lesions within a few weeks. The white appearance is due to optical phenomena associated with increased enamel porosity.

Tooth composition

There is good evidence to indicate that the enamel surface is more caries-resistant than the subsurface. Microradiographs of initial carious lesions frequently reveal marked demineralization of the subsurface enamel beneath an outermost layer that is only slightly affected (Fig 2-8).[91] Several hypotheses have been developed to explain this phenomenon. A pumping mechanism has been proposed whereby matter is transported from the inner enamel to the surface zone and from the surface zone to the saliva.[83] There is a net movement of inorganic mineral phase from the inner enamel to the oral cavity. The surface enamel appears unaltered simply because it is continuously being regenerated by precipitation of solid phases (dicalcium phosphate dihydrate, $CaHPO_4 \cdot 2H_2O$ and fluorapatite, $Ca_{10}[PO_4]_6F_2$, or more precisely, partially fluoridated hydroxyapatite, $Ca_{10}[PO_4]_6[OH]_{2-x}F_x$, where x is much smaller than 2). However, when "white spots" have been examined by scanning electron microscopy, the initial stage of such active carious lesions has been characterized by openings in the outer enamel surface through eroded focal holes.[120] Accordingly, the concept of a relatively unaffected surface layer, described in transverse sections examined by microradiography or light microscopy, needs revision in view of these surface defects, which represent signs of focal demineralization. By transmission electron microscopy, the enamel surface is seen to be indented by irregular destruction of apatite crystals. Small microdefects (0.2 to 2 μm), starting at the enamel surface and reaching the deeper enamel layer, have been observed[45] (see chapter 7). Surface enamel is harder than the underlying enamel.[92] These differences are likely to be related to the many differences between the composition of the surface and that of the rest of the enamel.[19] The surface enamel has more minerals and more organic matter but relatively less water. In addition, certain elements, including fluoride, chloride, zinc, lead, and iron, accumulate in the enamel surface, while other constituents, such as carbonate and magnesium, are sparse in surface as compared with subsurface enamel. Changes of the enamel, such as a decrease in density and

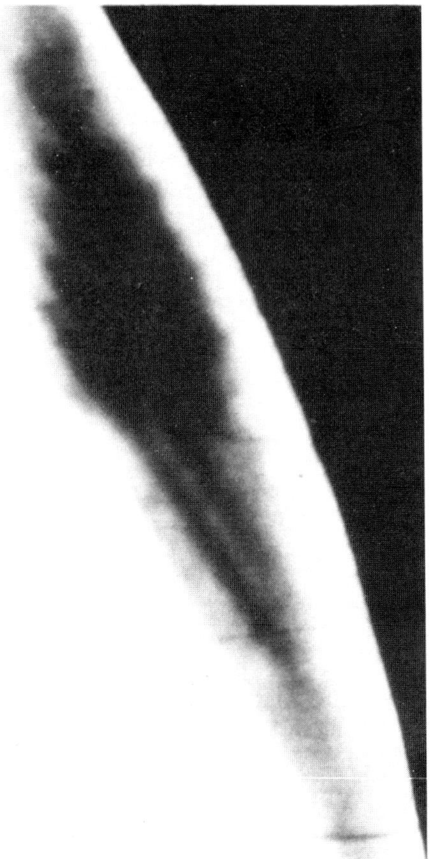

Fig 2-8 Microradiograph of white spot lesion of enamel. Compare the extensive demineralization of the subsurface enamel with the better mineralized surface layer (original magnification ×100).

permeability and an increase in nitrogen and fluoride content, occur with age. These alterations are part of the posteruptive "maturation" process whereby teeth become more resistant to caries with time. The concentration of fluoride of the surface layer of enamel increases as the fluoride concentration of the drinking water increases, and such enamel is less soluble in acids. Furthermore, the higher the fluoride concentration of the water supply, the lower the prevalence of caries. These aspects are dealt with in more detail in chapter 11 and elsewhere.[90] Analyses of teeth treated with topical fluoride indicate that a direct linear relationship does not exist between enamel fluoride deposition and caries prevention, although fluoride must be increased to obtain a clinically demonstrable benefit.[52]

Chapter review

Host saliva

- List the factor(s) in saliva that have some relationship to caries.
- Define xerostomia.
- List the pathological conditions associated with xerostomia.
- List the special precautions that should be taken with a patient suffering from xerostomia.
- Explain how postradiation caries differs from the usual type of caries.
- List some types of drugs that have xerostomic side effects.
- Describe when salivary secretion is the least in normal patients and why it is of clinical importance.
- State some of the differences between submandibular and parotid salivary secretion and describe how these affect caries and calculus formation.
- Define a buffer. Describe which is the most important buffering system in saliva.
- List the factors in saliva that have antibacterial properties.
- List the immunoglobulins found in saliva. Indicate which is the principal one and how it differs from its counterpart in serum, and say how one might raise the salivary antibody titer against cariogenic streptococci.
- List the categories of ingredients used in various saliva substitutes and state an example of each.

Host teeth

- Rank teeth in decreasing order of caries susceptibility.
- Compare the caries susceptibility of different surfaces of the same tooth.
- State the chemical difference between the enamel surface and the subsurface.
- State the importance of the bilateral symmetry of caries.
- Explain the chalky appearance of "white spot" lesions.

Selected readings

Bowen, W.H., Genco, R.J., and O'Brien, T.C. (eds) 1976. *Immunological Aspects of Dental Caries*. Washington, D.C.: Information Retrieval, Inc.

Genco, R.J. (ed) 1976. Immunological aspects of dental caries. *J Dent Res* 55:Sp. Issue.
Genco, R.J. 1979. Immune responses to oral organisms. Implications for dental caries and periodontal disease. *J Clin Periodontol* 6:Suppl. 22–31.
Kleinberg, I., Ellison, S.A., and Mandel, I.D. (eds) 1979. *Saliva and Dental Caries.* Sp. Suppl. Microbiol. Abstr. Washington, D.C.: Information Retrieval, Inc.
Krasse, B., Emilson, C.G., and Gahnberg, L. 1987. An anticaries vaccine: report on the status of research. *Caries Res* 21:255–276.
Lehner, T. 1982. Regulation of immune responses to streptococcal protein antigens involved in dental caries. *Immunol Today* 3:73–77.
Mandel, I.D. 1979. Dental caries. *Am Sci* 67:680–688.
McGhee, J.R., Mestecky, J., and Babb, J.L. (eds) 1978. *Secretory Immunity and Infection.* New York: Plenum Press.
McGhee, J.R., and Michalek, S.M. 1981. Immunobiology of dental caries. Microbial aspects and local immunity. *Ann Rev Microbiol* 35:595–638.
Mandel, I.D., and Wotman, S. 1976. The salivary secretions in health and disease. *Oral Sci Rev* 8:25–47.
Mergenhagen, S., and Scherp, H.W. (eds) 1973. *Comparative Immunology of the Oral Cavity.* Department of Health, Education, and Welfare publication No. 73–438. Washington, D.C.: U.S. Government Printing Office.
Roitt, I.M., and Lehner, T. 1983. *Immunology of Oral Diseases.* 2nd ed. Oxford: Blackwell Scientific Publications, pp. 345–374.
Rowe, N.H. (ed) 1972. *Salivary Glands and Their Secretion.* Proceedings of Symposium, Ann Arbor: University of Michigan.
Scherp, H.W. 1971. Dental caries. Prospects for prevention. *Science* 73:1199–1205.
Scully, C. 1981. Dental caries. Progress in microbiology and immunology. *J Infect* 3:107–133.
Sreebny, L. (ed) 1987. *The Salivary System.* Boca Raton: CRC Press.
Weatherell, J.A. 1975. Composition of dental enamel. *Br Med Bull* 31:115–119.

References

1. Adamson, M., and Carisson, J. 1982. Lactoperoxidase and thiocyanate protect bacteria from hydrogen peroxide. *Infect Immun* 35:20–24.
2. Aldous, J.A. 1964. Induced xerostomia and its relation to dental caries. *J Dent Child* 31:160–162.
3. Arnold, R.R., Mestecky, J., and McGhee, J.R. 1976. Naturally occurring secretory immunoglobulin A antibodies to *Streptococcus mutans* in human colostrum and saliva. *Infect Immun* 14:355–362.
4. Bahn, S.L., 1972. Drug-related dental destruction. *Oral Surg* 33:49–54.
5. Barletta, R.G., Robeson, J.P., and Curtiss, R. 1982. Properties of a *Streptococcus mutans* glucosyltransferase expressed in *Escherichia coli. J Dent Res* 61:Abstr. 1408, p. 335.
6. Bates, J.F., and Adams, D. 1968. The influence of mental stress on the flow of saliva in man. *Arch Oral Biol* 13:593–596.
7. Bateson, M.C., Gibberd, F.B., and Wilson, R.S. 1973. Salivary symptoms in Parkinson disease. *Arch Neurol* 29:274–275.
8. Berkenbilt, D.A., and Bahn, A.N. 1971. Development of antibodies to cariogenic streptococci in children. *J Am Dent Assoc* 83:332–337.
9. Bertram, V. 1967. Xerostomia. *Acta Odontol Scand* 25:Suppl. 49.
10. Bhoola, K.D., McNicol, M.W., Oliver, S., and Forna, J. 1969. Changes in salivary enzymes in patients with sarcoidosis. *N Engl J Med* 28:877–879.
11. Bowen, W.H., Cohen, B., Cole, M.F., and Colman, G. 1975. Immunization against dental caries. *Br Dent J* 139:45–58.
12. Brandtzaeg, P. 1971. Human secretory immunoglobulins, III. Immunochemical and physicochemical studies of secretory IgA and free secretory piece. *Acta Pathol Microbiol Scand* [B] 79:165–188.
13. Brandtzaeg, P., Fjellanger, I., and Gjeruldsen, S.T. 1970. Adsorption of immunoglobulin A onto oral bacteria. *J Bacteriol* 96:242–249.
14. Brandtzaeg, P., Fjellanger, I., and Gjeruldsen, S.T. 1970. Human secretory immunoglobulins, I. Salivary secretions from individuals with normal or low levels of serum

immunoglobulins. *Scand J Haematol* Suppl. 12, pp. 1–83.

15. Bratthall, D. 1970. Demonstration of five serological groups of streptococcal strains resembling *Streptococcus mutans*. *Odontol Rev* 21:143–152.
16. Bratthall, D., and Gibbons, R. 1975. Changing agglutination activities of salivary immunoglobulin A preparation against oral streptococci. *Infect Immun* 11:603–606.
17. Bratthall, D., and Köhler, B. 1976. *Streptococcus mutans* serotypes. Some aspects of their identification, distribution, antigenic shifts and relationship to caries. *J Dent Res* 55:C15–C21.
18. Brown, L.R., Dreizen, S., Handler, S., and Johnston, D.A. 1975. Effect of radiation-induced xerostomia in human oral microflora. *J Dent Res* 54:740–750.
19. Brudevold, F., and Söremark, R. 1964. Chemistry of the mineral phase of human enamel. In *Structural and Mineral Organization of Teeth*, A.E.W. Miles and R.C. Greulich (eds), New York: Academic Press.
20. Carlos, J.P. 1982. The prevention of dental caries. Ten years later. *J Am Dent Assoc* 104:193–197.
21. Carlsson, J. 1980. Bactericidal effect of hydrogen peroxide is prevented by lacto-peroxidase-thiocyanate system under anaerobic conditions. *Infect Immun* 29:1190–1192.
22. Carlsson, J., Grahnén, H., Jonsson, G., and Wikner, S. 1970. Establishment of *Streptococcus sanguis* in the mouths of infants. *Arch Oral Biol* 15:1143–1148.
23. Challacombe, S.J., Russell, M.W., Hawkes, J.E., Bergmeier, L.A., and Lehner, T. 1978. Passage of immunoglobulins from plasma to the oral cavity in rhesus monkeys. *Immunology* 35:923–931.
24. Charlton, G., Fitzgerald, R.J., and Keyes, P.H. 1971. Determination of saliva and dental plaque pH in hamsters with glass microelectrodes. *Arch Oral Biol* 16:649–654.
25. Charlton, G., Fitzgerald, R.J., and Keyes, P.H. 1971. Hydrogen ion activity in dental plaque of hamsters during metabolism of sucrose, glucose and fructose. *Arch Oral Biol* 16:655–662.
26. Clem, W.H., and Klebanoff, S.J. 1966. Inhibitory effect of saliva on glutamic acid accumulation by *Lactobacillus acidophilus* and the role of the lactoperoxidasethiocyanate system. *J Bacteriol* 91:1848–1853.
27. Cohen, B., Colman, G., and Russell, R.R.B. 1979. Immunization against dental caries. Further studies. *Br Dent J* 147:9–14.
28. Council on Dental Therapeutics. 1987. *Categorical Listing of Accepted Products*. Chicago: American Dental Association.
29. Curtiss, R. 1986. Genetic analysis of *Streptococcus mutans* virulence and prospects for an anti-caries vaccine. *J Dent Res* 65:1034–1045.
30. Daniels, T.E., Silverman, S., Michalski, J.P., Greenspan, J.S., Sylvester, R.A., and Talal, N. 1975. The oral component of Sjögren's syndrome. *Oral Surg* 39:875–885.
31. Dawes, C. 1970. Effects of diet on salivary secretion and composition. *J Dent Res* 49:1263–1272.
32. Dirksen, T.R., Little, M.F., and Bibby, B.G. 1963. The pH of carious cavities-II. The pH at different depths in isolated cavities. *Arch Oral Biol* 8:91–97.
33. Dobkin, A.B., and Purkin, N. 1960. The antisialogogue effect of phenothiazine derivatives. *Br J Anaesth* 32:57–59.
34. Dobkin, A.B., Wyant, G.M., and Assheim, G.M. 1958. Antisialogogue drugs in man. *Anaesthesia* 13:63–67.
35. Dreizen, S., Brown, L.R., Daly, T.E., and Drane, J.B. 1977. Prevention of xerostomia-related dental caries in irradiated cancer patients. *J Dent Res* 56:99–104.
36. Dreizen, S., Daley, T.E., Drane, J.B., and Brown, L.R. 1977. Oral complications of cancer radiotherapy. *Postgrad Med* 61:85–92.
37. Edgar, W.M., Bowen, W.H., and Cole, M.F. 1981. Development of rampant dental caries, and composition of plaque fluid and saliva in irradiated primates. *J Oral Pathol* 10:284–295.
38. Ericsson, Y. 1959. Clinical investigation of the salivary buffering action. *Acta Odontol Scand* 17:131–165.
39. Ericsson, Y. 1962. Salivary and food factors in dental caries development. *Int Dent J* 12:476–495.
40. Evans, R.T., and Mergenhagen, S.E. 1965. Occurrence of natural antibacterial antibody in human parotid fluid. *Proc Soc Exp Biol Med* 119:815–819.
41. Everhart, D.L., Grigsby, W.R., and Carter, W.H. 1972. Evaluation of dental caries experience and salivary immunoglobulins in whole saliva. *J Dent Res* 51:1487–1491.
42. Everhart, D.L., Grigsby, W.R., and Carter, W.H. 1973. Human dental caries experience related to age, sex, race and certain salivary properties. *J Dent Res* 52:242–

247.
43. Ferretti, J.J., Shea, C., and Humphrey, M.W. 1980. Cross-reactivity of *Streptococcus mutans* and human heart tissue. *Infect Immun* 30:69–73.
44. Finn, S.B., Klapper, C.E., and Volker, J.F. 1955. Intra-oral effects upon experimental hamster caries. In *Advances in Experimental Caries Research,* R.F. Sognnaes (ed), Washington, D.C.: American Association for the Advancement of Science, pp. 152–168.
45. Frank, R.M., Herdly, J., and Phillippe, E. 1965. Acquired dental defects and salivary gland lesions after irradiation for carcinoma. *J Am Dent Assoc* 70:868–883.
46. Frank, R.M., and Voegel, J.C. 1978. Dissolution mechanisms of the apatite crystals during dental caries and bone resorption. In *Molecular Basis of Biological Degradative Processes,* R.D. Berlin, H. Herrmann, I.H. Lepow, and J.M. Tanzer (eds), New York: Academic Press, pp. 277–311.
47. Gerstenberger, L., and Wencker-Hermstedt, E. 1976. Der synthetische speichel—ein zusatz zur praemedikation. *Anesthetist* 25:486–487.
48. Gibbons, R.J., de Stoppelaar, J.D., and Harden, L. 1966. Lysozyme insensitivity of bacteria indigenous to the oral cavity of man. *J Dent Res* 45:877–881.
49. Gilpin, M.L., Russell, R.D., and Morrissey, P. 1985. Cloning and expression of two *Streptococcus mutans* glucosyltransferases in *Escherichia coli* K-12. *Infect Immun* 49:414–416.
50. Glass, B.J., Van Dis, M.L., Langlais, R.P., and Miles, D.A. 1984. Xerostomia: diagnosis and treatment planning considerations. *Oral Surg* 58:248–252.
51. Grad, H., Grushka, M., and Yanover, L. 1985. Drug-induced xerostomia. *J Can Dent Assoc* 51:296–300.
52. Gron, P. 1978. Inorganic chemical and structural aspects of oral mineralized tissues. In *Textbook of Oral Biology,* J.H. Shaw, E.A. Sweeney, C.C. Cappuccino, and S.M. Meller (eds), Philadelphia: W.B. Saunders, pp. 484–507.
53. Guggenheim, B., Mühlemann, H.R., Regolati, B., and Schmid, R. 1970. The effect of immunization against streptococci or glucosyltransferases on plaque formation and dental caries in rats. In *Dental Plaque,* W.D. McHugh (ed), Edinburgh: E. & S. Livingstone, pp. 287–296.
54. Hayashi, J.A., Shklair, I.L., and Bahn, A.N. 1972. Immunization with dextransucrases and glucosidic hydrolases. *J Dent Res* 51:436–442.
55. Helms, J.F., Dodds, W.J., Soergel, K.H., Egide, M.S., and Wood, C.M. 1982. Acid neutralizing capacity of human saliva. *Gastroenterology* 83:69–74.
56. Hill, F.J. 1972. Rampant caries and the salivary glands. *Dent Pract Dent Rec* 22: 454–455.
57. Hoerman, K.C., Englander, H.R., and Shklair, I.L. 1956. Lysozyme. Its characteristics in human parotid and submaxillo-lingual saliva. *Proc Soc Exp Biol Med* 92:875–878.
58. Holt, R.G., Saito, S., Abiko, Y., Smorawinska, M., Hanson, J.B., and Curtiss, R. 1982. *Streptococcus mutans* genes that code for extracellular proteins in *Escherichia coli* K-12. *Infect Immun* 38:147–156.
59. Hughes, M., MacHardy, S.M., and Sheppard, A.J. 1983. Manufacture and control of a dental caries vaccine for parenteral administration to man. In *Glucosyltransferases, glucans, sucrose in dental caries,* R.J. Doyle and J.E. Ciardi (eds), Sp. Suppl. *Chemical sensors,* pp. 259–268.
60. Hughes, M., MacHardy, S.M., Sheppard, A.J., Davies, P., and Ivanyi, J. 1982. Use of monoclonal antibody for the preparation of a dental caries vaccine. *J Dent Res* 61:546, Abstr. 98.
61. Hughes, M., MacHardy, S.M., Sheppard, A.J., and Woods, N.C. 1980. Evidence for an immunological relationship between *Streptococcus mutans* and human cardiac tissue. *Infect Immun* 27:576–588.
62. Jenkins, G.N. 1978. *The Physiology of the Mouth.* 4th ed, Philadelphia: F.A. Davis, p. 317.
63. Kennedy, A.E., Shklair, I.L., Hayashi, J.A., and Bahn, A.N. 1968. Antibodies to cariogenic streptococci in humans. *Arch Oral Biol* 13:1275–1278.
64. Kermiol, M., and Walsh, R.F. 1975. Dental caries after radiotherapy of the oral regions. *J Am Dent Assoc* 91:838–845.
65. Kerr, A.C., and Wedderburn, D.L. 1958. Antibacterial factors in the secretions of human parotid and submaxillary glands. *Br Dent J* 105:321–326.
66. König, K.G., and Mühlemann, H.R. 1964. Further investigations into a possible effect of dietary lysozyme on caries incidence in rats. *Helv Odontol Acta* 8:22–24.
67. Kraus, F.W., and Konno, J. 1965. The salivary secretion of antibody. *Ala J Med Sci* 2:15–22.
68. Legler, D.W., McGhee, J.R., Lynch, D.P., Mestecky, J.F., Schaeffer, M.E., Carson, J.,

and Bradley, E.L. 1981. Immunodeficiency disease and dental caries in man. *Arch Oral Biol* 26:905–910.

69. Lehner, T., Challacombe, S.J., and Caldwell, J. 1975. An experimental model for immunological studies of dental caries in the rhesus monkey. *Arch Oral Biol* 20: 299–304.
70. Lehner, T., Challcombe, S.J., and Caldwell, J. 1975. An immunological investigation into the prevention of caries in deciduous teeth of rhesus monkeys. *Arch Oral Biol* 20:305–310.
71. Lehner, T., Wilton, J.M.A., and Ward, R.G. 1970. Serum antibodies in dental caries in man. *Arch Oral Biol* 15:481–490.
72. Leung, S.W. 1962. Saliva and dental caries. *Dent Clin North Am* July, pp. 347–355.
73. Levine, J.J., Aguire, A., Hatton, M.N., and Tabak, L.A. 1987. Artificial salivas: present and future. *J Dent Res* 66 (Spec. Iss.):693–698.
74. Llory, H., Dammron, A., Gionni, M., and Frank, R.M. 1972. Some population changes in oral anaerobic microorganisms, *Streptococcus mutans* and yeasts following irradiation of the salivary glands. *Caries Res* 6:298–311.
75. MacFarlane, T.W., and Mason, D.K. 1974. Changes in the oral flora in Sjögren's syndrome. *J Clin Pathol* 27:416–419.

75a. Mansson-Rahemtulla, B., Rahemtulla, F., Baldone, D.C., Pruitt, K.M., and Hjerpe, A. 1988. Purification and characterization of human salivary peroxidase. *Biochem* 27:233–239.

76. Markham, J.L., Knox, K.W., and Schamschula, R.G. 1973. Antibodies to teichoic acids in man. *Arch Oral Bol* 18:313–319.
77. Marlay, E. 1970. The relationship between dental caries and salivary properties at adolescence. *Aust Dent J* 5:412–422.
78. McGhee, J.R., and Michalek, S.M. 1981. Immunobiology of dental caries. Microbial aspects and local immunity. *Annu Rev Microbiol* 35:595–638.
79. McGhee, J.R., Michalek, S.M., Webb, J., Navia, J.M., Rahman, A.F.R., and Legler, D.W. 1975. Effective immunity to dental caries. Protection of gnotobiotic rats by local immunization with *Streptococcus mutans*. *J Immunol* 114:300–305.
80. Michalek, S.M., McGhee, J.R., Arnold, R.R., and Mestecky, J. 1978. Effective immunity to dental caries. Selective induction of secretory immunity by oral administration of *Streptococcus mutans* in rodents. *Adv Exp Med Biol* 107:261–269.
81. Michalek, S.M., McGhee, J.R., Mestecky, J., Arnold, R.R., and Bozzo, L. 1976. Ingestion of *Streptococcus mutans* induces secretory IgA and caries immunity. *Science* 192:1238–1240.
82. Michalek, S.M., McGhee, J.R., Navia, J.M., and Narkates, A.J. 1976. Effective immunity to dental caries. Protection of malnourished rats by local injection of *Streptococcus mutans*. *Infect Immun* 13:782–789.
83. Moreno, E.C., and Zahradnik, R.T. 1974. Chemistry of enamel subsurface demineralization in vitro. *J Dent Res* 53:226–235.
84. Morrison, M., and Steele, W.F. 1968. Lactoperoxidase, the peroxidase in the salivary gland. In *Biology of the Mouth*, P. Person (ed), Washington; D.C.: American Academy for the Advancement of Science, pp. 89–110.
85. Mühlemann, H.R., and König, K.G. 1962. The effect of lysozyme on experimental caries. *Helv Odontol Acta* 6:33–37.
86. Nakamoto, R.Y. 1979. Use of saliva substitute in post-radiation xerostomia. *J Prosthet Dent* 42:539–542.
87. *National Disease and Therapeutic Index Review*. 1971. 2:4.
88. Newbrun, E. 1961. Application of atomic absorption spectroscopy to the determination of calcium in saliva. *Nature* 192:1182–1183.
89. Newbrun, E. 1972. What is the relationship of saliva to dental caries? In *Salivary Glands and Their Secretion*, N.H. Rowe (ed), Ann Arbor: University of Michigan, pp. 22–37.
90. Newbrun, E. 1986. *Fluorides and Dental Caries*. 3rd ed. Springfield, Ill.: Charles C Thomas.
91. Newbrun, E., Brudevold, F., and Mermagen, H. 1959. A microradiographic evaluation of occlusal fissures and grooves. *J Am Dent Assoc* 58:26–31.
92. Newbrun, E., and Pigman, W. 1960. The hardness of enamel and dentine. *Aust Dent J* 5:210–217.
93. Orstavik, D., and Brandtzaeg, P. 1975. Secretion of parotid IgA in relation to gingival inflammation and dental caries experience in man. *Arch Oral Biol* 20:701–704.
94. Robertson, P.B., and Cooper, M.D. 1974. Oral manifestations of IgA deficiency. *Adv Exp Med Biol* 45:497–503.

95. Rudegren, J., Van Dijken, J., Mörnstad, H., and Von Knorring, L. 1985. Oral conditions in patients receiving long-term treatment with cyclic antidepressant drugs. *Swed Dent J* 9:55–64.
96. Schneyer, L.H., Pigman, W., Hanahan, L., and Gilmour, R.W. 1956. Rate of flow of human parotid, sublingual and submaxillary secretions during sleep. *J Dent Res* 35:109–114.
97. Schubert, M.M., and Izutsu, K.T. 1987. Iatrogenic causes of salivary gland dysfunction. *J Dent Res* 66 (Spec. Iss.):680–688.
98. Scully, C.M., Russell, M.S., and Lehner, T. 1980. Specificity of opsonizing antibodies to antigens of *Streptococcus mutans. Immunology* 41:467–473.
99. Shannon, I.L., Trodahl, J.N., and Starke, E.N. 1978. Remineralization of enamel by a saliva substitute designed for use by irradiated patients. *Cancer* 41:98–102.
100. Sirisinha, S. 1970. Reactions of human salivary immunoglobulins with indigenous bacteria. *Arch Oral Biol* 15:551–554.
101. Slowey, R.R., Eidelman, S., and Klebanoff, S.J. 1968. Antibacterial activity of the purified peroxidase from human parotid saliva. *J Bacteriol* 96:575–579.
102. Smith, D.J., and Taubman, M.A. 1978. Oral immunization of humans with *Streptococcus sobrinus* glucosyltransferase. *Infect Immun* 55:2562–2569.
103. Smith, D.J., Taubman, M.A., and Ebersole, J.L. 1979. Effect of oral administration of glucosyltransferase antigens on experimental dental caries. *Infect Immun* 26: 82–89.
104. Smith, D.J., Taubman, M.A., and Ebersole, J.L. 1980. Local and systemic antibody response to oral administration of glucosyltransferase antigen complex. *Infect Immun* 28:441–450.
105. Smith, D.J., Taubman, M.A., and Ebersole, J.L. 1982. Effects of local immunization with glucosyltransferase on colonization of hamsters by *Streptococcus mutans. Infect Immun* 37:656–661.
105a. Sreebny, L.M., and Schwartz, S.S. 1986. A reference guide to drugs and dry mouth. *Gerodontol* 5:75–99.
106. Stephan, R.M. 1971. Clinical study of etiology and control of rampant dental caries. 49th Gen. Session, International Association for Dental Research Abstr. 636, p. 211.
107. Sweeney, E.A., and Shaw, J.H. 1963. The effect of dietary lysozyme supplements on caries incidence in rats. *Arch Oral Biol* 8:775–776.
108. Tanzer, J.M., Hageage, G.J., and Larson, R.H. 1970. Inability to immunologically protect rats against smooth surface caries. 48th Gen. Meeting, International Association for Dental Research Abstr. 466, p. 165.
109. Tanzer, J.M., Hageage, G.J., and Larson, R.H. 1973. Variable experience in immunization of rats against *Streptococcus mutans*-associated dental caries. *Arch Oral Biol* 18:1425–1439.
110. Tatevossian, A., and Newbrun, E. 1981. Electrophoretic and immunoelectrophoretic studies of proteins in aqueous phase of human dental plaque. *Arch Oral Biol* 26: 275–280.
111. Taubman, M.A. 1973. Role of immunization in dental disease. In *Comparative Immunology of the Oral Cavity*, S. Mergenhagen and H.W. Scherp (eds), Department of Health, Education, and Welfare publication No. 73–438. Washington, D.C.: U.S. Government Printing Office, pp. 138–158.
112. Taubman, M.A., Ebersole, J.L., Smith, D.J., and Reger, R.C. 1980. The immunochemical approach to dental caries prevention. Secretory immune system adjuvant studies. *J Dent Res* 59:2163–2170.
113. Taubman, M.A., and Smith, D.J. 1974. Effects of local immunization with *Streptococcus mutans* on induction of salivary IgA antibody and experimental dental caries in rats. *Infect Immun* 9:1079–1091.
114. Taubman, M.A., Smith, D.J., and Ebersole, J.L. 1981. Conventional and specialized rodent models for studies of immune mechanisms and dental caries. Proceedings "Symposium on Animal Models in Cariology." J.M. Tanzer (ed), Sp. Suppl. Microbiol. Abstr., pp. 439–450.
115. Taubman, M.A., and Smith, D.J. 1977. Effects of local immunization with glucosyltransferase fractions from *Streptococcus mutans* on dental caries in rats and hamsters. *J Immunol* 118:710–720.
116. Tenovuo, J., Lehtonen, O.P., and Aaltonen, A.S. 1987. Serum and salivary antibodies against *Streptococcus mutans* in young children with and without detectable oral *S mutans. Caries Res* 21:289–296.
117. Tenovuo, J., and Pruitt, K.M. 1984. Relationship of the human salivary peroxidase system to oral health. *J Oral Pathol* 13:573–584.

118. Thomas, E.L., Bates, K.P., and Jefferson, M.M. 1981. Peroxidase antimicrobial system of human saliva. Requirements for accumulation of hypothiocyanite. *J Dent Res* 60:785–796.
119. Tourville, D., Bienenstock, J., and Tomasi, T.B., Jr. 1968. Natural antibodies of human serum, saliva and urine reactive with *Escherichia coli. Proc Soc Exp Biol Med* 128: 722–727.
120. Thylstrup, A., and Fejerskov, O. 1981. Surface features of early carious enamel at various stages of activity. In *Tooth Surface Interactions and Preventive Dentistry*, G. Rolla, T. Sonju, and G. Embery (eds), London: Information Retrieval, Inc, pp. 193–205.
121. Twetman, S., Linder, A., and Modeer, T. 1981. Lysozyme and salivary immunoglobulin A in caries-free and caries-susceptible pre-school children. *Swed Dent J* 5:9–14.
122. van de Rijn, I., Bleiweis, A.S., and Zabriskie, J.B. 1976. Antigens in *Streptococcus mutans* cross-reactive with human heart muscle. *J Dent Res* 55:C59–C64.
123. van de Rijn, I., and Zabriskie, J.B. 1976. Immunological relationship between *Streptococcus mutans* and human myocardium. In *Immonological Aspects of Dental Caries,* W.H. Bowen, R.J. Genco, and T.C. O'Brien (eds), Arlington, Va.: Information Retrieval, pp. 187–194.
124. Vissink, A., 'S-Gravenmade, E.J., Panders, A.K., Vermay, A., Petersen, J.K., Visch, L.L., and Schaub, M.B. 1983. A clinical comparison between commercially available mucin- and CMC-containing saliva substitutes. *Int J Oral Surg* 12:232–238.
125. Wagner, M. 1968. Specific immunization against dental caries in the gnotobiotic rat. In *Advances in Germfree Research and Gnotobiology*, M. Miyahawa and T.D. Luckey (eds), Cleveland: The Chemical Rubber Co, p. 264.
126. Williams, R.C., and Gibbons, R.J. 1972. Inhibition of bacterial adherence by secretory immunoglobulin A. Mechanism of antigen disposal. *Science* 177:697–699.
127. Winer, J.A., and Bahn, S. 1967. Loss of teeth with antidepressant drug therapy. *Arch Gen Psychiatry* 16:239–240.
128. Zengo, A.N., Mandel, I.D., Goldman, R., and Khurana, H.S. 1971. Salivary studies in human caries resistance. *Arch Oral Biol* 16:557–560.

Chapter 3

Microflora

If we compare the life-conditions of bacteria . . . with the conditions prevailing in the human mouth, it becomes evident that the oral cavity must be an excellent breeding-place for those organisms. . . . Within the last few years I have isolated more than one hundred different kinds of bacteria from the juices and deposits in the mouth. . . . We have been able to establish the fact that all micro-organisms of the human mouth which possess the power of exciting acid fermentation of foods may and do take part in producing the first stage of caries. . . . But whether there is any one bacterium which may always *be found in decayed dentine, and which might therefore be entitled to the name of* the *bacterium of tooth decay, or whether there are various kinds which occur with considerable constancy, we are not able to say.*

Willoughby D. Miller in
The Microorganisms of the Human Mouth
S.S. White Dental Mfg Co, 1890

Evidence of bacterial role in caries etiology

Although there are differences of opinion as to how and which microorganisms produce carious lesions, it is uniformly agreed that caries cannot occur without microorganisms. The overwhelming evidence implicating microorganisms in the etiology of caries is summarized below.

1. Germ-free animals do not develop caries.
2. Antibiotics fed to animals are effective in reducing the incidence and severity of caries.
3. Totally unerupted and unexposed teeth do not develop caries, yet when exposed to the oral environment and microflora can become carious. Rarely, impacted third molars with soft tissue covering are found to be carious, in which case a sinus tract to the oral cavity can be found.[1]
4. Oral bacteria can demineralize enamel and dentin in vitro and produce carieslike lesions.
5. Microorganisms have been histologically demonstrated invading carious enamel and dentin. They can be isolated and cultivated from carious lesions.

The classical germ-free animal studies of Orland et al[148,149] firmly established a principle that had been debated for more than a century, namely, that dental caries is a bacterial infection. These studies demonstrated that germ-free rats on a highly cariogenic diet containing sucrose did not develop caries. When the gnotobiotic rats on the same diet were infected with combinations of an enterococcus and a proteolytic bacillus (an unintentional contaminant) or an enterococcus and a pleomorphic bacterium, caries developed. This marked a new epoch in caries research. Various independent investigations have confirmed that germ-free animals do not develop caries, whereas gnotobiotic animals, when infected with one or more pure cultures of microorganisms, may develop caries.

The term gnotobiotic animal is used because etymologically it refers to an animal with a known microbiota (Greek: *gnosis* = positive knowledge). Gnotobiote, a wider definition, includes both germ-free or axenic (free from foreign organisms) animals and ex-germ-free animals deliberately inoculated with one or more types of microbes for experimental purposes. It does not include conventional animals deprived of a specific segment of their microflora by antibiotics, since the remaining microflora cannot be precisely defined.[72] Several organisms have been found capable of inducing carious lesions when used as monocontaminants in gnotobiotic rats. These include the mutans group of streptococci, a *Streptococcus salivarius* strain, *Streptococcus milleri, Streptococcus oralis,*[197] *Streptococcus sanguis* (several strains), *Peptostreptococcus intermedius,*[159] a *Lactobacillus acidophilus* strain, a *Lactobacillus casei* strain,[57,160] *Actinomyces viscosus,* and *Actinomyces naeslundii.*[63,87] However, not all of these organisms are equally virulent. Furthermore, in the same animal test system some streptococci and lactobacilli—such as *Lactobacillus fermentum, L acidophilus, Streptococcus lactis, Streptococcus faecalis, Streptococcus salivarius,* and *S sanguis*[53,54]—were not able to induce caries.

These findings show that:

1. Caries will not occur in the complete absence of microorganisms.
2. Caries can occur in rats that harbor only a single type of organism (monoinfected).
3. Most organisms are not cariogenic.

It is not known exactly what determines the cariogenicity of a microorganism. The streptococci with cariogenic potential are a somewhat heterogenous group of organisms. From the experiments on gnotobiotic rats, it is clear that neither all polysaccharide-forming organisms nor all acid-producing organisms are cariogenic.

There have been attempts to compare the relative cariogenic potency of streptococcal strains within a group known to induce caries. It is very difficult to definitely show innate differences in virulence between any types of pathogen. Named strains of microorganisms show minor variations in apparent cariogenicity simply by being grown in batch cultures, freeze dried, and retested. Large numbers of freshly isolated strains need to be studied before any comparative virulence can be established between different isolates of the mutans group of streptococci.

Localization of the oral flora related to caries

Careful evaluation of reports on caries indicates that different organisms

Table 3-1 Types of dental caries in animal model system

Type of caries	Etiological organism	Possible significance in human disease
Pit and fissure	*Streptococcus mutans*	Very significant
	Streptococcus sanguis	Not very significant
	Other streptococci	Not very significant
	Lactobacillus sp	Very significant
	Actinomyces sp	May be significant
Smooth surface	*Streptococcus mutans*	Very significant
	Streptococcus salivarius	Probably not significant
Root surface	*Actinomyces viscosus*	Very significant
	Actinomyces naeslundii	Very significant
	Other filamentous rods	Very significant
	Streptococcus mutans	Significant
	Streptococcus sanguis	May be significant
	Streptococcus salivarius	Probably not significant
Deep dentinal caries	*Lactobacillus* sp	Very significant
	Actinomyces naeslundii	Very significant
	Actinomyces viscosus	Significant
	Other filamentous rods	Very significant
	Streptococcus mutans	May be significant

display some selectivity as to which tooth surface they attack and suggests that there are at least four types of processes involved (Table 3-1).

Pit and fissure caries

This is the most common carious lesion found in modern humans. Many organisms can colonize in fissures, which provide mechanical retention for the bacteria. Gnotobiotic rats monoinfected with either *S mutans,*[43,44] *S salivarius,*[108] *S sanguis,* streptococcal species,[9,57] *L acidophilus,*[58] *L casei,*[160] *A viscosus,*[63,86] *A naeslundii,*[75] or *Actinomyces israelii*[75] develop fissure lesions. A wide variety of microbes may be able to initiate pit and fissure caries.

Smooth surface caries

A limited number of organisms have proved able to colonize smooth surfaces in large enough numbers to cause decay in test animals. *S mutans* is very significant in this respect and will be covered in detail in a subsequent section.

Root caries

In rodents, gram-positive filamentous rods, including *Actinomyces* species, have been associated with this type of lesion. Strains of *Nocardia* and *S sanguis,* besides causing enamel caries, may at times also cause root caries. In humans the mutans group of streptococci has been associated with surfaces with root caries when compared to intact root surfaces.

Deep dentinal caries

Because the environment in deep dentinal lesions is different from that at other locations, it is not unexpected that the flora here is also different. The predominant organism is *Lactobacillus,* which accounts for approximately one third of all bacteria.[52] Frequently isolated gram-positive anaerobic rods and filaments are *Arachnia, Bifidobacterium, Eubacterium,* and *Propionibacterium. Actinomyces, Rothia,* and *Bacillus* also occur in the forefront of deep dentinal lesions. The incidence of gram-positive facultative cocci is low.[47]

Flora of pits and fissures

One is obliged to use caution when extrapolating findings in the mono-infected gnotobiotic rat model system to naturally occurring caries in humans. Observations on humans in recent years, however, have generally confirmed the findings in animals. Very little is known about the microbiology of fissure lesions in humans, primarily because of the difficulty of sampling from the base of fissures (Fig 3-1).

An attempt has been made to monitor bacterial colonization using Mylar strips acting as "artificial fissures." These strips are inserted into specially designed inlays and may be removed for bacterial sampling or histological preparation.[127] Cultures from such artificial fissures reveal cocci as constituting 75% to 95% of the microorganisms. *S sanguis* is the predominant viable organism. *S mutans* and lactobacilli are low in newly formed plaque in fissures but increase over time.[190] Polyethylene strips do not exactly duplicate enamel-pellicle surfaces, and such factors may be of importance in favoring the colonization of specific organisms.

An alternative approach has been to use surgically removed impacted third molars cemented on a prosthesis and exposed for 0 to 5 days to the oral environment.[61] Detailed bacterial studies have not yet been done with this system, but preliminary findings indicate that cocci constitute about 80% of the viable organisms in the first 2 days. Rods and filaments increase to 12% in 5-day-old fissure plaque.

The large variation in the microflora in such sites indicates that each fissure is a separate ecological system. Generally, gram-positive cocci predominate (70% to 90% of the flora), especially *S sanguis,* whereas fusiforms, spirillae, and spirochetes are absent. *S mutans* has frequently been isolated in high numbers from plaque on smooth surface and fissure lesions. This will be discussed in more detail later.

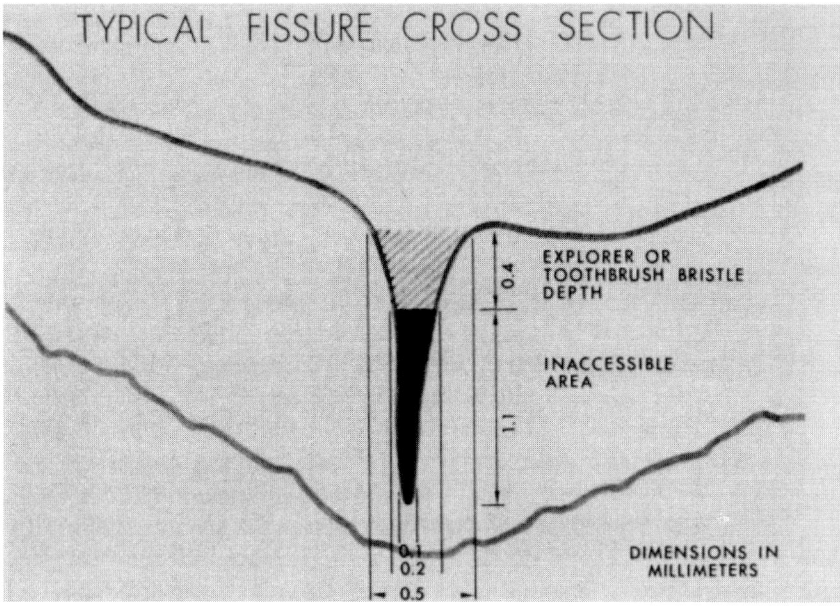

Fig 3-1 Cross section of an occlusal fissure showing the inability of an explorer or toothbrush bristle to reach the base.

Root caries

Root caries is a soft, progressive lesion of the root surface involving plaque and microbial invasion.[82] It can be distinguished from abrasion, erosion, and idiopathic resorption, which may also affect the root surface. It has been known by a variety of terms, including cemental caries, cervical caries, radicular caries, and even "senile" caries. Root caries is usually seen as a shallow (less than 2 mm deep), ill-defined, softened area, often discolored, and characterized by destruction of cementum with penetration of underlying dentin.[82,182] As it progresses, it extends circumferentially rather than in depth. Undetected lesions on the proximal surface may cause pulpal involvement (Fig 3-2). Heavy subgingival calculus frequently occurs apical to the lesion.[2] Accordingly, root caries is associated with periodontal disease.[161] Clinical surveys as well as examination of extracted teeth have shown that root caries:

1. Starts at or near the cementoenamel junction
2. Appears only after cementum is exposed and, therefore, becomes more prevalent with age
3. Occurs on facial, lingual, and proximal surfaces, the frequency of involvement of a specific surface being dependent upon the tooth type
4. Attacks mandibular molars most frequently, followed by mandibular

premolars and maxillary canines, the mandibular incisors being the least frequently involved teeth

5. Usually does not involve enamel

Examination of ancient skulls reveals that root caries was more common than enamel caries in ancient man (Egyptian, early Anglo-Saxon, North American Indian, pre-Columbian Peruvian). Similarly, in present-day primitive societies—such as among certain natives of the New Guinea highlands,[163] the islanders of Pukapuka, and aborigines of India—root caries has been observed as a major cause of tooth loss. In modern civilization, with water fluoridation, preventive dentistry programs, and improved dental restorative materials, the likelihood has increased that teeth will be retained longer. Consequently, there is more chance of gingival tissue recession as a result of periodontal disease. The exposed cemental surface is then potentially vulnerable to attack by root caries. Root caries is a significant problem among geriatric patients and patients who have undergone radiation therapy of the head and neck region (see Fig 2-2). There is an increase in the severity and prevalence of root caries with increasing age[104,134,194]; about 50% of the population between 40 and 49 years of age is affected[81,182] (Fig 3-3). In persons 20 to 64 years old, approximately one in nine surfaces with recession has root caries.[105]

Some of the organisms involved in root caries are different from those in other smooth surface lesions because the initial lesion is in cementum and dentin, not enamel. Bacteriological sampling of plaque covering caries of the root surface has yielded predominantly *A viscosus.*[186] However, other studies have found no difference in the prevalence of *A viscosus* on carious versus intact root surfaces. Microbial sampling of softened human dentin from root caries has also revealed the presence of other species of the genus *Actinomyces (A naeslundii, Actinomyces odontolyticus, Actinomyces eriksonii)* as well as *Rothia dentocariosa, Nocardia,* and *S mutans.*[101,186] Aerobic diphtheroidal organisms with characteristics similar to the genus *Arthrobacter* have been isolated from the advanced front of root caries.[181] The role of these various bacteria in root caries still needs clarification; no specific microorganism has been shown convincingly to be responsible for root surface caries.[145]

Experimental rodents have been useful in delineating some of the microbial parameters that appear to be involved in root caries. The presence of gram-positive filamentous organisms, such as *A viscosus,* was essential for the development of root caries in conventional animals.[102] In gnotobiotic rats, a variety of gram-positive organisms, such as *A naeslundii,*[172] *A viscosus,*[103] *S mutans,*[65] *S salivarius,*[108] *S sanguis,* and *Bacillus cereus,*[41] have been shown to produce root caries. The extent to which these organisms participate in the human disease is not clear. Certainly there is a unique bacterial flora associated with the cemental lesion.

The dental management of root surface caries may be mechanically difficult, particularly if proximal surfaces are involved or if the lesion has extended to involve multiple surfaces of the same tooth. Retention

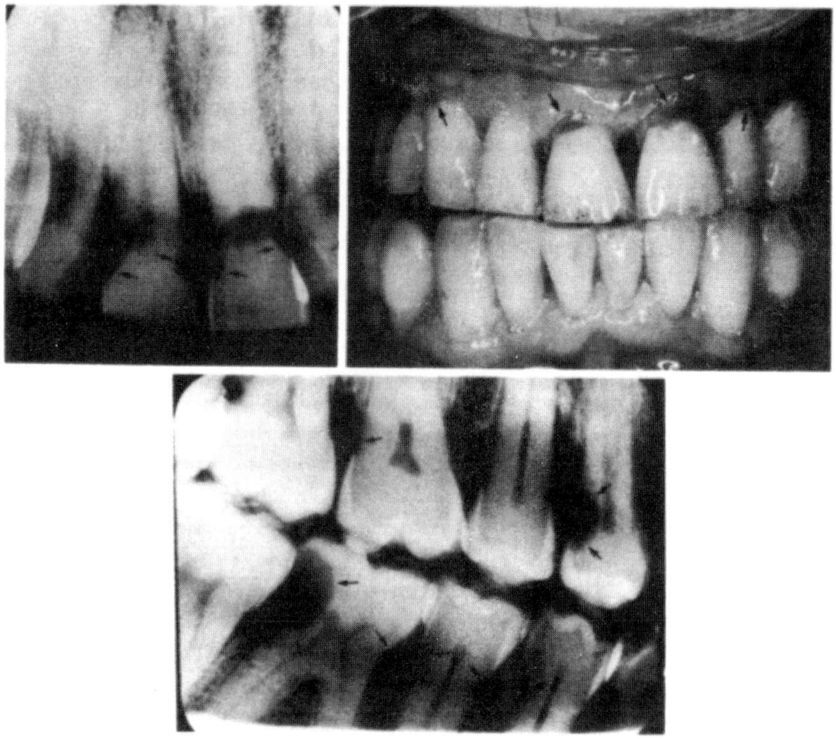

Fig 3-2 Root caries *(arrows)* in 39-year-old man free of coronal caries. Advanced interproximal lesions have already caused pulpal symptoms. (Courtesy of N. W. Chilton.)

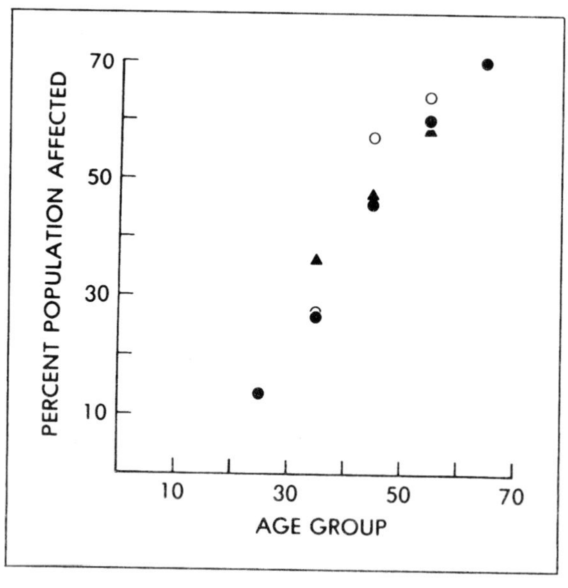

Fig 3-3 Prevalence of root caries in selected contemporary populations by age groups. (○) V.A. Hospital patients and staff; (▲) Insurance company employees; (●) Coast Guard base residents.

is a problem since there is no "box" into which to condense the restorative material. Materials that can be placed with little or no condensation are indicated.[3] Because cementum is much softer than enamel, it is difficult to finish such restorations. Fluoride in the drinking water reduces root surface caries in rats, although alveolar bone loss is not significantly decreased.[158] In humans, the lifelong consumption of fluoridated water significantly reduces the prevalence of root surface caries.[175] The key to the prevention of root surface caries may well lie with the control of periodontal disease.[2]

Transmissibility of the cariogenic flora

The specificity of the cariogenic flora has been demonstrated by animal experiments, clearly fulfilling one of Koch's postulates that the infectious agent should be able to produce the disease when transmitted to another animal.[59,109,148,149] The transmitted organisms were recovered from the mouths, feces, cavities, and plaques of newly infected animals. In 1960, Keyes[109] demonstrated that caries-inactive hamsters failed to develop extensive lesions unless they were caged with caries-rampant animals or were infected with fecal material from carious animals. Offspring of caries-rampant dams became caries-inactive if dams were treated with penicillin or erythromycin during pregnancy and lactation, indicating that the caries depended upon a transmittable antibiotic-sensitive flora.

The oral cavity houses a complex, mixed microflora, and early attempts at inoculation with organisms thought to be cariogenic gave equivocal results. In an adult animal, it may be necessary to depress the existing flora with an antibiotic before the establishment of cariogenic microorganisms can take place. Newborn animals, which do not require antibiotic suppression, will become infected if caged with infected adult animals (ie, transmission of the cariogenic flora). Alternatively, a caries-inducing flora can be transmitted by inoculating young animals with fecal or plaque material from caries-active animals or with pure cultures of cariogenic organisms (Fig 3-4).

Evidence of transmission of a specific cariogenic organism is readily apparent in gnotobiotic animals. In conventional animals, however, further proof is necessary to distinguish the infecting or "transmitted" organisms from the existing flora, which may appear to be similar. This has been demonstrated by using "tagged" or "labeled" mutants of microorganisms that have been made resistant to an antibiotic, and reisolating these mutants from the infected host animals. Some investigators have also used the technique of fluorescent antibodies prepared against a specific cariogenic strain to show that successful transmission of the cariogenic strain has occurred.

Implantation of *S mutans* in the human mouth has been attempted. Recovery of the "labeled" organisms was variable, and they were gradually lost over an extended period of time.[99,119] In these studies the failure of the labeled strains to become established in human plaques in high

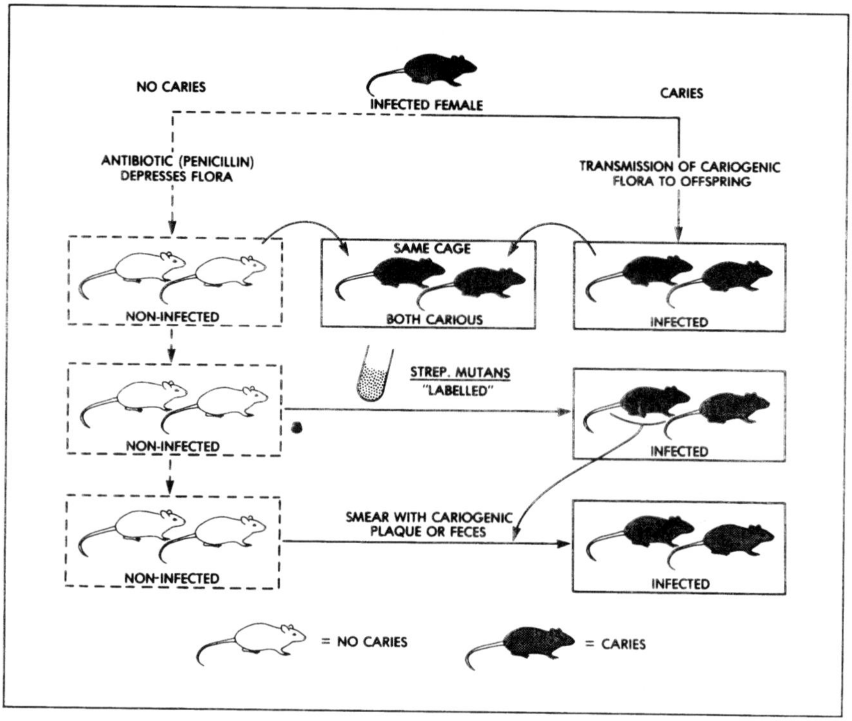

Fig 3-4 Transmission of cariogenic flora. Several generations of hamsters have been rendered caries-inactive by depressing the cariogenic microbiota. The infection has been reintroduced by contact with infected animals, by inoculation with a "labeled" streptomycin-resistant strain of *S mutans*, and also by transfer of plaque or fecal flora.

numbers for prolonged periods is not surprising, because adult subjects were used and their existing oral flora was not suppressed with antibiotics. When *S mutans* was implanted using dental floss, recovery of the organism was limited to the immediate area of implantation.[44] There appeared to be very little transfer to distant tooth surfaces.

Occasionally, marked differences have been seen in the pattern of caries on the left versus right side of the mouth. This is further reflected in the highly localized distribution of *S mutans*, which may constitute a much higher proportion of the plaque on the affected side.[184]

Bacterial interactions

Although innumerable species of organisms have been isolated from the oral cavity, many are only transient inhabitants. The ecological balance established in the gingival crevice, the tooth surfaces, and other regions in the mouth may depend on several factors, such as local supply of nutrients and adhesion of bacteria to pellicle or epithelial cells. The availability of essential bacterial nutrients is different in occlusal fissures from that in the gingival crevice, where there is a flow of gingival fluid exudate. Specific microorganisms preferentially bind to the epithelial cells of the oral mucosa.[67,122] Once established, such organisms may either favor or hinder the accumulation of other types of organisms at the same site.

The normal oral flora of Osborne-Mendel rats causes some fissure caries. If infected with *S mutans* and fed the same diet, these rats develop appreciably more fissure lesions. This suggests a symbiotic relationship between the indigenous flora and the superimposed cariogenic strain. Often, however, infecting animals with a combination of organisms may actually decrease the amount of caries. For example, if the normal flora is depressed and rats are infected with *S mutans* plus three other organisms, a pronounced interaction between the inoculating organisms occurs (Table 3-2). The rats infected with *S mutans* alone develop a much higher smooth surface caries score than those infected with *S mutans* plus other organisms.[116] Smooth surface caries is also reduced (Table 3-2) in gnotobiotic rats infected with *S mutans* and specific pathogen-free flora.

Similarly, *Veillonella alcalescens,* when introduced with *S mutans* or *S sanguis* into gnotobiotic rats, reduces the cariogenicity of the streptococci alone.[138] *Veillonella* will not ferment glucose or other carbohydrates,[155,156] but growing cultures can utilize lactate to form the weaker propionic and acetic acids. This may explain the observed decrease in caries of rats infected with veillonellae in combination with streptococci, in spite of enhanced plaque formation. In other words, it is the *composition* of the plaque microflora rather than just the *quantity* of plaque that determines pathogenicity.

An interaction between the two dominant streptococcal groups found in plaque has been observed.[26] *S sanguis* grows in a chemically defined medium free of *p*-aminobenzoic acid, while a strain of *S mutans* does not grow in this medium. In a mixed culture of *S sanguis* and *S mutans* in the *p*-aminobenzoic acid-free medium, both organisms will grow. Presumably *S sanguis* supplies the necessary growth factor to *S mutans* so that the interaction would be characterized as syntrophism.

An apparently inverse relationship has been observed between *S mutans* and *S sanguis* isolated from plaque. When patients followed a strict carbohydrate-free diet, the percentage of *S mutans* found in plaque decreased to a very low or undetectable level, whereas the percentage of *S sanguis* rose significantly. On resuming a normal diet supplemented with sucrose, the percentage of *S mutans* increased markedly and the percentage of *S sanguis* returned to about the original level.[178]

Lactobacilli constitute a minor component of dental plaque. They are usually confined to sites on teeth where there are already clinically detectable carious lesions. Deep in the carious dentin, lactobacilli, mostly *L casei,* may constitute half of the recoverable flora.[47] Such sites are known to provide an acidic milieu while fermentable carbohydrates are available and, therefore, selectively favor proliferation of aciduric lactobacilli. This represents an example of bacterial succession.

Table 3-2 Comparison of caries produced by *Streptococcus mutans* alone or in combination with other organisms

Rat system	Conventional animals (erythromycin-depressed flora)*		Gnotobiotic†	
Inoculation	*S mutans*	*S mutans* Gram-negative rod Gram-positive rod Gram-positive coccus	*S mutans*	*S mutans* SPF‡ feces
Smooth surface caries score	24	8	14.3	5.0

* König et al.[115]
† Hoeven et al.[87]
‡ Specific pathogen-free.

Another example of bacterial interaction is evidenced by bacteriocins, which are bactericidal proteins synthesized by certain bacterial strains that contain extra chromosomal elements called bacteriocinogens. Bacteriocins are active against some strains of the same or closely related species, but not against unrelated species (Fig 3-5). Several types of bacteriocins have been detected from streptococci indigenous to the oral cavity.[107] The bacteriocin from *S mutans* (serovar *c*) has been studied in detail and found to be a basic protein with a molecular weight of 4,800. It is relatively stable when subjected to a wide range of pH, to heat, and to several digestive enzymes.[97] Its lethal activity appears to be due to its ability to bind to proteins of cell walls and cell membranes, disrupting the integrity of the cell membrane and releasing cellular DNA.[187]

Some bacteriocins, when added to rodent diet or instilled directly into the hamster's cheek pouch, have been shown to reduce oral levels of *S mutans* and to reduce caries in these animals.[60]

What is involved in such bacterial interactions is not yet clear. Careful reconstruction of the normal flora by introducing two or more strains in combination, using the gnotobiotic system, should further clarify the complex situation within dental plaque.

Bacteriology of smooth surface dental plaque

In direct smears, the early plaque is dominated by cocci and rods, most of which are gram-positive. With time the percentage of cocci in the plaque decreases rapidly, and after 7 days filaments and rods constitute about 50% of the organisms in plaque. The ecological term for this is *succession.*

On culture, a more detailed picture can be obtained, although the same general trend is observed. Streptococci are the predominant organisms in both old and young plaques. Subsequently, there is a shift in the relative proportions, and in older plaques filamentous organisms (*Veillonella* and *Actinomyces* species) form fairly large groups. Lactobacilli

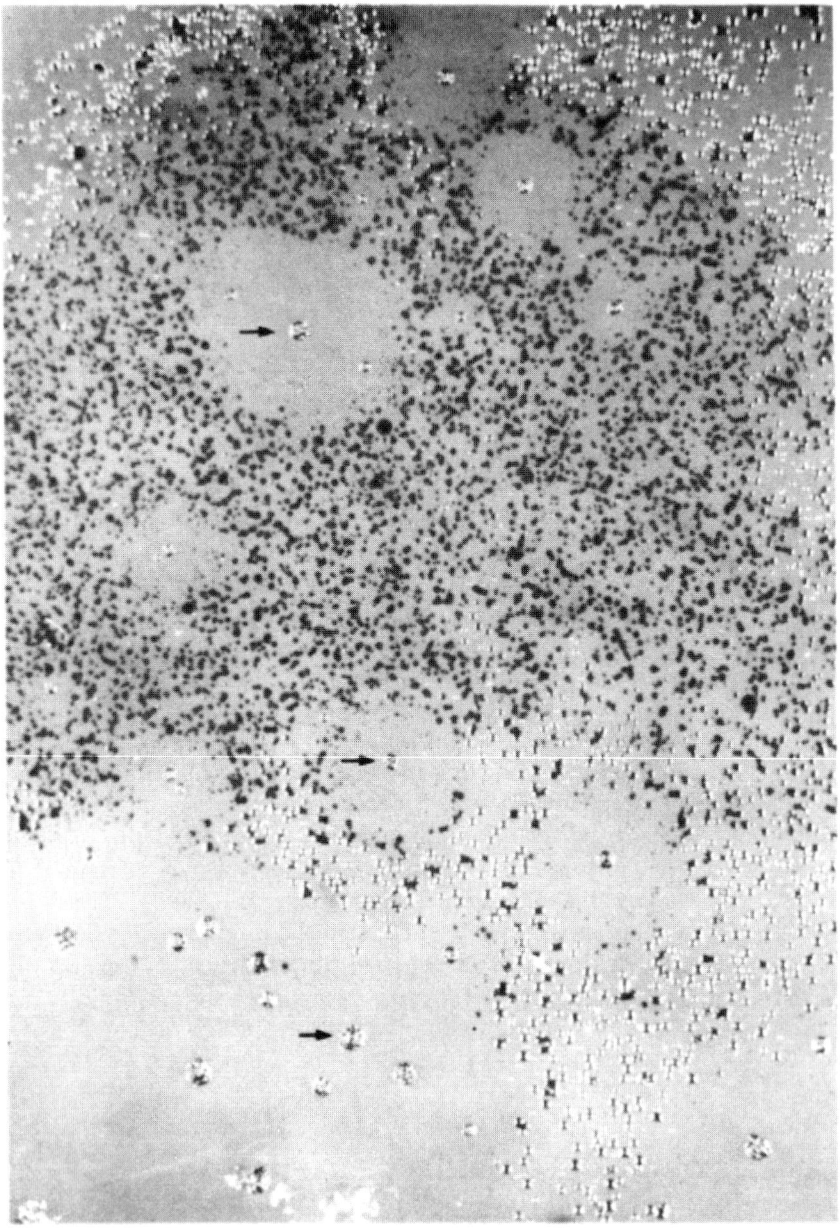

Fig 3-5 Bacteriocin production by *S mutans*, serotype c *(arrows)*. Note the zones of inhibition against other species of streptococci from dental plaque. Growth on mitis-salivarius agar containing bacitracin (MSB) in 85% N_2, 10% H_2, and 5% CO_2 at 37°C for 48 hours.

comprise less than 1% of the plaque flora. Because of their low numbers, a selective medium is employed to quantify them.

There is an orderly progression in the growth of dental plaque with shifts in the relative proportions of different microbial populations due to varying affinities of different bacteria for the dynamically changing plaque surface. Other factors within the plaque, such as pH, nutrient availability, and oxidation-reduction potential, will also contribute to the bacterial shifts.[128]

One of the problems in identifying and culturing the microorganisms in plaque is that no single culture environment can be used to isolate the multiplicity of microbes that can grow in plaque. Some organisms grow only in the absence of oxygen; others require both oxygen and carbon dioxide. Current attempts to increase the viable count recovery of organisms from human plaque samples are based on culturing in the absence of oxygen, using a variety of media.

Filamentous organisms have long been recognized in plaque and carious dentin. These organisms include *Leptothrix buccalis, Fusobacterium nucleatum, Bacterionema matruchotii,* several *Actinomyces* species, *Rothia dentocariosa,* and *A viscosus.* A fibrillar or "hairy" outer surface has been found on both *A viscosus* and *A naeslundii.* These fibrils may provide a mechanism that enables the cells to stay in contact with one another and with the tooth surface.[70] The role of fibrils in the etiology of enamel caries has not been established. However, as mentioned previously, certain of these filamentous organisms initiate root caries in rodents.

Oral streptococci

Irrespective of the age of plaque and the previous diet, the predominant organisms are gram-positive cocci of the genus *Streptococcus,*[152,173] which form about 50% of the total colony-forming units recoverable from young plaque. These streptococci have been divided into various groups,[23,51,200] based on their colonial morphology and physiological characteristics. Oral streptococci have been primarily isolated on mitis-salivarius agar, a useful selective medium that permits isolation from mixed flora and provides good colonial differentiation.

S sanguis

This is one of the predominant groups of streptococci colonizing on the teeth. Formerly it was called *Streptococcus s.b.e.* because of its involvement in subacute bacterial endocarditis. Certain strains within this group are minimally cariogenic in animals, but most strains are not. Caries from this strain occurs primarily in sulci and is significantly less extensive than that from *S mutans,* which causes smooth surface caries as well. *S sanguis* grows as small zoogleal colonies with a firm consistency and forms extracellular polysaccharides in sucrose broth. The colony morphology does not permit a sharp selection of *S sanguis* only. On blood agar, *S sanguis* causes α (green) hemolysis. *S sanguis* grown aerobically has relatively complex nutritional requirements for amino acids.[24] It is not clear how these requirements are met on the tooth surface. Under anaerobic conditions its requirements may be simpler. By using a sensitive immunofluorescent technique, investigators have found *S sanguis* in all plaques tested and on some tongues, but not in any throat specimens.[62]

S mutans

In 1924 Clarke isolated a streptococcus that predominated in many human carious lesions and that he named *Streptococcus mutans* because of its varying morphology. Clarke[32] noted that *S mutans* adhered closely to tooth surfaces in artificially induced caries. For the next 40 years, *S mutans* was virtually ignored, until the 1960s when it was "rediscovered" and its prevalence in plaque confirmed. It has further been shown that these specific streptococci almost invariably induced strong to moderate caries activity if implanted in suitable animal model systems (monkey, gerbil, rat, or hamster).

Characteristics of this group of streptococci have been described.[45,50,74] They are nonmotile, catalase-negative, gram-positive cocci in short or medium chains. On mitis-salivarius agar they grow as highly convex to pulvinate (cushion-shaped) colonies. These colonies are opaque; the surface resembles frosted glass. Hemolysis of blood agar is variable and may be α (green) or γ (no change), and occasionally β (clear).[51]

Colony morphology is divergent, depending on the culture medium. Although the most common morphology on solid media is that of rough colonies, smooth and mucoid variants have been found in about 7% of the isolates in one study. These *S mutans* variants also possess caries-inducing properties, and when re-isolated from infected animals they may resume the original rough colonial form.[46] The appearance of rough, smooth, and mucoid variants grown on mitis-salivarius agar, mitis-salivarius agar with sulfonamide, or trypticase yeast sucrose agar is shown in Fig 3-6.

When cultured with sucrose, they form polysaccharides that are insoluble or can be precipitated with one part ethanol. This property of forming insoluble extracellular polysaccharides from sucrose is regarded as an important characteristic contributing to the caries-inducing properties of *S mutans*.[167] Mutants of *S mutans*, which lack the ability to synthesize insoluble glucans or to stick to glass surfaces, do not cause smooth surface caries.[179,188]

S mutans ferments mannitol and usually sorbitol. Except for certain vitamin requirements, it is not as fastidious in its growth requirements as are most streptococci. The organisms can use ammonia as the sole source of nitrogen. Carlsson[25] speculates that this gives *S mutans* an ecological advantage. These organisms appear to be well adapted for growth in the deepest parts of the microbial aggregations on the teeth, where the anaerobic environment and ammonia may be sufficient to permit survival without exogenous amino acids.

Unlike other oral streptococci, most strains of *S mutans* can be cultured

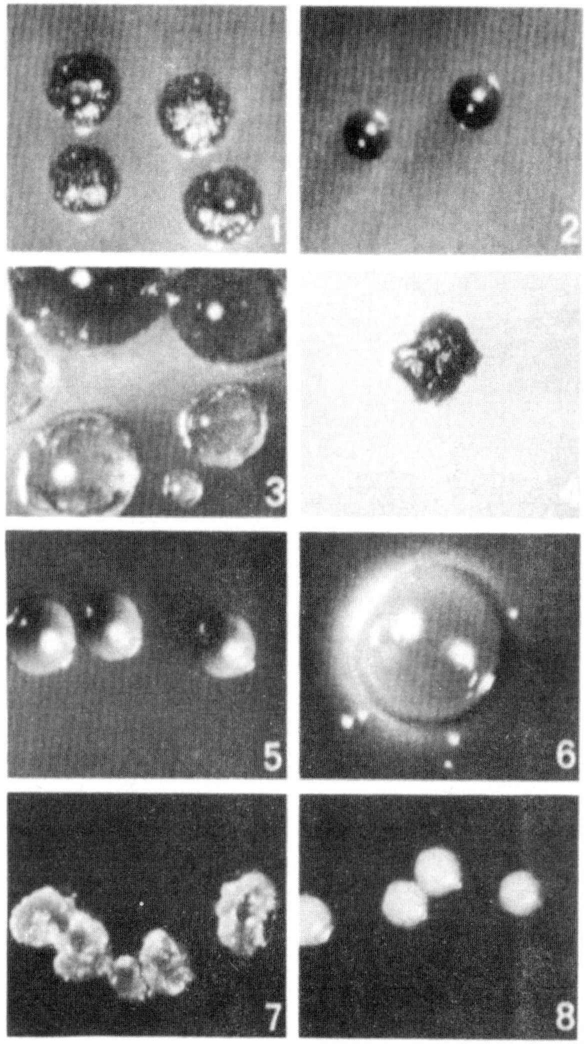

Fig 3-6 Appearance of different colonial variants of *S mutans:* *(1)* rough; *(2)* smooth; *(3)* mucoid variants on mitis-salivarius agar incubated at 37°C for 24 hours in 95% N_2 and 5% CO_2, and 24 hours at room temperature; *(4)* rough; *(5)* smooth; *(6)* mucoid variants on mitis-salivarius agar with sulfonamide incubated 48 hours in 95% N_2 and 5% CO_2; *(7)* rough; *(8)* smooth variants on trypticase yeast sucrose agar incubated 96 hours in 94% H_2 and 6% CO_2. (Courtesy of S. Edwardsson.[46])

in the presence of noninhibitory (ie, low) concentrations of sulfonamide. This property has been utilized as a basis for a selective culture medium for isolating *S mutans.*[22] An even better selective medium is mitis-salivarius agar containing 20% sucrose and 0.2 units/ml bacitracin[71] (MSB), which suppresses most other streptococci but permits growth of all but two serotypes of *S mutans.* The principal advantage of MSB is that it allows the isolation of the species even when present in low numbers relative to the total population.

S mutans exhibits several important properties:

1. It synthesizes insoluble polysaccharides from sucrose.
2. It is a homofermentative lactic acid former.

Table 3-3 Summary of some basic differences within the "mutans group" of streptococci

Species		*mutans*		*rattus*		*sobrinus*		*cricetus*	*ferus*
Serovar	c	e	f	b	d	g	h	a	c
Genotype, mol % G + C		36–38		42–43		44–45		43–44	44
Antigenic serovar determinant	Glucose-(α) (1-4)glucose	Glucose-(β) (1-4)glucose	Glucose-(α) (1-6)glucose	(α)galactose	Galactose-(β) (1-6)glucose	(β)galactose	ND	Glucose-(β) (1-6)glucose	ND
Cell wall carbohydrate		Glucose, rhamnose		Galactose, rhamnose		Glucose, galactose, rhamnose		Glucose, galactose, rhamnose	Glucose, rhamnose
Fermentation									
Mannitol	+	+	+	+	+	+	+	+	+
Sorbitol	+	+	+	+	+/−	+/−	−	+	+
Raffinose	+	+	+	+	−	−	−	+	−
Melibiose	+	+/−	+	+	−	−	+	+	N.D.
NH_3 from arginine	−	−	−	+	−	−	−	−	−
Growth in bacitracin†	+	+	−	+	−	+	−	−	−

*G + C = guanosine + cytosine.
β†0.2 U/ml.
ND = Not determined.

3. It colonizes on tooth surfaces.
4. It is more aciduric than other streptococci.

However, these are not unique characteristics that can be correlated with cariogenicity. Nor is there any single physiological test that can be used to identify *S mutans*. In other words, mannitol fermenters and polysaccharide formers have also been found among noncariogenic strains (eg, enterococci, *S faecalis, S sanguis*).[118] Cariogenic and noncariogenic streptococci grown on glucose in liquid media produce similar fermentation end products and similar amounts of acid.[42,98] On solid media, however, acid accumulation by *S mutans* is substantially greater than that of other oral streptococci.[147]

Cariogenic strains of *S mutans* contain lysogenic bacteriophage,[73,83,111] which has not been isolated from noncariogenic strains. Noncariogenic mutants of *S mutans* are unable to adhere to glass and have decreased ability to form insoluble polysaccharide. If these mutants are infected with lysogenic phages, they are transformed, acquiring the ability to adhere and form abundant insoluble polysaccharide.

Because DNA is the molecule that determines the structure of all other molecules, it is to be expected that the various genotypes differ in other respects such as isozyme patterns, aldolases, invertases, glucosyltransferases, a few biochemical reactions,[165] and even morphology. *S mutans* isolates can be grouped into three "chemotypes" based on differences in the composition of the cell wall. At least seven serovars of *S mutans* have been found[16] (Table 3-3). Compared to *S sanguis, S mutans* is more aciduric and can reproduce in a culture medium at a pH as low as 4.3.[176]

S mutans forms a homogeneous group, based on physiological, ecological, and morphological characteristics,[23,45,74,200] and has been recognized as a distinct species by the National Communicable Disease Center. However, analysis of the guanosine and cytosine content and hybridization studies on the homologies of the DNA isolated from strains of *S mutans* revealed significant differences.[34,35,164] These cariogenic organisms, though phenotypically similar, are genetically heterogeneous and were therefore divided into five genotypes or "geno species." However, because their nucleic acid base content and sequence are too disparate, these "mutans-like" organisms have been divided into separate species, namely *S mutans* (36 to 38 mol % guanosine (G) + cytosine (C), ie, guanosine + cytosine); *Streptococcus rattus* (41 to 43 mol % G + C); *Streptococcus cricetus* (43 mol % G + C); *Streptococcus sobrinus* (44 to 45 mol % G + C); and *Streptococcus ferus* (44 mol % G + C).[37-39,164,169] Of the "mutans-group" *S mutans, S rattus,* and *S cricetus* have been accepted and appear on the Approved Lists of Bacterial Names.[169] *S mutans* and *S sobrinus* are most commonly found in human plaque. *S cricetus* and *S rattus* are less common in humans, and *S ferus* only occurs in rats.

Serological classification of mutans group

Serological techniques have been very useful in classifying the β-hemolytic streptococci on the basis of immunological reactivity. Lancefield has classified these organisms into 17 groups and 55 types. The cell wall polysaccharide is responsible for the group specificity, whereas the type specificity is due to a protein constituent of the cell wall termed the M protein. Classification is carried out on the basis of the reaction of acid extracts of the bacteria with type-specific or group-specific antisera.

Because early attempts at classification of cariogenic streptococci indicated that extracts of these organisms did not react with any of the Lancefield grouping antisera,[59] development of a de novo classification scheme for them was necessary. Initially, Zinner and Jablon[200] were able to identify two serologically distinct types, the prototypes of which were *S mutans* strains HS and FA-1. In subsequent experiments, Bratthall[12,13] succeeded in defining five serovars of *S mutans* that have been designated a through e. Groups a through d are unique for *S mutans*, whereas group e is defined on the basis of its cross-reactivity with Lancefield Group E antiserum.[12] This serological classification has been supported by DNA-DNA hybridization experiments.[36] Perch et al[150] identified two additional serovars of *S mutans* denoted f and g. In monkeys a new serovar h of *S mutans* has been isolated from dental plaque.[5] Other oral streptococci have not yet been similarly classified systematically.

The organisms used for the production of group-specific antisera must be grown in a medium devoid of sucrose, because the presence of this component results in the production of a dextran capsule that gives rise to antidextran antibodies in addition to the group-specific antibodies.[12] However, even in the absence of sucrose, the antisera give broad bands when reacted with Lancefield extracts in double immunodiffusion experiments,[1] suggesting that multiple antigenic components are involved.[12] This contention is also supported by comparative immunoelectrophoresis and immunofluorescence experiments.[12,13,15] Thus, immunoelectrophoresis of extracts of groups b and d reveals two major arcs,[12,13] and at least two weaker antigens can be observed in extracts of groups a and b.[12]

Comparative immunoelectrophoretic analyses of extracts of *S salivarius* and *S sanguis*, using antisera to *S mutans* groups a and b, have demonstrated that *S salivarius* contains components that are cross-reactive with *S mutans* groups a and b, whereas *S sanguis* extracts cross-react with antisera to group b.[13] These cross-reactivities are with components other than those responsible for the group specificities. Using immunofluorescent techniques, Bratthall[15] also demonstrated cross-reactions between *S mutans* groups a and d as well as those mentioned above. Although the molecular basis of these cross-reactions is not entirely understood, the recent studies of Chorpenning et al[31] and Wicken and Knox[196] suggest that one of the cross-reactive components may be the polyglycerophosphate backbone of the cell wall teichoic acids.

A detailed study of *S mutans*, isolated by different investigators, separated 60 strains into five serological groups on the basis of specific antigens.[13] Fifty of the strains, including most of those isolated from human plaque or carious lesions, belonged to one serological group (serovar c). On the basis of common strains, the serological[13] and genetic groups[35] are identical (see Table 3-3). Dental plaque samples from 14 areas in 10 countries were analyzed with fluorescein-conjugated and absorbed antisera against five serological variants of *S mutans,* groups a, b, c, d, and e. The results show that *S mutans* of groups c, d, and e have a wide distribution and are found in all areas. Groups a and b were found less frequently.

Fluorescein-conjugated antisera against *S mutans* is prepared from sera after repeated intravenous injection of antigen (washed heated cells). These antisera against *S mutans* react not only with *S mutans* but also with *S sanguis, S salivarius,* and *Streptococcus mitis.* Through absorption it is possible to prepare specific antisera against some of the different antigens of *S mutans* (a, b, and d). Plaque samples are then studied by phase contrast microscopy and fluorescence of a smear that has been reacted with the specific antisera.[14] Using this technique, *S mutans* has been found to constitute 2%[191] and 7.3% of the direct cell counts of dental plaque, with a range of 0.7% to 27.8%.[49] There is tremendous variation from site to site, even in the same mouth, in the proportion of *S mutans* on tooth surfaces.

It is not clear whether one serovar of *S mutans* is more virulent than another. In one comparison of five strains, *S mutans* AHT (serovar a) showed more severe buccal lesions, whereas *S mutans* 6715 (serovar d) caused more proximal caries in gnotobiotic rats. *S mutans* LM7 (serovar e) exhibited the lowest level of caries.[137] However, the test strains were stock laboratory cultures, which tend to decrease in virulence with repeated transfer. A more valid measure of virulence would require isolation of fresh strains from humans or maintenance in gnotobiotic host rats. Monkeys in which serovar e was the predominant strain of *S mutans* developed significantly more caries when fed a high sucrose diet than those in which serovars c and h predominated.[4] In humans, *S mutans* serovar d may be more cariogenic than other serovars, since this organism has been isolated more frequently from the plaque of caries-active persons than from those who are caries-free or have very little caries.[88, 95,136]

Biochemical composition of *S mutans* cell wall

The structural elements of the cell wall of oral streptococci have not been extensively delineated. *S mutans* possesses *(1)* an outer capsule of glucan or levan when grown in the presence of sucrose, and *(2)* a cell wall polysaccharide. This is composed either of rhamnose, glucose, and galactose, or galactose and rhamnose, or glucose and rhamnose (which is the most common type found). The exact qualitative and quantitative composition of the cell wall depends on the strain.[10,79] In addition to these components, the cell walls possess a peptidoglycan and glycerol teichoic acid. Many of these various cell wall macromolecular components are also present at the cell surface, as shown diagrammatically in

Fig 3-7, and are of potential importance in any attempts at developing anti-*S mutans* vaccines.

The biochemical nature of the cell wall macromolecules containing the *S mutans* group-specific antigenic determinants has been investigated. Slade and associates studied the cell wall antigens responsible for group specificities a, b, c, d, e, and f.[76,77,123,124,174] The group a antigen is a polysaccharide, the specificity of which depends on a D-glucose sequence.[141] The same molecule also contains an antigenic site that reacts with group d antisera, the specificity of which depends on a terminal D-galactose. The group b antigen has been isolated and separated into two forms: a polysaccharide and a glycoprotein.[142] Galactose and galactosamine are found in both fractions, and rhamnose is the major constituent (47%) of the polysaccharide.[142]

S mutans with the group c antigen is the most common of the biotypes (over 90% of isolates).[106,151] Extracts of *S mutans*, strain Ingbritt, using trichloroacetic acid, gave two antigens, both of which contain rhamnose (66% to 69%) and glucose (27% to 29%).[123]

The group d antigen is a polysaccharide that cross-reacts with group a antisera.[124] As with the group a polysaccharide, the dual specificities reside on the same molecule.[124] The antigenic determinant responsible for the group d specificity is D-galactose. The specificity of *S mutans* group e resides in the oligosaccharide sequence D-glucose-L-rhamnose-L-rhamnose[174]; the major type-specific antigen is composed of rhamnose (56%), glucose (37%), protein (5%), and phosphorus (0.5%).[77] Type f cell wall antigen is composed of about equal amounts of rhamnose and glucose.[76]

In contrast to the above observations, van de Rijn and Bleiweis[192] and Vaught and Bleiweis[193] have conducted experiments that indicate the antigenic determinants of *S mutans*, groups a and b, reside in the cell wall glycerol teichoic acid. The specificities of both group-specific antigens appear to be due to a β-galactoside linkage.[192,193] However, in agreement with Mukasa and Slade,[142] Vaught and Bleiweis also found a polysaccharide in extracts of group b cells that contains the antigenic determinants.[193]

The *S mutans* group-specific antigens are sugars, and the antigenic determinants have been identified. However, elucidation of the precise nature of the specific macromolecules on which they reside requires further experimentation.

Ecology of *S mutans*

Accumulated evidence of the ecology of *S mutans* indicates that this organism can survive in the mouth only when solid surfaces such as teeth or dentures are present.[30] Microorganisms whose colonies resemble *S mutans* and *S sanguis* morphologically were not detected in the mouths of newborn monkeys until teeth had erupted,[33] and the situation was similar in infants' mouths.[29] On the other hand, *S salivarius*, whose pre-

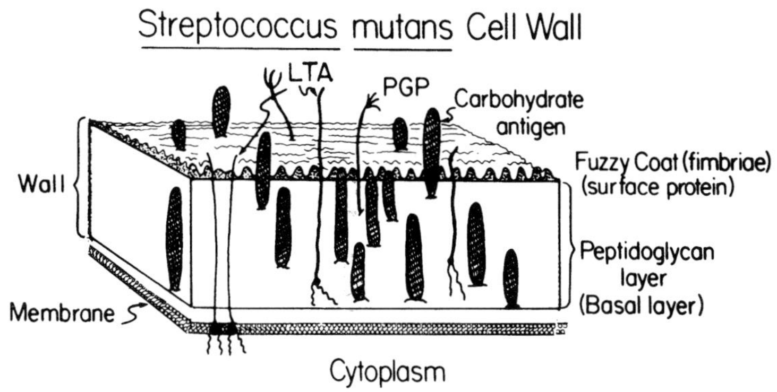

Fig 3-7 Diagrammatic representation of the cell wall of *Streptococcus mutans*. Carbohydrate, serotype antigen, and lipoteichoic acid *(LTA)* with its component polyglycerol phosphate *(PGP)* portion are interspersed in the peptidoglycan layer and also protrude from the cell surface. The fatty acid portion of *LTA* may be associated with the cytoplasmic membrane or may extend from the surface of the cell. (Courtesy of J. R. McGhee and S. Hamada.)

ferred habitat is the tongue, establishes itself early in the mouth of the newborn.[28] Although the favorite habitat of *S mutans* is the tooth surface, it does not uniformly colonize all tooth surfaces but instead localizes on certain surfaces.[44,66]

The exact mechanism(s) by which *S mutans* can adhere to and accumulate on the surfaces of teeth is unknown. It has been thought that *S mutans* is a pathogen because of its ability to produce extracellular glucans from sucrose. Many bacteria, however, can synthesize polysaccharides such as glucans or dextrans and yet are unable to produce carious lesions. Other factors may, therefore, be involved in the virulence of *S mutans*. *S mutans* contains tightly and possibly covalently bound polypeptide molecules that may serve as factors in the attachment of the bacteria to smooth surfaces.[144]

Studies of plaque from humans indicated that *S mutans* is pandemic in many parts of the world.[68,106,120,162,177] It has been isolated from populations of diverse ethnic and socioeconomic background. In cross-sectional studies,* *S mutans* is found in large numbers, proportions, or both, in plaque isolated from caries-active populations, and more frequently in plaque overlying carious lesions than in plaque from sound tooth surfaces. Longitudinal investigations† also support a role for *S mutans* in the development of decay, although some teeth can have high proportions of *S mutans* without becoming carious.

S mutans levels in plaque can be influenced by a variety of factors, including diet (especially sucrose ingestion),[139] topical fluoride therapy,

*References 20, 84, 91, 125, 145, 166.
†References 17, 80, 95, 121, 133, 195.

systemic use of antibiotics, salivary *S mutans* levels of other family members, and possibly oral hygiene. In addition, salivary factors (both composition and flow rate), microbial interactions in the plaque, and host immunological experience could affect the degree of infection. Because of these numerous complicating factors, unequivocal demonstration of the etiological role of *S mutans* in human decay is unlikely.[133] Nevertheless, numerous independent studies have found a strong statistical relationship between caries and the occurrence of *S mutans* in plaque. This holds both for typical coronal caries and also for rampant caries involving the deciduous anterior teeth, so-called nursing bottle caries.[8,92] Such observations implicate *S mutans* as an important odontopathogen but do not rule out the possibility that other acidogenic-aciduric plaque organisms can exert a cariogenic challenge.

Human salivary concentrations of *S mutans* range from undetectable to 10^6 to 10^7 colony-forming units (CFU)/ml, with a mean concentration of about 10^5 CFU.[90] Salivary contamination of cups and glasses or eating utensils such as spoons may account for the transmission of *S mutans* from parent to child.[112] There is good evidence implicating the child's mother as the principal vector, especially mothers with high concentrations of *S mutans* in their plaque and saliva (more than 10^5 CFU/ml).[8,93] Mothers with these high salivary concentrations of *S mutans* are more likely to infect their infants than mothers with low salivary concentrations.[8,114] Furthermore, if highly infected mothers are treated (in a preventive program consisting of dietary counseling, professional tooth cleaning, oral hygiene instruction, topical fluoride application, excavation of large carious lesions, plus daily use of 1% chlorhexidine gel for 5 minutes over a 2-week period) to reduce their levels of *S mutans,* their children are significantly less likely to develop decay than are children of highly infected untreated mothers.[113] Toothbrushes and occasionally toothpaste may become infected with *S mutans* [183]; intrafamilial spread by this route has not been proven. However, studies using the bacteriocin typing technique suggest that some strains of *S mutans* are transmitted from one family member to another, particularly from mother to infant.[6,153,154] Intraoral spread of *S mutans* within the same individual does not easily occur but could be accomplished by an infected dental explorer[131,185] or by improper use of dental floss.

In several instances, *S mutans* has been cultured from the blood of patients with the typical clinical picture of subacute bacterial endocarditis.[78,143] Usually some type of dental procedure was involved previously, and the patient had already had valvular heart disease. All types of *S mutans* are highly susceptible to penicillin. Subacute bacterial endocarditis due to *S mutans* can be treated successfully with penicillin therapy. Patients allergic to penicillin can be treated with lincomycin or cephalothin.

S salivarius

These colonies grow as large, heaped, mucoid, or gummy colonies on mitis-salivarius agar. In sucrose broth they form a water-soluble polymer of fructose known as levan, as well as insoluble glucans. They have been found in the plaque, throat, nasopharynx, and oral mucosa, but their natural habitat is the dorsum of the tongue. They can be recovered from the mouths of infants shortly after birth. *S salivarius* can colonize on the teeth of hamsters, resulting in moderate caries activity. In humans they have only a minor degree of cariogenic significance and have virtually never been implicated in systemic disease.[171] On blood agar they cause no hemolysis (γ).

S mitior

S mitior is a heterogeneous species. On mitis-salivarius agar it forms soft, circular, black-brown colonies. It does not form extracellular polysaccharides from sucrose but forms intracellular polysaccharides, which can be demonstrated by iodine staining. Intracellular polysaccharide synthesis is not unique for this group but is common to almost all carbohydrate-fermenting species found in plaque. On blood agar most strains produce a green (α) coloration of the plate. The proportion of this group of the total streptococci varies among subjects; however, it is found most regularly on the nonkeratinized mucosa, particularly the cheek, lip, and ventral tongue surfaces.[11]

Miscellaneous streptococcal species

Streptococci *(S milleri, S oralis)* with colonial and physiological characteristics different from those of the previous groups are consistently found in dental plaque. In fact, some streptococci isolated from dental plaque cannot be adequately categorized. For example, *S milleri* is reasonably homogeneous on the basis of physiological tests but is heterogeneous based on serology and DNA homology. *S milleri* does not produce extracellular glucans from sucrose but is cariogenic in gnotobiotic animals.

In summary, *S mutans* and *S sanguis* preferentially grow on human teeth, that is, in plaque, and *S salivarius* grows on the tongue. It has been suggested that plaque-forming strains may evolve from non-plaque-forming strains by natural selection of the more adhesive extracellular polysaccharide-forming microorganisms.[189] Another proposed explanation is that these streptococci have the specific ability to utilize the adsorbed glycoproteins on the tooth surface.[117] Gibbons and Spinnell[69] have reported that a high molecular weight fraction in submandibular saliva can cause oral microorganisms to stick together and that saliva-coated enamel particles can bind bacterial cells. Large differences in the degree of adsorption and in the susceptibility to agglutination exist among the various oral microorganisms. The selectivity of this process may explain the relative presence or absence of various types of oral bacteria in the initial phase of plaque formation.

Oral lactobacilli

Lactobacilli are gram-positive, non-spore-forming rods that generally grow best under microaerophilic conditions. Isolation and enumeration of oral lactobacilli have been facilitated by use of a selective agar medium (Rogosa), which suppresses the growth of most other oral organisms by its low pH (5.4). Rogosa agar has a high concentration of acetate and other salts and contains a surface tension depressant.

Lactobacilli are found mostly as transients in the mouths of infants.[27] Lactobacilli represent about 1% of the oral flora; *L casei* and *L fermentum* are the most common oral species.[135] The population of oral lactobacilli is influenced by dietary habits. A favorite habitat of lactobacilli is in the dentin of deep carious lesions.[47]

Lactobacilli and caries

Lactobacilli, or organisms resembling lactobacilli, have been reported in the oral cavity ever since Miller enunciated the chemoparasitic theory (for a historical review see Burnett et al[19]). In 1925, Bunting and his collaborators[18] claimed that *Bacillus acidophilus* was the specific etiological factor responsible for the initiation of caries. Subsequent investigators have isolated other types of lactobacilli besides *L acidophilus* in saliva, plaque, and carious lesions. Small anaerobic lactobacilli *(Lactobacillus minutus)* have been isolated consistently from pockets of patients with chronic periodontitis.[140] The genus *Lactobacillus* includes many species with a broad range of guanosine + cytosine content (35 to 53 mol %). The following are those most commonly encountered in the mouth:

Homofermentative	**Heterofermentative**
L casei	*L fermentum*
L acidophilus	*Lactobacillus brevis*
Lactobacillus plantarum	*Lactobacillus buchneri*
Lactobacillus salivarius	*Lactobacillus cellobiosus*

In isolates of lactobacilli from human carious dentin, the homofermentative outnumber the heterofermentative variety.[21,168]

The idea that lactobacilli played the major role in the carious process dominated dental literature for about 35 years. It was argued that lactobacilli are both acidogenic and aciduric and could, therefore, multiply in the low pH of plaque and carious lesions. Using selective culture media, counts of lactobacilli in the saliva could be correlated with the prevalence of dental caries. Furthermore, the growth site of lactobacilli was reported to correspond to sites of clinically diagnosed carious lesions. When such lesions were restored, most of the growth sites of the lactobacilli were removed.

Acceptance of the doctrine that lactobacilli were the etiological agents of dental caries was not universal, however. As more information on the microbial composition of dental plaque became available, it was found that lactobacilli constitute only a minor fraction (1/10,000) of the plaque flora.[64] The amount of acid that can be formed by the relatively small number of lactobacilli present in plaque is almost insignificant in comparison with that produced by other acidogenic oral organisms.[180] The heavier growth of lactobacilli at active carious lesions does not necessarily establish their causative role, although they could be secondary contributors to the carious process.[129] An alternative explanation is that plaque conditions that are conducive to caries also favor colonization by lactobacilli. In humans, lactobacilli can be isolated from the saliva, tooth surfaces, dorsum of the tongue, vestibular mucosa, and hard palate. *L acidophilus* is most frequently isolated from saliva. Lactobacilli have a relatively low affinity for the tooth surface.[91] The establishment of oral lactobacilli coincides with the development of carious lesions; *L casei* is the predominating lactobacillus in dental plaque and carious dentin. Fitzgerald[55] interprets such data to mean that lactobacilli are more a consequence than a cause of caries initiation.

Evidence implicating certain streptococci as the infectious and transmittable agent in dental caries of experimental animals has undermined the belief that lactobacilli initiate dental caries. In gnotobiotic animals, some strains of lactobacilli induced dental caries. In such cases, the lesions were restricted to the occlusal sulcal regions.[56]

Oral *Actinomyces*

Actinomyces is a gram-positive, nonmotile, non-spore-forming organism occurring as rods and filaments that vary considerably in length. Filaments are usually long and slender and may be branching.[8,146] The species that have been found in the oral cavity are:

Facultative anaerobic	**Anaerobic**
A naeslundii	*A israelii*
A viscosus	*Actinomyces meyeri*
	A odontolyticus

All species of *Actinomyces* ferment glucose, producing mostly lactic acid, lesser amounts of acetic and succinic acid, and traces of formic acid. Most interest has centered on *A viscosus* and *A naeslundii* because of their ability to induce root caries, fissure caries, and periodontal destruction when inoculated into gnotobiotic rats.[63,75,103,126,172] *A viscosus* has been separated into two, and *A naeslundii* into four, serological types.

Actinomyces is a good plaque former, capable of adhering to wires[110] and forming tenacious deposits on the teeth of infected animals.[86, 99] It is the most common group of organisms isolated from the subgingival microflora and from plaque of human root surface caries.[186,198] It is found in the supragingival plaque of all children and comprises about 50% of all cells present.[191] *A naeslundii* predominates in the tongue, salivary flora, and in the plaque of young children, while plaque from teenagers and adults has a higher proportion of *A viscosus*.[48] *A viscosus* is one of the first species to recolonize the supragingival surface of a cleaned adult tooth.[173] High numbers of *A viscosus* have been associated with gingivitis.[130,171]

A viscosus forms extracellular levans and heteropolysaccharides consisting of hexosamine and hexose.[85,94,157]

Summary

Bacteria are essential for the development of a carious lesion. The microflora associated with pit and fissure caries, smooth surface caries, root caries, and deep dentinal caries are not the same. A number of different organisms are capable of inducing caries in animals, depending on the experimental conditions.

In humans there have been no *direct* demonstrations of cariogenicity of any microorganisms. There is considerable *indirect* evidence of an epidemiological nature that there is a strong worldwide association of *S mutans* in plaque with caries incidence and prevalence. Tests of human isolates have shown that *S mutans* is usually more cariogenic in animals receiving sucrose diets than other plaque organisms. Thus, the principal evidence supporting *S mutans* as the causative organism in human dental caries is derived from results of epidemiological studies in humans and pathogenicity studies in animals, neither of which are conclusive.

Because many factors may influence the formation, composition, and metabolism of dental plaque, one can expect caries in humans may be caused by several types of microorganisms. This does not negate the possibility that caries is a specific microbial disease, but it does require that etiological specificity must be defined in terms of the organisms involved and the environmental conditions at the site.

Chapter review

- List the evidence that microorganisms are involved in the carious process.
- Define a gnotobiotic animal.
- List the most important microorganisms that are cariogenic *(1)* in fis-

sures, *(2)* on smooth surfaces, *(3)* on roots of teeth, *(4)* in deep dentinal lesions.

- Indicate how to determine if an organism is cariogenic.
- Specify the main groups of streptococci found in the mouth and their preferred habitat (intraorally).
- List separately the characteristics common to most strains of *S mutans, S sanguis, S salivarius,* and oral lactobacilli.
- State the species of *Actinomyces* found in dental plaque and their properties.
- Define the transmissibility of oral flora.
- Indicate how cariogenic organisms can be transmitted to and recognized in conventional animals.
- Give some specific examples of bacterial interaction in dental plaque.
- List some of the properties of cariogenic streptococci. Indicate whether they are unique to cariogenic organisms.
- List examples of modes of transmission of *S mutans* from person to person and intraorally (in the same person).
- Explain the presence of lactobacilli in deep carious dentin.
- List what is known concerning root caries.

Selected readings

Bowen, W.H. 1974. Microbiological aspects of dental caries. *Adv Caries Res* 2:xxv–xxxii.

Doyle, R.J., and Ciardi, J.E. (eds) 1983. *Chemistry and biology of glucosyltransferases.* Washington, D.C.: Information Retrieval, Inc.

Gibbons, R.J. 1972. Ecology and cariogenic potential of oral streptococci. In *Streptococci and Streptococcal Disease,* L.W. Wannamaker and J.M. Matson (eds), New York: Academic Press, pp. 371–385.

Gibbons, R.J., and van Houte, J. 1975. Dental caries. *Annu Rev Med* 26:121–136.

Hamada, S., Michalek, S.M., Kiyono, H., Menaker, L., and McGhee, J.R. (eds) 1986. *Molecular Microbiology and Immunobiology of Streptococcus mutans.* Amsterdam: Elsevier Science Publishers.

Hamada, S., and Slade, H.D. 1980. Biology, immunology, and cariogenicity of *Streptococcus mutans. Microbiol Rev* 44:331–384.

Hardie, J.M. 1986. Oral streptococci. In *Bergey's Manual of Systematic Bacteriology,* P.H.A. Sneath (ed), Baltimore: Williams & Wilkins, 2:1054–1063.

Houte, J. van. 1980. Bacterial specificity in the etiology of dental caries. *Int Dent J* 30:305–326.

Ikari, N. (ed) 1973. *Streptococcus mutans and Dental Caries.* Department of Health, Education, and Welfare Publication No. (NIH) 74-286. Bethesda, Md.: National Caries Program, National Institute of Dental Research.

Loesch, W.J. 1986. Role of *Streptococcus mutans* in human dental decay. *Microbiol Rev* 50:353–380.

Loesche, W. 1978. *Oral Bacteriology.* Ann Arbor: University of Michigan Press.

Marsh, P., and Martin, M. 1984. *Oral Microbiology.* 2nd ed. Washington, D.C.: American Society of Microbiology.

McGhee, J.R., Michalek, S.M., and Cassell, G.H. 1982. *Dental Microbiology*. Philadelphia: Harper and Row, pp. 679–713.
Newman, M.G., and Nisengard, R. (eds) 1988. *Oral Microbiology and Immunology*. Philadelphia: W.B. Saunders.
Schuster, G.S (ed) 1983. *Oral Microbiology and Infectious Disease*. 2nd students' ed. Baltimore: Williams & Wilkins, pp. 162–233.
Stiles, H.M., Loesche, W.J., and O'Brien, T.C. (eds) 1976. *Microbial Aspects of Dental Caries*. Sp. Suppl. Microbiol. Abstr. Washington, D.C.: Information Retrieval, Inc.

References

1. Baab, D.A., Morton, T.H., and Page, R.C. 1984. Caries and periodontitis associated with an unerupted third molar. *Oral Surg* 58:428–430.
2. Banting, D.W., and Courtright, P.N. 1975. The distribution and natural history of carious lesions on the roots of teeth. *J Can Dent Assoc* 41:45–59.
3. Banting, D.W., and Ellen, R.P. 1976. Carious lesions on the roots of teeth. A review for the general practitioner. *J Can Dent Assoc* 42:496–502.
4. Beighton, D., Cohen, B., and Hayday, H. 1983. The association between dental caries incidence and two *Streptococcus mutans* populations in monkeys *Macaca fascicularis*. *Caries Res* 17:125–130.
5. Beighton, D., Russell, R.R.B., and Hayday, H. 1981. The isolation and characterization of *Streptococcus mutans* serotype h from dental plaque of monkeys *(Macaca fascicularis)*. *J Gen Microbiol* 124:271–279.
6. Berkowitz, R.J., and Jordan, H.V. 1975. Similarity of bacteriocins of *Streptococcus mutans* from mother and infant. *Arch Oral Biol* 20:725–730.
7. Berkowitz, R.J., Turner, J., and Green, P. 1981. Maternal salivary levels of *Streptococcus mutans* and primary oral infection of infants. *Arch Oral Biol* 26:147–149.
8. Berkowitz, R.J., Turner, J., and Hughes, C. 1984. Microbial characteristics of the human dental caries associated with prolonged bottle-feeding. *Arch Oral Biol* 29:949–951.
9. Blackmore, D.K., Drucker, D.B., and Green, R.M. 1970. Caries induction in germ-free rats by streptococci isolated from dental abscesses in man. *Arch Oral Biol* 15:1377–1379.
10. Bleiweis, A.S., Craig, R.A., Coleman, S.E., and van de Rijn, I. 1971. The streptococcal cell wall. Structure, antigenic composition, and reactivity with lysozyme. *J Dent Res* 50:1118–1129.
11. Bowden, G.H., Hardie, J.M., and Fillery, E.D. 1976. Antigens for *Actinomyces* species and their value in identification. *J Dent Res* 55:A192–A204.
12. Bratthall, D. 1969. Immunodiffusion studies on the serological specificity of streptococci resembling *Streptococcus mutans*. *Odontol Revy* 20:231–243.
13. Bratthall, D. 1970. Demonstration of five serological groups of streptococcal strains resembling *Streptococcus mutans*. *Odontol Revy* 21:143–152.
14. Bratthall, D. 1972. Demonstration of *Streptococcus mutans* strains in some selected areas of the world. *Odontol Revy* 23:401–410.
15. Bratthall, D. 1972. Immunofluorescent identification of *Streptococcus mutans*. *Odontol Revy* 23:181–186.
16. Bratthall, D., and Köhler, B. 1976. *Streptococcus mutans* serotypes. Some aspects of their identification, distribution, antigenic shifts and relationship to caries. *J Dent Res* 55:C15–C21.
17. Brown, L.R., Dreizen, S., and Handler, S. 1976. Effects of selected caries preventive regimens on microbial changes following irradiation-induced xerostomia in cancer patients. In *Microbial Aspects of Dental Caries*, H.M. Stiles, W.W. Loesche, and T.C. O'Brien (eds), Sp. Suppl. Microbiol. Abstr., vol. 1, Washington, D.C.: Information Retrieval, Inc., pp. 257–290.
18. Bunting, R.W., and Palmerlee, F. 1925. The role of *Bacillus acidophilus* in dental caries. *J Am Dent Assoc* 12:381–411.
19. Burnett, G.W., Scherp, H.W., and Schuster, G.S. 1976. *Oral Microbiology and Infectious Diseases*. 4th ed. Baltimore: Williams & Wilkins, pp. 287–290.
20. Burt, B.A., Loesche, W.J., Eklund, S.A., and Earnest, R.W. 1983. Stability of *Streptococcus mutans* and its relationship to caries in a child population over two years.

Caries Res 17:532–542.
21. Camilleri, G.E., and Bowen, W.H. 1963. Classification of lactobacilli isolated from human carious dentin. *J Dent Res* 42:1104–1105.
22. Carlsson, J. 1967. A medium for isolation of *Streptococcus mutans*. *Arch Oral Biol* 12:1657–1658.
23. Carlsson, J. 1968. A numerical taxonomic study of human oral streptococci. *Odontol Revy* 19:137–160.
24. Carlsson, J. 1970. Chemically defined medium for growth of *Streptococcus sanguis*. *Caries Res* 4:297–304.
25. Carlsson, J. 1970. Nutritional requirements of *Streptococcus mutans*. *Caries Res* 4:305–320.
26. Carlsson, J. 1971. Growth of *Streptococcus mutans* and *Streptococcus sanguis* in mixed culture. *Arch Oral Biol* 16:963–966.
27. Carlsson, J., Grahnén, H., and Jonsson, G. 1975. Lactobacilli and streptococci in the mouth of children. *Caries Res* 9:333–339.
28. Carlsson, J., Grahnén, H., Jonsson, G., and Wikner, S. 1970. Early establishment of *Streptococcus salivarius* in the mouths of infants. *J Dent Res* 49:415–418.
29. Carlsson, J., Grahnén, H., Jonsson, G., and Wikner, S. 1970. Establishment of *Streptococcus sanguis* in the mouths of infants. *Arch Oral Biol* 15:1143–1148.
30. Carlsson, J., Söderholm, G., and Almfeldt, I. 1969. Prevalence of *Streptococcus sanguis* and *Streptococcus mutans* in the mouths of persons wearing full dentures. *Arch Oral Biol* 14:243–252.
31. Chorpenning, F.W., Cooper, H.R., and Rosen, S. 1975. Cross-reactions of *Streptococcus mutans* due to cell wall teichoic acid. *Infect Immun* 12:586–591.
32. Clarke, J.K. 1924. On the bacterial factor in the aetiology of dental caries. *Br J Exp Pathol* 5:141–147.
33. Cornick, D.E.R., and Bowen, W.H. 1971. Development of the oral flora in newborn monkeys *(Macaca irus)*. *Br Dent J* 130:231–234.
34. Coykendall, A.L. 1970. Base composition of deoxyribonucleic acid isolated from cariogenic streptococci. *Arch Oral Biol* 15:365–368.
35. Coykendall, A.L. 1971. Genetic heterogenicity in *Streptococcus mutans*. *J Bacteriol* 106:192–196.
36. Coykendall, A.L. 1974. Four types of *Streptococcus mutans* based on their genetic and biochemical characteristics. *J Gen Microbiol* 83:327–338.
37. Coykendall, A.L. 1976. On the evolution of *Streptococcus mutans* and dental caries. In *Microbial Aspects of Dental Caries*, H.M. Stiles, W.W. Loesche, and T.C. O'Brien (eds) Sp. Suppl. Microbiol. Abstr. 3:703–712.
38. Coykendall, A.L. 1977. Proposal to elevate the subspecies of *Streptococcus mutans* to species status, based on the molecular composition. *Int J Syst Bacteriol* 27:26–30.
39. Coykendall, A.L. 1983. *Streptococcus sobrinus* nom. rev. and *Streptococcus ferus* nom., rev.: Habitat of these and other Mutans Streptococci. *Int J Syst Bacteriol* 33:883–885.
40. Coykendall, A.L., and Gustafson, K.B. 1986. Taxonomy of *Streptococcus mutans*. In *Molecular Microbiology and Immunobiology of Streptococcus mutans*, S. Hamada et al (eds), Amsterdam: Elsevier Science Publishers, pp. 21–28.
41. Crawford, A.C.R., Socransky, S.S., Smith, E., and Phillips, R. 1977. Pathogenicity testing of oral isolates in gnotobiotic rats. *J Dent Res* 56 (Sp. Issue B, Abstr. 275):B120.
42. Drucker, D.B., and Melville, T.H. 1968. Fermentation end-products of cariogenic and non-cariogenic streptococci. *Arch Oral Biol* 13:563–570.
43. Duany, L.F., Zinner, D.D., and Landy, J.J. 1971. Bone loss and caries in rats infected with human streptococci. *J Dent Res* 50:460–465.
44. Edman, D.C., Keene, H.J., Shklair, I.L., and Hoerman, K.C. 1975. Dental floss for implantation and sampling of *Streptococcus mutans* from approximal surfaces of human teeth. *Arch Oral Biol* 20:145–148.
45. Edwardsson, S. 1968. Characteristics of caries-inducing human streptococci resembling *Streptococcus mutans*. *Arch Oral Biol* 13:637–646.
46. Edwardsson, S. 1970. The caries-inducing property of variants of *Streptococcus mutans*. *Odontol Revy* 21:153–157.
47. Edwardsson, S. 1974. Bacteriological studies on deep areas of carious dentine. *Odontol Revy* 25:Suppl. 32.
48. Ellen, R.P. 1976. Establishment and distribution of *Actinomyces viscosus* and *Actinomyces naeslundii* in the human oral cavity. *Infect Immun* 14:1119–1124.
49. Emilson, C.G., Köhler, B., and Bratthall, D. 1975. Immunofluorescent determination of the relative proportions of *Streptococcus mutans* in human plaque. A comparison with cultural techniques. *Arch Oral Biol* 20:81–86.

50. Facklam, R.R. 1974. Characteristics of *Streptococcus mutans* isolated from human dental plaque and blood. *Int J Syst Bacteriol* 24:313–319.
51. Facklam, R.R. 1977. Physiological differentiation of viridans streptococci. *J Clin Microbiol* 5:184–201.
52. Fairbourn, D.R., Charbeneau, G.T., and Loesche, W.J. 1980. Effect of improved Dycal and IRM on bacteria in deep carious lesions. *J Am Dent Assoc* 100:547–552.
53. Fitzgerald, R.J. 1963. Gnotobiotic contribution to oral microbiology. *J Dent Res* 42:549–552.
54. Fitzgerald, R.J. 1968. Dental caries in gnotobiotic animals. *Caries Res* 2:139–146.
55. Fitzgerald, R.J. 1968. Plaque microbiology and caries. *Ala J Med Sci* 5:239–246.
56. Fitzgerald, R.J., Adams, B.O., and Fitzgerald, D.B. 1981. Cariogenicity of human plaque lactobacilli in gnotobiotic rats. *J Dent Res* 60:919–926.
57. Fitzgerald, R.J., Jordan, H.V., and Stanley, H.R. 1960. Experimental caries and gingival pathological changes in the gnotobiotic rat. *J Dent Res* 39:923–935.
58. Fitzgerald, R.J., Jordan, H.V., and Stanley, H.R. 1966. Dental caries in gnotobiotic rats infected with a variety of *Lactobacillus acidophilus*. *Arch Oral Biol* 11:473–476.
59. Fitzgerald, R.J., and Keyes, P.H. 1960. Demonstration of the etiologic role of streptococci in experimental caries in the hamster. *J Am Dent Assoc* 61:9–19.
60. Fitzgerald, R.J., Morhart, R.E., Marquez, C., and Adams, B.O. 1986. Inhibition of caries in hamsters treated with staphylococcin 1580. *Infect Immun* 54:288–290.
61. Folke, L.E.A., Sveen, O.B., and Tlott, E.K. 1973. A new methodology for study of plaque formation in natural human fissures. *Scand J Dent Res* 87:411–414.
62. Forsum, U., and Holmberg, K. 1974. Identification of *Streptococcus sanguis* by defined immunofluorescence. *Caries Res* 8:105–112.
63. Frank, R.M., Guillo, B., and Llory, H. 1972. Caries dentaires chez le rat gnotobiote inoculé avec *Actinomyces viscosus* et *Actinomyces naeslundii*. *Arch Oral Biol* 17:1249–1253.
64. Gibbons, R.J. 1964. Bacteriology of dental caries. *J Dent Res* 43:1021–1028.
65. Gibbons, R.J., Berman, K.S., Knoettner, P., and Kapsimalis, B. 1966. Dental caries and alveolar bone loss in gnotobiotic rats infected with capsule forming streptococci of human origin. *Arch Oral Biol* 11:549–560.
66. Gibbons, R.J., Depoala, P.F., Spinell, D.M., and Skobe, Z. 1974. Interdental localization of *Streptococcus mutans* as related to dental caries experience. *Infect Immun* 9:481–488.
67. Gibbons, R.J., and Houte, J. van. 1971. Selective bacterial adherence to oral epithelial surfaces and its role as an ecological determinant. *Infect Immun* 3:567–573.
68. Gibbons, R.J., and Loesche, W.J. 1967. Isolation of cariogenic streptococci from Guatemalan children. *Arch Oral Biol* 12:1013–1014.
69. Gibbons, R.J., and Spinell, D.M. 1970. Salivary-induced aggregation of plaque bacteria. In *Dental Plaque*, W.D. McHugh (ed), Edinburgh: E. and S. Livingstone, pp. 207–215.
70. Girard, A.E., and Vacius, B.H. 1974. Ultrastructure of *Actinomyces viscosus* and *Actinomyces naeslundii*. *Arch Oral Biol* 19:71–79.
71. Gold, O.G., Jordan, H.V., and Houte, J. van. 1973. A selective medium for *Streptococcus mutans*. *Arch Oral Biol.* 18:1357–1364.
72. Green, R.M., Blackmore, D.K., and Drucker, D.B. 1973. The role of gnotobiotic animals in the study of dental caries. *Br Dent J* 134:537–540.
73. Greer, S.B., Hsiang, W., Musil, G., and Zinner, D.D. 1971. Virus of cariogenic streptococci. *J Dent Res* 50:1594–1604.
74. Guggenheim, B. 1968. Streptococci of dental plaque. *Caries Res* 2:147–163.
75. Guillo, G., Klein, J.P., and Frank, R.M. 1973. Fissure caries in gnotobiotic rats infected with *Actinomyces naeslundii* and *Actinomyces israelii*. *Helv Odontol Acta* 17:2–30.
76. Hamada, S., Gill, K., and Slade, H.D. 1976. Chemical and immunological properties of the type f polysaccharide antigen of *Streptococcus mutans*. *Infect Immun* 14:203–211.
77. Hamada, S., and Slade, H.D. 1976. Purification and immunochemical characterization of type e polysaccharide antigen of *Streptococcus mutans*. *Infect Immun* 14:68–76.
78. Harder, E.J., Wilkowske, C.J., Washington, J.A., and Geraci, J.E. 1974. *Streptococcus mutans* endocarditis. *Ann Intern Med* 80:364–368.
79. Hardie, J.M., and Bowden, G.H. 1974. Cell wall and serological studies on *Streptococcus mutans*. *Caries Res* 8:301–316.
80. Hardie, J.M., Thompson, P.L., South, R.J., Marsh, P.D., Bowden, G.H., McKee, A.S., Fillery, E.D., and Slack, G.L. 1977. A longitudinal epidemiological study on dental plaque and the development of caries. Interim results after two years. *J Dent Res* 56(Sp. Issue C):C90–C98.

81. Hazen, S.P., Chilton, N.W., and Mumma, R.D., Jr. 1972. The problem of root caries. 3. A clinical study. International Association for Dental Research Scientific Proceedings, 50th Gen. Session, Program and Abstracts of Papers, Abstr. 689, p. 219.
82. Hazen, S.P., Chilton, N.W., and Mumma, R.D., Jr. 1973. The problem of root caries. 1. Literature review and clinical description. *J Am Dent Assoc* 86:137–144.
83. Higuchi, M., Rhee, G.H., Araya, S., and Higuchi, M. 1977. Bacteriophage deoxyribonucleic acid-induced mutation of *Streptococcus mutans*. *Infect Immun* 15:938–944.
84. Hoerman, K.C., Keene, H.J., Shklair, I.L., and Burmeister, J.A. 1972. The association of *Streptococcus mutans* with early carious lesions in human teeth. *J Am Dent Assoc* 85:1349–1352.
85. Hoeven, J.S. van der. 1974. A slime-producing microorganism in dental plaque of rats, selected by glucose feeding. *Caries Res* 8:193–210.
86. Hoeven, J.S. van der, Mikx, F.H.M., König, K.G., and Plasschaert, A.J.M. 1974. Plaque formation and dental caries in gnotobiotic and SPF Osborne-Mendel rats associated with *Actinomyces viscosus*. *Caries Res* 8:211–233.
87. Hoeven, J.S. van der, Mikx, F.H.M., Plasschaert, A.J.M., and König, K.G. 1972. Methodological aspects of gnotobiotic caries experimentation. *Caries Res* 6:203–210.
88. Hoover, C.O., Newbrun, E., Mettraux, G., and Graf, H. 1980. Microflora and chemical composition of dental plaque from subjects with hereditary fructose intolerance. *Infect Immun* 28:853–859.
89. Hoshino, E. 1985. Predominant obligate anaerobes in human carious dentin. *J Dent Res* 64:1195–1198.
90. Houte, J. van, and Green, D.B. 1974. Relationship between the concentration of bacteria in saliva and the colonization on teeth in humans. *Infect Immun* 9:624–630.
91. Houte, J. van, Gibbons, R.J., and Pulkkinen, A.J. 1972. Ecology of oral lactobacilli. *Infect Immun* 6:723–729.
92. Houte, J. van, Gibbs, G., and Butera, C. 1982. Oral flora of children with "nursing bottle caries." *J Dent Res* 61:382–385.
93. Houte, J. van, Yanover, L., and Brecher, S. 1981. Relationship of levels of the bacterium *Streptococcus mutans* in saliva of children and their parents. *Arch Oral Biol* 26:381–386.
94. Howell, A., and Jordan, H.V. 1967. Production of extracellular levan by *Odontomyces viscosus*. *Arch Oral Biol* 12:571–573.
95. Huis in't Veld, J.H.J., van Palenstein Helderman, W.H., and Backer Dirks, O. 1979. *Streptococcus mutans* and dental caries in humans. A bacteriological and immunological study. *Antonie Van Leeuwenhoek* 45:25–33.
96. Ikeda, T., Sandham, H.J., and Bradley, E.L. 1973. Changes in *Streptococcus mutans* and lactobacilli in plaque in relation to the initiation of dental caries in negro children. *Arch Oral Biol* 18:555–566.
97. Ikeda, T., Iwanami, T., Hirasawa, M., Watanabe, C., McGhee, J.R., and Shiota, T. 1982. Purification and certain properties of a bacteriocin from *Streptococcus mutans*. *Infect Immun* 35:861–868.
98. Jordan, H.V. 1965. Bacteriological aspects of experimental dental caries. *Ann NY Acad Sci* 131:905–912.
99. Jordan, H.V., Englander, H.R., Engler, W.O., and Kulczyk, S. 1972. Observations on the implantation and transmission of *Streptococcus mutans* in human beings. *J Dent Res* 51:515–518.
100. Jordan, H.V., Englander, H.R., and Lim, S. 1969. Potentially cariogenic streptococci in selected population groups in the western hemisphere. *J Am Dent Assoc* 78:1331–1335.
101. Jordan, H.V., and Hammond, B.F. 1972. Filamentous bacteria isolated from human root surface caries. *Arch Oral Biol* 17:1333–1342.
102. Jordan, H.V., and Keyes, P.H. 1964. Aerobic, gram-positive, filamentous bacteria as etiological agents of experimental periodontal disease in hamsters. *Arch Oral Biol* 9:401–414.
103. Jordan, H.V., Keyes, P.H., and Bellack, S. 1972. Periodontal lesions in hamsters and gnotobiotic rats infected with *Actinomyces* of human origin. *J Periodont Res* 7:21–28.
104. Jordan, H.V., and Sumney, D.C. 1973. Root surface caries. Review of the literature and significance of the problem. *J Periodontol* 44:158–163.
105. Katz, R.V., Hazen, S.P., Chilton, N.W., and Mumma, R.D. 1982. Prevalence and intraoral distribution of root caries in an adult population. *Caries Res* 16:265–271.
106. Keene, H.J., Shklair, I.L., Mickel, G.J., and Wirthlin, M.R. 1977. Distribution of *Streptococcus mutans* biotypes in five human populations. *J Dent Res* 56:5–10.
107. Kelstrup, J., and Gibbons, R.J. 1969. Bacteriocins from human and rodent strep-

tococci. *Arch Oral Biol* 14:251–258.

108. Kelstrup, J., and Gibbons, R.J. 1970. Induction of dental caries and alveolar bone loss by a human isolate resembling *Streptococcus salivarius*. *Caries Res* 4:360–377.
109. Keyes, P.H. 1960. The infectious and transmissible nature of experimental dental caries. *Arch Oral Biol* 1:304–320.
110. Keyes, P.H., and McCabe, R.M. 1973. The potential of various compounds to suppress microorganisms in plaques produced in vitro by a streptococcus or an actinomycete. *J Am Dent Assoc* 86:396–400.
111. Klein, J.P., and Frank, R.M. 1973. Mise en évidence de virus dans les bacteries cariogenes de la plaque dentaire. *J Biol Buccale* 1:79–85.
112. Köhler, B., and Bratthall, D. 1978. Intrafamilial levels of *Streptococcus mutans* and some aspects of the bacterial transmission. *Scand J Dent Res* 86:35–42.
113. Köhler, B., Andréen, I., and Jonsson, B. 1984. The effect of caries-preventive measures in mothers on dental caries and the oral presence of the bacteria *Streptococcus mutans* and lactobacilli in their children. *Arch Oral Biol* 29:879–883.
114. Köhler, B., Bratthall, D., and Krasse, B. 1983. Preventive measures in mothers influence the establishment of the bacterium *Streptococcus mutans* in their infants. *Arch Oral Biol* 28:225–231.
115. König, K.G., Guggenheim, B., and Mühlemann, H.R. 1965. Modifications of the oral flora and their influence on dental caries in the rat. II. Inoculation of a cariogenic streptococcus and its effect in relation to varying time of depression of the indigenous flora. *Helv Odontol Acta* 9:130–134.
116. König, K.G., and Mühlemann, H.R. 1964. Further investigations into a possible effect of dietary lysosome on caries incidence in rats. *Helv Odontol Acta* 8:22–24.
117. Krasse, B. 1970. A review of the bacteriology of dental plaque. In *Dental Plaque*, W.D. McHugh (ed), Edinburgh: E. and S. Livingstone, pp. 199–205.
118. Krasse, B., and Carlsson, J. 1970. Various types of streptococci and experimental caries in hamsters. *Arch Oral Biol* 15:25–32.
119. Krasse, B., Edwardsson, S., Svensson, I., and Trell, L. 1967. Implantation of caries inducing streptococci in the human oral cavity. *Arch Oral Biol* 12:231–236.
120. Krasse, B., Jordan, H.V., Edwardsson, S., Svensson, I., and Trell, L. 1968. The occurrence of certain "caries-inducing" streptococci in human dental plaque material. *Arch Oral Biol* 13:911–918.
121. Lang, N.P., Hotz, P.R., Gusberti, F.A., and Joss, A. 1987. Longitudinal clinical and microbiological study on the relationship between infection with *Streptococcus mutans* and the development of caries in humans. *Oral Microbiol Immunol* 2:39–47.
122. Liljemark, W.F., and Gibbons, R.J. 1972. Proportional distribution and relative adherence of *Streptococcus miteor (mitis)* on various surfaces in the human oral cavity. *Infect Immun* 6:852–859.
123. Linzer, R., Gill, K., and Slade, H.D. 1976. The chemical composition of *Streptococcus mutans* type c antigen. Comparison to type a, b, and d antigens. *J Dent Res* 55:A109–A115.
124. Linzer, R., and Slade, H.D. 1974. Purification and characterization of *Streptococcus mutans* group d cell wall polysaccharide antigen. *Infect Immun* 10:361–368.
125. Littleton, N.W., Kakehashi, S., and Fitzgerald, R.J. 1970. Recovery of specific "caries-inducing" streptococci from carious lesions in the teeth of children. *Arch Oral Biol* 15:461–463.
126. Llory, H., Guillo, B., and Frank, R.M. 1971. A cariogenic *Actinomyces viscosus*. A bacteriological and gnotobiotic study. *Helv Odontol Acta* 15:134–138.
127. Löe, H., Karring, T., and Theilade, E. 1973. An in vivo method for the study of the microbiology of occlusal fisures. *Caries Res* 7:120–129.
128. Loesche, W.J. 1975. Bacterial succession in dental plaque. Role in dental disease. *Microbiology* 44:132–136.
129. Loesche, W., and Syed, S.A. 1973. The predominant cultivable flora of carious plaque and carious dentine. *Caries Res.* 7:201–206.
130. Loesche, W.J., and Syed, S.A. 1978. Bacteriology of human experimental gingivitis. Effect of plaque and gingivitis score. *Infect Immun* 21:830–839.
131. Loesche, W.J., Svanberg, M.L., and Pape, H.R. 1979. Intraoral transmission of *Streptococcus mutans* by a dental explorer. *J Dent Res* 58:1765–1770.
132. Loesch, W.J., Walenga, A., and Loos, P. 1973. Recovery of *Streptococcus mutans* and *Streptococcus sanguis* from a dental explorer after clinical examination of single human teeth. *Arch Oral Biol* 18:571–575.
133. Loesche, W.J., Eklund, S., Earnest, R., and Burt, B. 1984. Longitudinal investigation of bacteriology of human fissure decay: epidemiological studies in molars shortly

after eruption. *Infect Immun* 46:765–772.

134. Lohse, W.G., Carter, H.G., and Brunelle, J.A. 1977. The prevalence of root surface caries in a military population. *Military Med* 141:700–703.
135. London, J. 1976. The ecology and taxonomic status of the lactobacilli. *Annu Rev Microbiol* 30:279–301.
136. Masuda, N., Tsutsumi, N., Sobue, S., and Hamada, H. 1979. Longitudinal survey of the distribution of various serotypes of *Streptococcus mutans* in infants. *J Clin Microbiol* 10:497:502.
137. Michalek, S.M., McGhee, J.R., and Navia, J.M. 1975. Virulence of *Streptococcus mutans*. A sensitive method for evaluating cariogenicity in young gnotobiotic rats. *Infect Immun* 12:69–75.
138. Mikx, F.H.M., Hoeven, J.S. van der, König, K.G., and Guggenheim, B. 1972. Establishment of defined microbial ecosystems in germ-free rats. *Caries Res* 6:211–223.
139. Minah, G.E., Solomon, E.S., and Chu, K. 1985. The association between dietary sucrose consumption and microbial population shifts at six oral sites in man. *Arch Oral Biol* 30:397–401.
140. Moore, W.E.C., Holdeman, L.V., Cato, E.P., Good, I.J., Smith, E.P., Ranney, R.R., and Palcanis, K.G. 1984. Variation in periodontal floras. *Infect Immun* 46:720–726.
141. Mukasa, H., and Slade, H.D. 1973. Extraction, purification and chemical and immunological properties of the *Streptococcus mutans* group a polysaccharide cell wall antigen. *Infect Immun* 7:190–198.
142. Mukasa, H., and Slade, H.D. 1973. Structure and immunological specificity of the *Streptococcus mutans* group b cell wall antigen. *Infect Immun* 7:578–585.
143. Neefe, L.I., Chretien, J.H., Deloha, E.C., and Garagusi, V.F. 1974. *Streptococcus mutans* endocarditis. *J Am Med Assoc* 230:1298–1299.
144. Nesbitt, W.E., Staat, R.H., Rosan, B., Taylor, K.G., and Doyle, R.J. 1980. Association of protein with the cell wall of *Streptococcus mutans*. *Infect Immun* 28:118–126.
145. Newbrun, E., Matsukubo, T., Hoover, C.I., Graves, R.C., Brown, A.T., Disney, J.A., and Bohannan, H.M. 1984. Comparison of two screening tests for *Streptococcus mutans* and evaluation of their suitability for mass screening and private practice. *Community Dent Oral Epidemiol* 12:289–295.
146. Nyvad, B., and Fejerskov, O. 1982. Root surface caries: clinical, histopathological and microbiological features and clinical implications. *Internat Dent J* 32:312–326.
147. Onose, H., and Sandham, H.J. 1976. pH changes during culture of human dental plaque streptococci on mitis-salivarius agar. *Arch Oral Biol* 21:291–296.
148. Orland, F.J., Blayney, J.R., Harrison, R.W., Reyniers, J.A., Trexler, P.C., Ervin, R.F., Gordon, H.A., and Wagner, M. 1955. Experimental caries in germ-free rats inoculated with enterococci. *J Am Dent Assoc* 50:259–272.
149. Orland, F.J., Blayney, J.R., Harrison, R.W., Reyniers, J.A., Trexler, P.C., Wagner, M., Gordon, H.A., and Luckey, T.D. 1954. The use of germ-free animal techniques in the study of experimental dental caries. I. Basic observations on rats reared free of all microorganisms. *J Dent Res* 33:147–174.
150. Perch, B., Kjems, E., and Ravn, T. 1974. Biochemical and serological properties of *Streptococcus mutans* from various sources. *Acta Pathol Microbiol Scand* Sect B, 82:357–370.
151. Qureshi, J.V., Goldner, M., le Riche, W.H., and Hargreaves, J.A. 1977. *Streptococcus mutans* serotypes in young schoolchildren. *Caries Res* 11:141–152.
152. Ritz, H.L. 1967. Microbial population shifts in developing human dental plaque. *Arch Oral Biol* 12:1561–1568.
153. Rogers, A.H. 1977. Evidence for the transmissibility of human dental caries. *Aust Dent J* 22:53–56.
154. Rodgers, A.H. 1980. Bacteriocin typing of *Streptococcus mutans* strains isolated from family group. *Aust Dent J* 25:279–283.
155. Rogosa, M. 1964. The genus *Veillonella*. I. General cultural, ecological and biochemical considerations. *J Bacteriol* 87:162–170.
156. Rogosa, M., Krichevsky, M.I., and Bishop, F.S. 1965. Truncated glycolytic system in *Veillonella*. *J Bacteriol* 90:164–171.
157. Rosan, B., and Hammond, B.F. 1974. Extracellular polysaccharides of *Actinomyces viscosus*. *Infect Immun* 10:304–308.
158. Rosen, S., Doff, R., McDaniel, T., and App, G.R. 1977. Root surface caries. Experimental animal model and inhibition by fluoride. *J Dent Res* 56:(Sp. Issue B, Abstr. 638) B211.
159. Rosen, S., and Kolstad, R.A. 1977. Dental caries in gnotobiotic rats inoculated with a strain of *Peptostreptococcus intermedius*. *J Dent Res* 56:187.

160. Rosen, S., Lenny, W.S., and O'Malley, J.E. 1968. Dental caries in gnotobiotic rats inoculated with *Lactobacillus casei*. *J Dent Res* 47:358–363.
161. Schamschula, R.G., Barnes, D.E., Keyes, P.H., and Gulbinat, W. 1974. Prevalence and interrelationships of root surface caries in Lufa, Papua, New Guinea. *Community Dent Oral Epidemiol* 2:295–304.
162. Schamschula, R.G., and Charlton, G. 1971. A study of caries etiology in New South Wales schoolchildren. I. The streptococcal flora of plaque and caries prevalence. *Aust Dent J* 16:77–82.
163. Schamschula, R.G., Keyes, P.H., and Hornabrook, R.W. 1972. Root surface caries in Lufa, New Guinea. I. Clinical observations. *J Am Dent Assoc* 85:603–608.
164. Schleifer, K.H., Kilpper-Bälz, R., Kraus, J., and Gehring, F. 1984. Relatedness and classification of *Streptococcus mutans* and "mutans-like" streptococci. *J Dent Res* 63:1047–1050.
165. Shklair, I.L., and Keene, H.J. 1974. A biochemical scheme for the separation of five varieties of *Streptococcus mutans*. *Arch Oral Biol* 19:1079–1081.
166. Shklair, I.L., Keene, H.J., and Simonson, L.G. 1972. Distribution and frequency of *Streptococcus mutans* in caries active individuals. *J Dent Res* 51:882.
167. Shklair, I.L., Leonard, E.P., and Bruton, W.F. 1979. *S mutans* glucan production and proximal caries activity in rats. *J Dent Res* Sp. Issue A 58:377.
168. Shovlin, F.E., and Gillis, R.E. 1969. Biochemical and antigenic studies of lactobacilli isolated from deep dentinal caries. I. Biochemical aspects. *J Dent Res* 48:356–360.
169. Skerman, V.B.D., McGowan, V., and Sneath, P.H.A. (eds) 1980. Approved list of bacterial names. *Int J Syst Bacteriol* 30:225–420.
170. Slack, J.M., and Gerencser, M.A. 1975. *Actinomyces, Filamentous Bacteria: Biology and Pathogenicity*. Minneapolis: Burgess.
171. Slots, J., Möenbo, D., Langebaek, J., and Frandsen, A. 1978. Microbiota of gingivitis in man. *Scand J Dent Res* 86:174–181.
172. Socransky, S.S., Hubersak, C., and Propas, D. 1970. Induction of periodontal destruction in gnotobiotic rats by a human oral strain of *Actinomyces naeslundii*. *Arch Oral Biol* 15:993–995.
173. Socransky, S.S., Manganiello, A.D., Propas, D., Oram, V., and Houte, J. van. 1977. Bacteriological studies of developing supragingival dental plaque. *J Periodont Res* 12:90–106.
174. Soprey, P., and Slade, H.D. 1971. Chemical structure and immunological specificity of the streptococcal group d cell wall polysaccharide antigen. *Infect Immun* 3:653–658.
175. Stamm, J.W., and Banting, D.W. 1980. Comparison of root caries prevalence in adults with life-long residence in fluoridated and nonfluoridated communities. *J Dent Res* 59:(Sp. Issue A, Abstr. 552.): 405.
176. Stoppelaar, J.D. de. 1971. *Streptococcus mutans, Streptococcus sanguis* and dental caries. Thesis. University of Utrecht, The Netherlands.
177. Stoppelaar, J.D. de, Houte, J. van, and Backer Dirks, O. 1969. The relationship between extracellular polysaccharide-producing streptococci and smooth surface caries in 13-year old children. *Caries Res* 3:190–199.
178. Stoppelaar, J.D. de, Houte, J. van, and Backer Dirks, O. 1970. The effect of carbohydrate restriction on the presence of *Streptococcus mutans, Streptococcus sanguis* and iodophilic polysaccharide-producing bacteria in human dental plaque. *Caries Res* 4:114–123.
179. Stoppellaar, J.D. de, König, K.G., Plasschaert, A.J.M., and Hoeven, J.S. van der. 1971. Decreased cariogenicity of a mutant of *Streptococcus mutans*. *Arch Oral Biol* 16:971–975.
180. Strålfors, A. 1950. Investigations into the bacterial chemistry of dental plaques. *Odontol Tidsk* 58:155–341.
181. Sumney, D.L., and Jordan, H.V. 1974. Characterization of bacteria isolated from human root surface carious lesions. *J Dent Res* 53:343–351.
182. Sumney, D.L., Jordan, H.V., and Englander, H.R. 1973. The prevalence of root surface caries in selected populations. *J Periodontol* 44:500–504.
183. Svanberg, M. 1978. Contamination of toothpaste and toothbrush by *Streptococcus mutans*. *Scand J Dent Res* 86:412–414.
184. Svanberg, N., and Krasse, B. 1978. Asymmetrical dental caries and *Streptococcus mutans*. *J Am Dent Assoc* 96:1025–1027.
185. Svanberg, M., and Loesche, W.J. 1978. Intraoral spread of *Streptococcus mutans*. *Arch Oral Biol* 23:557–561.
186. Syed, S.A., Loesche, W.J., Pape, H.L., and Grenier, E. 1975. Predominant cultivable

flora isolated from human root surface plaque. *Infect Immun* 11:727–731.

187. Takada, K., Ikeda, T., Mitsui, I., and Shiota, T. 1984. Mode of inhibitory action of bacteriocin produced by *Streptococcus mutans* C3603. *Infect Immun* 44:370–378.
188. Tanzer, J.M., Freedman, M.L., Fitzgerald, R.J., and Larson, R.H. 1974. Diminished virulence of glucan synthesis-defective mutants of *Streptococcus mutans*. *Infect Immun* 10:197–203.
189. Tanzer, J.M., and McCabe, R.M. 1968. Selection of plaque-forming streptococci by the serial passage of wires through sucrose-containing broth. *Arch Oral Biol* 13:139–143.
190. Theilade, E., Larson, R.H., and Karring, T. 1973. Microbiological studies of plaque in artificial fissures implanted in human teeth. *Caries Res* 7:130–138.
191. Thomson, L.A., Little, W.A., Bowen, W.H., Sierra, L.I., Aguirrer, M., and Gillespie, G. 1980. Prevalence of *Streptococcus mutans* serotypes, *Actinomyces*, and other bacteria in the plaque of children. *J Dent Res* 59:1581–1589.
192. van de Rijn, I., and Bleiweis, A.S. 1973. Antigens of *Streptococcus mutans*. I. Characterization of serotype-specific determinant from *Streptococcus mutans*. *Infect Immun* 7:795–804.
193. Vaught, R.M., and Bleiweis, A.S. 1974. Antigens of *Streptococcus mutans*. II. Characterization of an antigen resembling a glycerol teichoic acid in walls of strain BHT. *Infect Immun* 9:60–67.
194. Vehkalahti, M., Rajala, M., Tuominen, R., and Paunio, I. 1983. Prevalence of root caries in the adult Finnish population. *Community Dent Oral Epidemiol* 11:188–190.
195. Walter, R.G. 1982. A longitudinal study of caries development in initially caries-free naval recruits. *J Dent Res* 61:1405–1407.
196. Wicken, A.J., and Knox, K.W. 1975. Lipoteichoic acids. A new classification of bacterial antigen. *Science* 187:1161–1167.
197. Willcox, M.D.P., Drucker, D.B., and Green, R.M. 1987. Relative cariogenicity and in vivo plaque-forming ability of the bacterium *Streptococcus oralis* in gnotobiotic WAG/RIJ rats. *Arch Oral Biol* 32:455–457.
198. Williams, B.L., Pantalone, R.M., and Sherris, J.C. 1976. Subgingival microflora and periodontitis. *J Periodont Res* 11:1–18.
199. Williams, R.E.O. 1973. Benefit and mischief from commensal bacteria. *J Clin Pathol* 26:811–818.
200. Zinner, D., and Jablon, J.M. 1968. Human streptococcal strains in experimental caries. In *Art and Science of Dental Caries Research*, R.S. Harris (ed), New York: Academic Press, pp. 87–108.

Chapter 4

Substrate: Diet and Caries

Oh, I wish I'd looked after me Teeth

Oh, I wish I'd looked after me teeth,
And spotted the perils beneath,
All the toffees I chewed,
And the sweet sticky food,
Oh, I wish I'd looked after me teeth.

I wish I'd been that much more willin'
When I had more tooth there than fillin'
To pass up gobstoppers,
From respect to me choppers
And to buy something else with me shillin'.

When I think of the lollies I licked,
And the liquorice allsorts I picked,
Sherbet dabs, big and little,
All that hard peanut brittle,
My conscience gets horribly pricked.

by Pam Ayres, from *Some of me Poetry*,
Arrow Books, 1972

Influence of diet on the caries process

Before discussing the role of diet, it is important to define certain terms. *Diet* refers to the customary allowance of food and drink taken by any person from day to day. Thus, the diet may exert an effect on caries locally in the mouth by reacting with the enamel surface and by serving as a substrate for cariogenic microorganisms. *Nutrition* concerns the assimilation of foods and their effect on metabolic processes of the body. Nutrition can act only through a systemic route and therefore influences the host during tooth development. With the exception of the well-established caries-reducing effect of systemic fluoride, it has not been conclusively shown that human teeth are more or less susceptible to caries depending on the exposure to various nutritional conditions in early life and before eruption.

Since the time of the early Greek philosophers, the diet has been suspected of influencing the etiology of caries. Human volunteers do not subject themselves readily to strictly controlled diets for extended periods (at least 2 to 3 years). Therefore, positive proof of the diet's role in human caries has not been easily established. In an attempt to identify which foods may be particularly cariogenic, many studies have depended on information obtained from the patient's dietary history.[12,91,156,159] A dietary history can be quite useful for educating and motivating the patient.[107] However, the reliability and accuracy of such an anamnestic history for measuring the contribution of diet to the prevalence of caries is questionable. Above all, such studies usually lack scientifically acceptable control groups. Nevertheless, a certain pattern has emerged which indicates that patients with rampant caries frequently include sucrose-containing foods in their diet. Sucrose has been indicated as "the arch criminal" in the etiology of caries.[104]

Epidemiological observations of caries and diet

Circumstantial evidence linking sucrose consumption and prevalence of caries can readily be found in several epidemiological surveys. The prevalence of caries among native populations such as Australian Aborigines, New Zealand Maoris, Eskimos, Ghanaians, Tristan da Cunhans, etc, was very low prior to their exposure to European-type diets. Native diets did not contain any sucrose other than the relatively small amounts found in fruits and vegetables. Staple carbohydrate foods included cassava, yam, maize, millet, and potatoes. As their diets changed to include products containing sugar, caries prevalence increased.

In England, which imports most of its sucrose, records of the last 100 years show a steady increase in per capita consumption, or disappearance,* of sucrose, from about 20 lb/year in 1820 to over 100 lb/year today.[102] Present disappearance of sucrose in the United States is about the same. This represents 15% to 20% of an individual's caloric requirements. Concomitant with this increased disappearance of sucrose has been an almost parallel rise in the prevalence of caries.[54] Conversely, surveys in Europe and Japan have demonstrated that caries was dramatically reduced during periods of wartime food restrictions, when the disappearance of sugar, syrup, and all sugar products was reduced.[75,127,134,143,149]

The common features in each of these countries were the severe rationing of sucrose and the decreased between-meal eating. It has been proposed that the decrease in caries during and after World War II was due to influences (nutritional) exerted during tooth formation rather than simply lack of sucrose substrate (dietary) locally for the oral flora. Marthaler[92] has pointed out that teeth that had already formed, as well as those still forming during 1941 to 1946, had less decay. On the other hand, matrix formation and mineralization of first molars during periods of maximal sugar restriction did not endow these teeth with any unique caries resistance. In the postwar years, as rationing eased and sugar became more readily available, the caries rate rose again. These findings

*Estimating per capita sugar "consumption" by the method of dividing sugar supplies by population yields a value that exceeds the actual consumption of sugar per capita, as calculated from dietary recall questionnaires or interviews. Therefore, the values obtained by this method are better termed "disappearance."

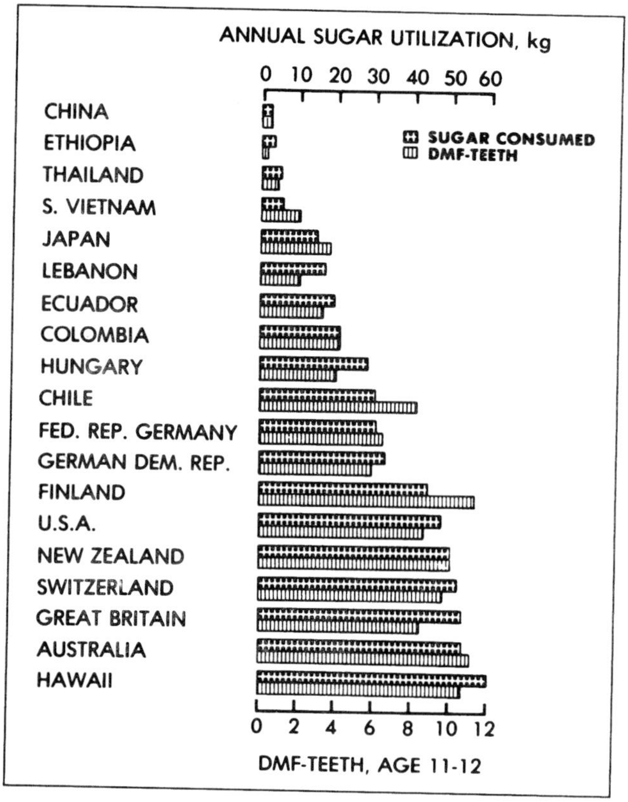

Fig 4-1 Cumulative dental decay prevalence, expressed as DMF permanent teeth, in children ages 11 to 12. Corresponding annual 1959 per capita sucrose utilization data for 18 countries and the state of Hawaii, from the Food and Agriculture Organization of the United Nations. (Courtesy of Dr T. Marthaler.[94])

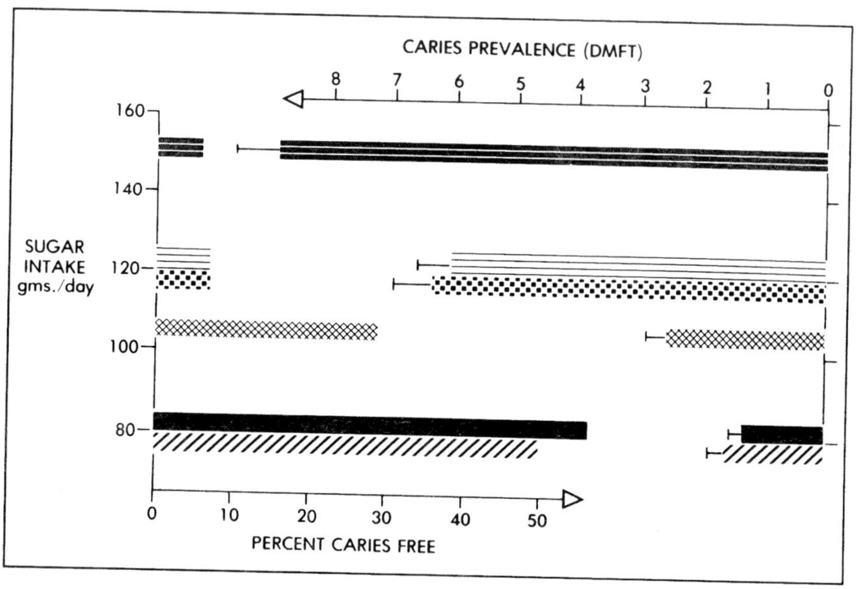

Fig 4-2 Relationship between dental caries and mean sugar intake (g/day) for South African males (16 to 17 years old) of four different ethnic groups. There is a direct relationship between percent population caries-free and sugar intake. (Drawn from the data of Retief et al.[111])

on the effects of wartime dietary restrictions indicate that the caries process can be influenced by diet.

Subsequently, data from 18 countries was compiled on sugar disappearance and average numbers of decayed, missing, and filled (DMF) teeth of children 10 to 12 years old (Fig 4-1).[94] These data revealed a highly significant correlation (r = 0.95 by linear regression analysis) between sugar disappearance and dental caries experience. Analysis of data derived from the World Health Organization's Global Oral Epidemiology Bank also revealed a significant positive relationship (r = 0.72) between sugar supplies and dental caries for 12-year-old children in 47 populations.[37,136] A high prevalence of caries, or low percentage of persons free from caries, was found among teenage South Africans with a high sugar intake (Fig 4-2). Conversely, rural blacks of similar age eating less sugar had less caries and more caries-free mouths.[111,153] This interpretation of the South African survey is contrary to the conclusions of the investigators but is supported by the overall data.

Interventional human studies

Vipeholm

Vipeholm is a mental institution in southern Sweden. Adult patients followed for several years on a nutritionally adequate diet, were found to develop caries at a slow rate. Subsequently, the patients were divided into nine groups to compare the effects of various modifications of carbohydrate intake. Sucrose was included in the diet as toffee, chocolate, caramel, in bread, or in liquid form. Caries increased significantly when sucrose-containing foods were ingested between meals. In addition, not only the frequency but also the form in which sucrose was ingested was important. Sticky or adhesive forms of sucrose-containing foods, which can maintain high sugar levels in the mouth, were more cariogenic than those forms that were rapidly cleared.[52]

The Vipeholm study demonstrated that it was possible to increase the average sugar consumption (from about 30 to 330 g/day) with very little increase in caries (0.27 to 0.43 new carious surfaces/year) *provided* the additional sugar was consumed at meals in solution. These observations on an institutional population, however, should not be misinterpreted, because the conditions were artificial. Where there is a free choice and access to sugar-containing foods and beverages, such items are more often eaten between meals, so that in general an increase in the amount of sugary foods and drinks consumed will lead to more decay. Undoubtedly, the minimal sucrose content required for cariogenicity will vary with the stickiness or oral clearance and the frequency of ingestion of that food item.

Hopewood House

Interesting findings on the effect of diet on dental caries have emerged from the study of institutionalized children at Hopewood House in Bowral, NSW, Australia. This was a children's home located in the country that was founded in 1942 by a businessman who had recovered his own health by a drastic reorganization of his dietary habits. He had sufficient wealth to attempt to put his dietary theories into practice. Babies were either born at the home or taken into it in the first few weeks of life, and the population gradually increased to 80 children.

From the very beginning, sugar and other refined carbohydrates (eg, white bread) were excluded from the children's diet. Carbohydrates were given in the form of whole-meal bread, soya beans, wheat germ, oats, rice, potatoes, and some treacle and molasses. Dairy products, fruit, raw vegetables, and nuts featured prominently in the typical menu. Although this was a vegetarian diet, it nevertheless provided an adequate amount of proteins, fats, minerals, and vitamins.

Dental surveys of these children during the ages of 5 and 13 revealed an average def (decayed, extracted, filled deciduous teeth) and DMFT

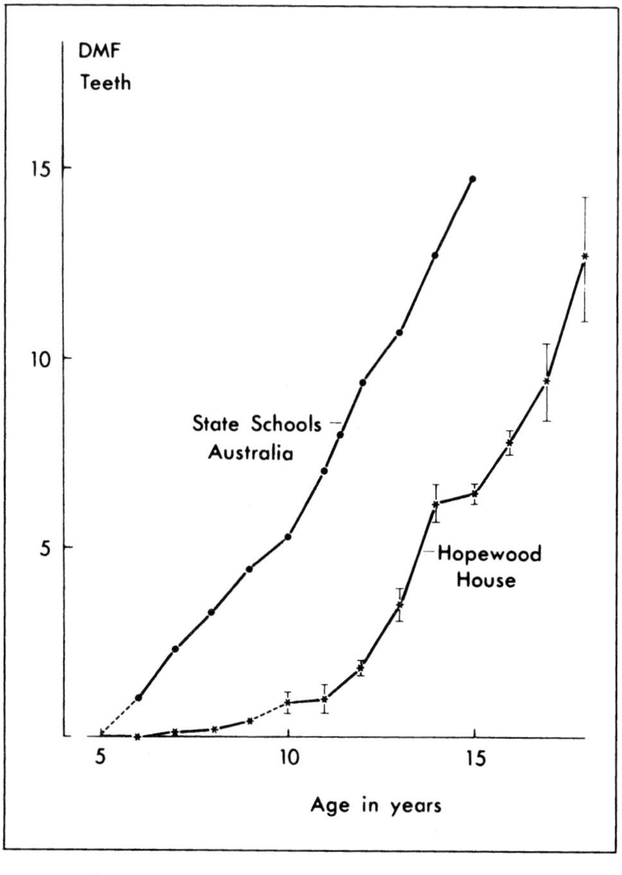

Fig 4-3 Plot of the mean number of DMF teeth per child versus chronological age in state schools of Australia and in children of Hopewood House (with standard error of means). Note the extremely low caries increment of the institutionalized children while under strict dietary control and the steep increase in caries experience when dietary supervision was no longer in effect—at above 13 years of age. (Courtesy of T. Marthaler.[92])

score of 1.1, or about 10% of the caries prevalence in the general population of that age group. It should be noted that the water supply contained insufficient fluoride (0.1 ppm) and that the children's oral hygiene was poor; about 75% of them suffered from gingivitis. It follows that caries can be reduced to a minimal level by dietary means alone in spite of unfavorable hygiene and fluoride levels. However, it must be recognized that this applies to an institutionalized population and is not valid for other situations. In fact, there is an important postscript to the Hopewood House study. As the children grew older they were relocated and no longer adhered to the original diet that had limited caries almost completely. A steep increase of DMFT experience occurred in the children above 13 years of age,[55] corresponding to the deviation in the dietary habits (Fig 4-3). This indicates that these teeth had not acquired any permanent resistance to caries. The reason that the teeth had not decayed during the prepuberty period was that the local oral environment was favorable and that few, if any, cariogenic foods were ingested.

Special population groups

Hereditary fructose intolerance

With the exception of the Vipeholm and Hopewood House studies, most investigations on the relationship of diet to human caries prevalence have relied on information obtained from dietary history. The limitations of this approach have already been mentioned. Nature, however, has provided a group of subjects who observe a strict dietary pattern because of hereditary fructose intolerance (HFI).

Hereditary fructose intolerance, first described in 1956[24] is a rare, autosomal recessive disorder of fructose metabolism. Intolerance to fructose results from drastically reduced activity (2% to 5% of normal) of fructose 1-phosphate aldolase in the liver, lower renal cortex, and small bowel. This enzyme splits fructose 1-phosphate into two 3-carbon fragments that are subsequently metabolized by the Embden-Meyerhof pathway. Besides this primary enzyme defect, there are secondary alterations and/or competitive enzyme inhibition(s) of fructose 1,6-diphosphate aldolase, fructokinase, and phosphorylase-a caused by intracellular depletion of inorganic phosphate and accumulation of fructose 1-phosphate (Fig 4-4).[74] After intake of fructose, persons with HFI become nauseated, vomit, and sweat excessively; malaise, tremor, coma, and convulsions may develop. Most of these symptoms can be attributed to a secondary hypoglucosemia resulting from a block in glycogenolysis. These acute symptoms are first noticed at weaning when infants are fed foods containing sucrose or fructose. Small children with HFI who are chronically exposed to fructose do not thrive, they experience hepatomegaly, jaun-

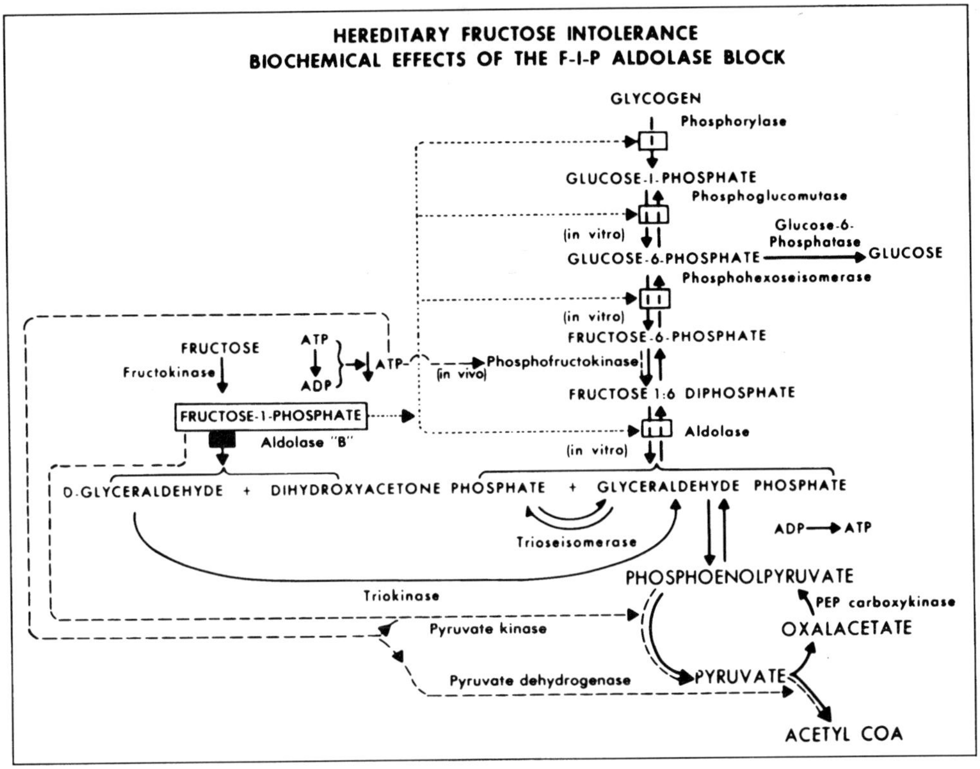

Fig 4-4 Embden-Meyerhof pathway shows enzyme defect (fructose 1-phosphate aldolase) in hereditary fructose intolerance and secondary enzyme inhibitions (. . . .) caused by accumulation of fructose 1-phosphate and depletion of inorganic phosphate.

dice, hyperbilirubinemia, albuminuria, and aminoaciduria.[38] If HFI is diagnosed and the children survive early life, they learn to avoid all sweets, cakes, candies, and most fruits. However, they eat glucose, galactose, lactose, and starch-containing foods such as milk, dairy products, bread, semolina and oat cereals, noodles, spaghetti, rice, and potatoes.

Although most persons with HFI have been examined by physicians rather than dentists, it has often been noted that their teeth are "in extraordinarily good condition."[38] Unlike an equivalent age group of the general population, approximately half of all people with HFI are free of caries.* Caries, when present, is restricted to pits and fissures and is usually not found in smooth enamel surfaces.[95,103,106]

In a detailed study of 17 persons with HFI, their diet was recorded several times over a 2-year period. It was found that their total sucrose intake was approximately 5% that of control subjects and their caries score (DMFS) less than 10% that of control subjects (Table 4-1). No

*References 2, 13, 28, 39, 60, 87, 88.

Table 4-1 Comparison of caries prevalence, oral hygiene, daily sucrose consumption, and plaque microbiota for HFI and control subjects

	HFI subjects	Control subjects
Mean age (yr)	29.1	26.5
Caries prevalence		
DMFT score	2.1	14.3
DMFS score	3.3	36.1
Persons caries-free	59%	0%
Oral hygiene		
Plaque index	1.2	1.2
Oral hygiene index	1.7	1.8
Sucrose consumption		
Sucrose-containing items ingested/day (frequency)	0.83	4.32
Sucrose intake/person/day	2.5g	48.2g
Plaque microbiota		
S mutans in plaque (isolation frequency)	26%	72%
Lactobacilli in plaque (isolation frequency)	10%	40%

significant differences were found in the oral hygiene status (plaque or oral hygiene indices) of the two groups. Highly significant differences in the proportion of *Streptococcus mutans* and lactobacilli were found between the plaque of the HFI group and that of the control population group.[61] The low prevalence of caries in persons with HFI indicates that starchy foods per se do not produce decay, whereas sugary foods do. These observations also emphasize that the plaque microflora is directly influenced by the type of dietary sugar ingested.

Industrial risk

Workers in industries such as bakeries and candy factories are exposed daily to air polluted with sugar dust, which may exceed 200 mg/m^3. They also consume relatively large amounts of sugar-containing food at their work. Epidemiological surveys of such workers have shown a significantly higher caries prevalence (DMFT 15.59 ± 5.97) than among workers in the textile industry (DMFT 9.14 ± 4.75).[1] Similarly, employees in a chocolate factory have been shown to have a higher prevalence of dental caries than comparable employees at a shipyard.[109]

Sugar cane cutters *(macheteros)* habitually chew raw sugar cane and consume large quantities of raw sugar cane juice *(guarapo)*.[32] Epidemiological surveys comparing Cuban sugar cane workers with a similarly aged population of textile workers have shown the adverse effects of these habits in terms of dental decay and illustrate the fact that raw sugar can be as deleterious to dental health as refined sugar.[81]

Noninterventional human studies

In the previously described populations, a diet was imposed either by the institution (Vipeholm, Hopewood House) or by the subjects (HFI) that was considerably different with respect to intake of sugary foods than the diet of the general population. Under such circumstances it is not difficult to demonstrate a clear-cut relationship between dietary sugars and dental caries. In noninterventional studies, where the subjects are free to choose whatever diet they please, the correlation between caries increment and dietary factors is low. One reason for this is that in recent studies the caries incidence has been low, total sugar consumption has been relatively high, and there has been little variation in many dietary habits among the children studied. Longitudinal studies, over 2 and 3 years, of adolescent school children in England and the United States, involved multiple dietary intake questionnaires, the data from which were analyzed by computer.[15,119] Children with high caries increments ingested significantly more snacks, and a significantly higher proportion of total caloric intake was obtained from snack carbohydrate and snack sugars. Weight of sugar intake and concentration of sugar in foods and snacks were all positively correlated to caries, but the correlation was relatively small (r = 0.1 to 0.14). It can be concluded that consumption of sugar remains an etiological factor, particularly in the incidence of smooth surface caries.

Assessment of cariogenic potential of foodstuffs

Background

Food composition and dietary habits can affect caries activity both favorably and unfavorably. Foods and beverages serve as substrates for fermentation by the plaque microflora, which form organic acids, thereby promoting demineralization of tooth structure and directly affecting caries activity. Food composition and dietary habits also influence the type and proportions of specific cariogenic microorganisms found in the dental plaque,[61,63,141] thereby indirectly affecting caries activity. Because of the multifactorial nature of caries etiology, the fact that humans eat a mixed diet, and evidence that the sequence of eating may affect the cariogenic potential of foods; the precise cariogenicity of any one food cannot be predicted accurately in human subjects. Furthermore, compliance is extremely hard to obtain in clinical trials. Human volunteers, even if testing foods that are considered noncariogenic, do not subject themselves readily to strictly controlled diets. Therefore, we depend upon animal and in vitro testing of cariogenic potential.

A number of different approaches have been used in attempting to develop reliable methods for measuring the caries-inducing potential of individual foods. These include *(1)* in vitro models of caries, such as adhesiveness of foods, enamel demineralization, production of titratable acid, and an artificial mouth; *(2)* monitoring of plaque pH changes, whereby acidogenicity is measured either in vivo or by a combination of in vivo and in vitro techniques; and *(3)* animal testing, to measure cariogenicity of individual foods fed to rodents under standardized conditions.[5,8,146] An ideal test for measuring cariogenicity of a food or beverage would take into account all the various factors known to be involved in the carious process (host and microflora as well as substrate). However, since it is improbable that a single test can serve this purpose, a combination of tests has been proposed to assess the cariogenic potential of foods.[6,29,90,96] Better still, a sequence or cascade of testing may be simpler and more practical. In the initial screening, foods are tested to determine if they have any cariogenic potential at all; if so, further tests can quantify the cariogenic potential as low or high.[140] Using currently accepted methods (primarily plaque pH measurements and animal testing), foods can be categorized as having *(1)* no cariogenic potential, *(2)* low cariogenic potential, or *(3)* high cariogenic potential.

The first category would include any foods that do not lower plaque pH significantly, as compared with a negative control such as sorbitol. The second category would include foods that are acidogenic in plaque pH tests but, when assessed in an animal model, cause less than 40% of the caries of a positive control diet such as sucrose. The third category would include foods that when fed to animals, cause as much or more caries as a positive sucrose control diet. A large group of foods falls into an intermediate category between low and high cariogenic potential and cannot be ranked because of considerable overlap of standard deviations when tested repeatedly in the rat model.

In vitro caries models

Various types of artificial mouths have been used for testing the cariogenicity of individual foods. In the crudest form, the food is mixed with an inoculum of salivary flora, and the supposed caries-producing capacity of the food is determined based on the amount of acids formed. Such a technique has several obvious shortcomings in that the in vitro model is remote from the real life situation. The salivary flora is not representative of the plaque microbiota, nor is there a continuous salivary flow. A related method has been to measure enamel demineralization by the amount of phosphorus-32 dissolved from radioactive bovine enamel by a mixture of food and saliva.[7] Generally, the results of such in vitro tests have not matched the findings of cariogenicity observed in animal tests, plaque pH measurements, or human clinical and epidemiological experience.

In vivo/in vitro caries models

The Intraoral Caries Test (ICT)[80] and the Iodine Permeability Test

(IPT)[14] use blocks of bovine enamel mounted on a prosthesis that is worn intraorally. Plaque is grown on the surface of the enamel, which is then exposed to a solution of the test food either extra- or intraorally. The extent of demineralization/remineralization (usually compared with a positive control such as sucrose solution) is measured by changes in enamel hardness (ICT) or permeability to iodine (IPT). Both these tests have limitations (eg, they test foods only in solution and depend on patient compliance) and have therefore not been used widely for assessing cariogenic potential.

Adhesiveness of foods

Adhesiveness refers to a firm attachment between the food and the tooth surface. However, intraoral retention of food depends not only on adhesion but also on cohesion, the tendency of food to stick to itself. Another property of food, its tackiness, has been invoked.[17] Adhesion is considered as occurring when there is pressure applied to the food; it relates primarily to interproximal and occlusal sites where the food is under masticatory force. Tackiness is the ability of a food to stick to the tooth surface when only minimal force is involved in making the contact between the food and the tooth; this property may be important in the retention of food on the buccal, labial, and lingual surfaces.

Because food clearance is thought to be an important property influencing cariogenicity, there have been attempts to rank or classify foods by in vivo measurements of oral sugar clearance[90] or intraoral food retention.[6] Subsequently it was recognized that much food was retained on mucous membranes, whereas only food retained on the teeth was considered significant in cariogenicity.[18,19] The adhesiveness of 77 foods on teeth has been measured in vitro.[17] The adhesion test involved measurement of the tensile force required to break a bond between mixtures of food and saliva and the enamel surface of teeth. Certain foods have high adhesiveness by this method (more than 600 g/cm^2) and also contain sugar. These include corn flakes and milk, sugar-coated flakes, toffee, chocolate, caramel, cupcake, chocolate cake, plain cake, cherry, date, apple, and tomato. However, there are obvious limitations to relying on in vitro measurements of adhesiveness in attempting to categorize this property of foods. Unfortunately, good data for making these judgments are unavailable.

Plaque pH measurements

Acid production by plaque bacteria causes a rapid decrease in pH after the ingestion of a fermentable substrate. Based on in vitro studies, it has been proposed that when the pH drops below a level of approximately 5.5 (the so-called critical pH), demineralization of enamel can occur.

Methods used to measure plaque pH include sampling, touch electrodes, and built-in electrodes.

In the plaque sampling method, plaque is removed from the teeth at intervals after ingestion of the test food, and the pH is measured outside of the mouth. Some of the limitations of this technique are that the plaque is disturbed each time a sample is collected, the sample represents a pooling of plaque from different sites, and measurement is intermittent rather than continuous.

One finding of particular interest emerging from observations of plaque pH patterns is that the sequence of ingesting different foods at one meal can influence the plaque pH response. For example, eating salted peanuts, cheese, egg, and crispbread after a lump of sucrose, pears in syrup, or sugared coffee can minimize the usual fall in plaque pH and cause a rapid return to resting plaque pH.[42,69,116-118] These observations imply that it is very unlikely that a particular food can be precisely ranked in terms of cariogenicity, because its cariogenicity will be modified by the other foods consumed.

The touch electrode method employs microelectrodes that are placed within the plaque on the tooth surface at intervals after food ingestion. This technique allows direct readings of pH on the plaque surface. Investigations with antimony and glass electrodes have provided useful data. In general, this method provides information similar to that obtained by plaque sampling. It also disrupts the plaque structure, permitting soluble substrates like sugars to enter and organic acids to exit around the electrode rather than having to diffuse through the plaque.

The method using built-in electrodes is more complex because it requires miniature electrodes built into a prosthesis consisting of either a partial denture or a crown.[67,70,123] Plaque is allowed to accumulate directly on these indwelling electrodes, and pH readings can be made continuously by either wire or radio telemetry. Originally this technique employed glass electrodes that have a slow response (about 30 seconds) to pH changes. Recently, Japanese investigators invented a hydrogen ion-sensitive field effect transistor electrode that is extremely small and has low electric resistance and rapid response time (about 10 seconds). The pH-sensitive tips have an area of 1 mm^2, and the surface is covered with silicon nitride, Si_3N_4.[66] Another improvement has been the development of an indwelling bimetallic (palladium/palladium oxide) wire electrode that also rapidly responds to pH changes, is highly versatile, and promises to be useful in the technology of plaque pH measurement.[86]

Determination of a product's acidogenicity based on plaque pH changes more nearly represents the odontolytic process than other in vivo measurements, but it still does not measure cariogenicity per se. This is the method employed by the Swiss health authorities to classify foods for labeling. If a food or beverage does not cause the plaque pH to fall below 5.7 during a 30-minute interval after ingestion, it is "safe for teeth" *(Zahnschonend)*. This critical limit of pH 5.7 is arbitrary and only valid when indwelling electrodes are used, thereby leaving plaque structure and diffusion characteristics undisturbed.[35]

Plaque pH measurements after consumption of many sugar-containing foods (eg, chocolate, caramel toffee, candy, ice cream, biscuits, cream caramel, meringue, breakfast cereal), beverages (eg, fresh fruit juices, reconstituted fruit drink concentrates, carbonated beverages, sports drinks), chewing gums, and sugar-based pharmaceutical products (eg, throat lozenges, vitamin preparations) have all been demonstrated to lower the plaque pH below the critical limit and are highly acidogenic.[9,68] In contrast, many products using nonnutritive sweeteners (cyclamate, mannitol, saccharin, sorbitol, xylitol, starch-hydrolysates) such as chewing gums, candies, toffees, and diet beverages are nonacidogenic when measured by plaque pH biotelemetry.

Determining sucrose content

The sucrose content of foods and beverages varies greatly (Table 4-2). Because animal tests have shown some relationship between sucrose content of foods and cariogenicity, some consumer groups have urged the Food and Drug Administration to require disclosure of the percentage sucrose content on food labels together with a statement: "Frequent use contributes to tooth decay and other problems." Conversely, a seal of approval indicating that a particular item "contains no sugar and produces no cavities" has been suggested. Although such proposals have merit, they tend to oversimplify the diet-dental caries relationship.

Table 4-2 Sucrose content of often-ingested foods, drinks, and liquid medicinals

Class	% sucrose content	
	Mean	Range
Diet soft drinks	0.0	0–0.06
Cheeses	0.0	0–0.18
Luncheon meats	0.1	0–0.90
Breads	0.1	0–3.44
Fresh fruits and vegetables	2.0	0–8.66
Canned juices	2.5	0–8.1
Crackers and wafers	4.2	0–32.03
Conventional soft drinks	4.3	1.0–9.8
Snack puddings	9.7	1.8–15.4
Ice cream products	15.1	8.76–21.02
Dry breakfast cereals	25.1	1.0–68.0
Candies	38.9	20.0–60.9
Chocolate		
plain	56	30–60
milk	45	
milk—nut and raisin	32	
Liquid medicinals (vitamin drops, cough syrups, etc)	~50	10–80
Mints	68.6	39.7–98.6

The physical form, consistency, and frequency of intake, as well as the sugar content, are major determinants of the cariogenicity of foods.

Experimental caries of animals

Serious moral and legal problems arise, as does the practical difficulty of the long time required, when caries is deliberately induced in human subjects in order to study factors involved in cariogenicity. It is extremely difficult to secure large enough groups that can be scientifically controlled. Accordingly, many investigators use animals for experiments on dental caries, and much useful information has come out of these studies. Rodents (hamsters and rats) have been the favorite species because they are small and, therefore, economical, and particularly because caries can be produced in them within a few weeks. In contrast, primates, such as humans or monkeys, usually take from 6 to 18 months to develop clinically detectable lesions.

Objections may be raised to applying conclusions from animal experiments directly to humans. Certainly there are differences, for example, in the composition of the saliva and the morphology of the teeth, between rodents and primates. Even between rodent species there are certain genetic differences and variations in eating patterns.[78] Nevertheless, there are also pronounced similarities in the caries process in animals and man as far as cariogenic flora and cariogenic diet are concerned.

Stephan[139] has compared the cariogenicity of a wide range of human foods and refreshments fed to rats ad libitum in addition to their basic diet. This basic diet (581 S), consisting of dried skim milk powder and whole dried liver substance, is noncariogenic when fed to the rats twice per day for 1 hour. Cheeses also were noncariogenic, a finding confirmed by subsequent studies.[114] In fact, cheddar cheeses exert cariostatic activity when fed in conjunction with an otherwise cariogenic diet. This fits previously described observations on the effect of cheese on plaque pH. Sucrose gave by far the highest caries score. Some of the findings are shown in Table 4-3. Foods producing a caries score greater than 10 were considered significantly cariogenic. It may come as a surprise that certain fruits (apples, bananas, some grapes) fall in this category. These fruits contain from 10% to 15% (wt/wt) available sugars (eg, glucose, fructose, and sucrose), whereas citrus fruits (oranges, grapefruits, and mandarins) contain 7% to 8% sugars.[31,84] Some fruits, such as berries (boysenberries, gooseberries, loganberries, raspberries, currants, strawberries), some grapes, cherries, and pears, contain less than 2% sucrose. The sucrose content of fruits and vegetables depends on the species, ripeness, storage, etc.

This should not be interpreted as condemning fresh fruits, but it should be recognized that they, too, contain fermentable sugars, and, therefore, one needs to brush thoroughly after eating them. Apples do not "clean the teeth," and eating them will not remove plaque.[93] The ad libitum feeding behavior of rats being offered highly cariogenic foods cannot be directly related to human dietary habits, because most people do not have continuous access to food. However, patients with unusual dietary habits are occasionally encountered. For example, one patient, a 51-year-old man in an age group where one would not normally expect a high caries increment, had a high caries rate and considerable recurrent caries. He did not eat sweets, candies, or foods with added sugar. A detailed diet history revealed that the patient worked in an apple orchard and habitually ate 15 to 20 apples a day. Rats develop marked food preferences, such as for Coca Cola, which they will drink frequently when provided. Nevertheless, one can draw conclusions about the non-cariogenic or "safe" food items, which include corn chips, peanuts, milk, lettuce, and cabbage. These should be kept readily available in the home for children to eat as between-meal snacks. Most vegetables have a low content of available sugar, between 0.5% and 4.5%, with about equal amounts of glucose and fructose and only small amounts of sucrose. Beet roots, celeriac, and canned peas are exceptions, because sucrose accounts for more than 90% of their total available sugar.[135]

Table 4-4, a comparison of the relative cariogenicity of different between-meal snacks fed to rats ad libitum, reveals a parallelism between the cariogenicity and the amount of sucrose contained in the diet.[71] Other ingredients and physical texture, in the case of the biscuits, also seemed to be important. The cariogenicity of bread is determined by the garnishing.

Table 4-3 Comparison of caries score with sucrose and total sugar content of human foods fed to rats ad libitum*

Food†	Sucrose (%)	Total sugar (%)	Caries score
Sucrose	99.5	100	62.1
Milk chocolate	42	55	34.1
Dates	47	84	32.7
10% sucrose water	10	10	32.3
Raisins	14	70	30.9
Cola	3	11	29.6
Candy mints (Lifesavers)	78	89	24.7
Chocolate sandwich cookie (Oreo)	35	35	23.8
Bananas	9	20	21.0
Apples	3	11	19.4
Honey graham crackers	16	18	19.2
Caramels	64	77	16.0
Chewing gum (Wrigley's)	55	59	14.0
Figs	0.1	73	10.3
Soda crackers	0	<1	0.3
Milk	0	5	0
Sorbitol	0	0	0

*Adapted from Stephan.[139]
†Rats fed diet 581 (noncariogenic) for 1 hour twice a day. Test food was continuously available.

Table 4-4 Cariogenicity of snack foods fed rats ad libitum*

Food	Sucrose (%)	Total sugar (%)	Carious fissure lesions	Carious buccolingual lesions
Milk chocolate & rice crispies	42	50	12.9	43
Chocolate wafers	30	35	11.2	30
Biscuit, whole meal flour	20	22	8.0	5
Biscuit, white flour	14	19	10.6	2
Bread and jam	7	15	3.0	1.5
Biscuit, "sugar-free"	1	3	2.6	0
Bread and cheese	0.4	3	3.1	0

*Adapted from Ishii et al.[71]

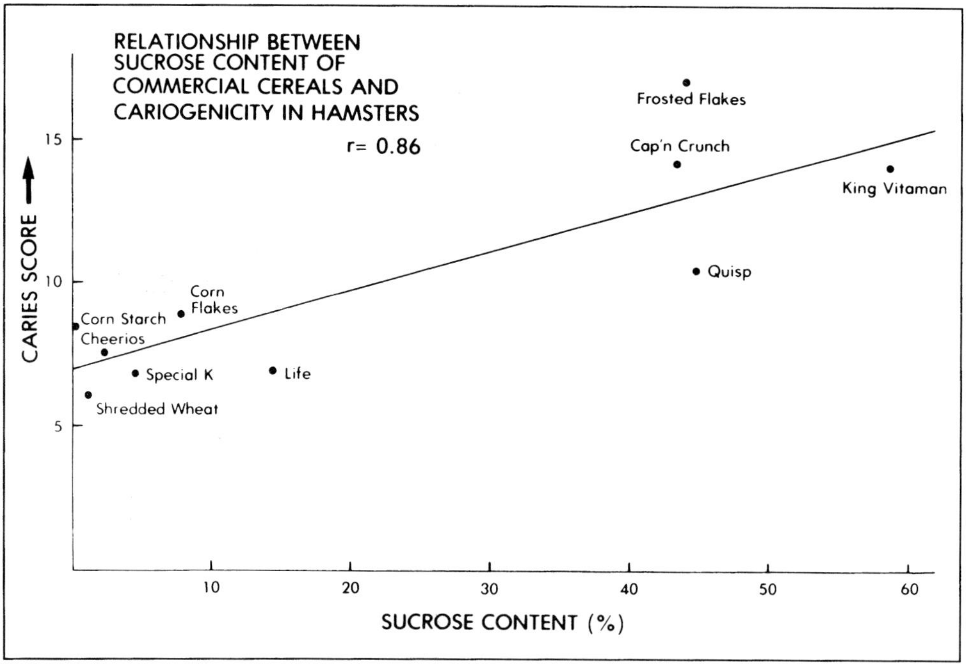

Fig 4-5 Relationship between sucrose content (wt %) of commercially available cereals (constituting 33% of total diet fed ad libitum) and caries score in hamsters.

When hamsters were fed various commercial breakfast cereals ad libitum as 33% of their total diet, smooth surface caries developed proportionately to the sucrose content of the cereal (Fig 4-5).[100,128] The correlation coefficient of this relationship is +0.86; the regression line was drawn by method of least squares.

The relationship between the sucrose content of the food or of the total diet and the resulting caries is not necessarily linear, but it is direct. Other animal studies have shown that the concentration of sucrose in

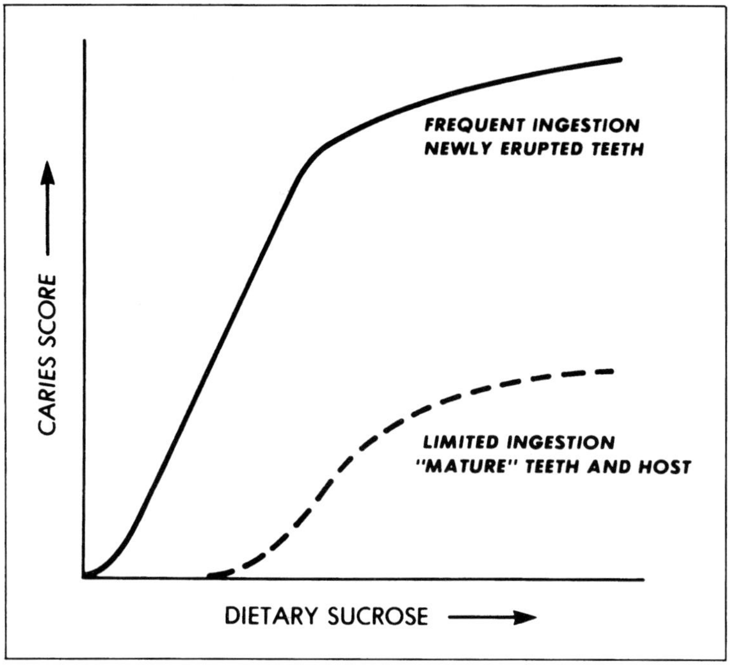

Fig 4-6 Proposed relationship between caries score and dietary sucrose intake in humans. In young children with newly erupted teeth and frequent sucrose ingestion, the S-shaped curve shifts to the left *(solid line)*. In older persons with "mature" enamel and limited sucrose ingestion, the curve shifts to the right and does not reach as high a caries score *(broken line)*.

the diet strongly influences the incidence of smooth surface and fissure caries, and this is a direct relationship.[59,65] The relationship between dietary sucrose and caries probably approximates an S-shaped curve, rising steeply when the sucrose-containing food is eaten frequently, when newly erupted teeth are at risk, and when the immune response is immature,[85] as in young children (Fig 4-6). Animal data support this contention. Following this sharp rise in caries, the curve eventually tends to flatten out, so that increasing the sucrose content of the diet beyond a certain level does not increase caries to any appreciable extent. This may explain why in some human trials, in which only one sugary food item was varied while the rest of the diet still had a high sucrose content, no significant differences in caries were found.[44,115,138,155] If the sucrose-containing foods are eaten less frequently, if the teeth have had time to "mature," if the host has developed an immune response to the cariogenic flora,[85] or if most susceptible surfaces have already decayed or been restored, as in some adults, then it may take a higher concentration of sucrose in the foods to cause caries, and the resulting caries may not be as extensive. Nevertheless, the direct relationship between the sucrose content of the food and its cariogenicity is still maintained.

Cariogenicity of sucrose and other carbohydrates

The foregoing findings concerning the role of sucrose in the etiology of caries are based on epidemiological grounds and controlled human and animal studies. Other animal studies, instead of comparing common human dietary items, have compared the cariogenicity of different carbohydrates—starches, sucrose, maltose, lactose, fructose, and glucose—usually added to the animals' diet in a powdered form. Under such conditions, sucrose more than any other carbohydrate invariably induces the most smooth-surface-type lesions.[10,45,50,126]

This is especially so if the animals are infected with a cariogenic microorganism such as *S mutans*.[21,33,48,145] However, if comparisons are made on the basis of fissure-type (sulcal) lesions, the distinction between different carbohydrates is not always as clear cut,[113,130,145] so that some investigators have disputed the importance of sucrose as a caries inducer vis-à-vis the other sugars.[83] But humans do not eat diets consisting of 60% to 70% powdered carbohydrate, and the relevance of such animal studies can be questioned. The principal carbohydrates available in human diets are starches, sucrose, and some lactose, not glucose, fructose, or maltose. In both the United States and Europe, wheat, potatoes, and sucrose provide about 90% of the total carbohydrate consumed. From a clinical point of view, therefore, the significant comparison is between starches and sucrose, and in this case there can be no doubt that sucrose is the "bad guy." In many human foods, such as cakes and pastries, sucrose coexists in a mixture with cooked starch. Tests in rats whose frequency of eating was carefully controlled show that a 1:1 mixture of sucrose and cooked wheat starch is more cariogenic than sucrose alone, and it is considerably more cariogenic than cooked wheat starch alone.[36] This higher cariogenicity seems to be due to the slower oral clearance of sucrose when mixed with sticky cooked starch.

The key role of sucrose as a dietary substrate in the caries process on smooth surfaces can be explained on biochemical grounds. Smooth surface caries depends on the growth of dental plaque. Several independent investigations have clearly demonstrated the presence of extracellular polysaccharides, both glucans and levans, in plaque (Fig 4-7) (see Guggenheim[47] and Newbrun[103]). The glucans, particularly the water-insoluble fraction, can serve as structural components of the plaque matrix, in effect "gluing" certain bacteria to the teeth. The soluble levans and some of the soluble glucans are degradable by the plaque flora[124] and may function as transient reserves of fermentable carbohydrates, thereby prolonging the duration of acid production. These polysaccharides are synthesized by enzymes, which for the most part are extracellular or bound to the cell surface and show a high specificity for sucrose (and sometimes raffinose) as a substrate. Unlike intracellular bacterial, mammalian, or plant polysaccharide syntheses, which require sugar 1-phosphate or nucleoside diphosphate-sugar intermediates, this extracellular synthesis transfers glucose or fructose units directly to the growing polymer. Polysaccharide is built up by extrusion from the enzyme. Glucose units are transferred from sucrose to the active site of the enzyme and then to the growing polymer chain. The enzyme conserves the relatively high energy of the link between the two anomeric carbons,

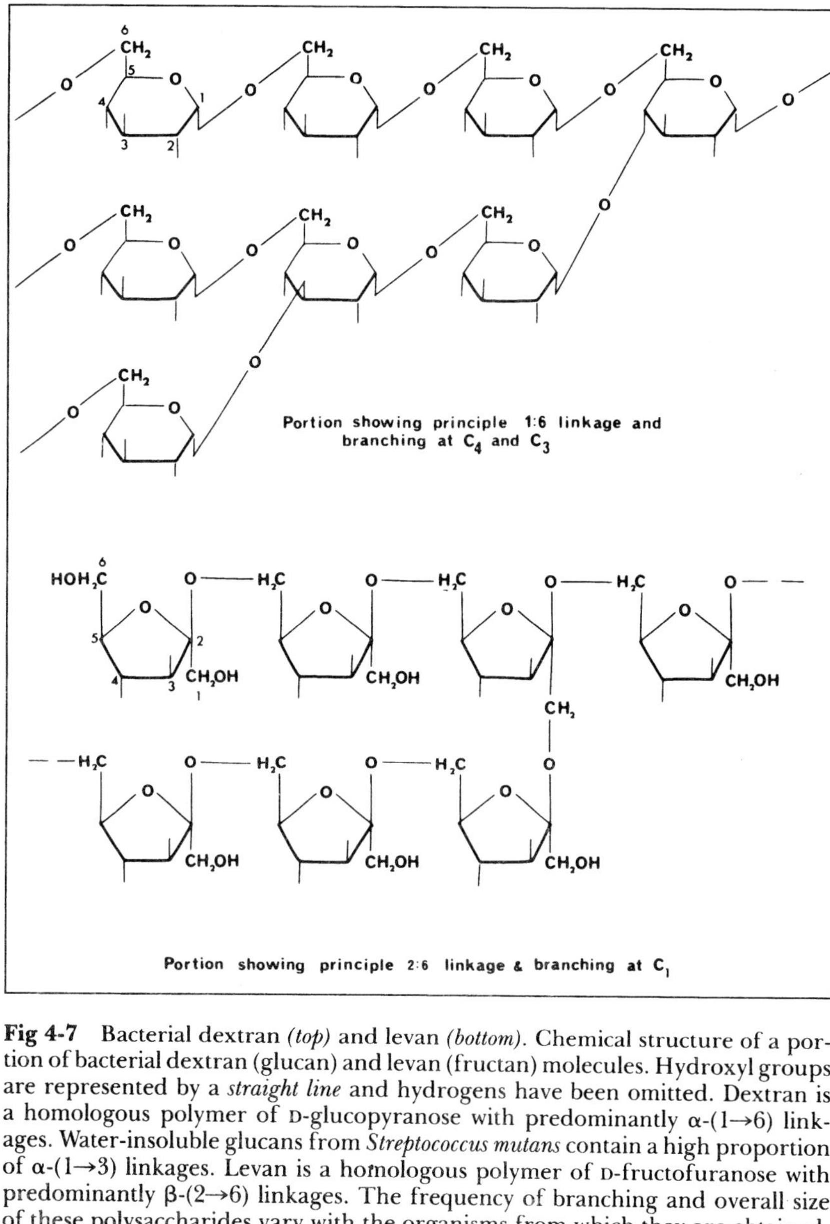

Fig 4-7 Bacterial dextran *(top)* and levan *(bottom)*. Chemical structure of a portion of bacterial dextran (glucan) and levan (fructan) molecules. Hydroxyl groups are represented by a *straight line* and hydrogens have been omitted. Dextran is a homologous polymer of D-glucopyranose with predominantly α-(1→6) linkages. Water-insoluble glucans from *Streptococcus mutans* contain a high proportion of α-(1→3) linkages. Levan is a homologous polymer of D-fructofuranose with predominantly β-(2→6) linkages. The frequency of branching and overall size of these polysaccharides vary with the organisms from which they are obtained.

C1 of glucose and C2 of fructose, found in sucrose (Fig 4-8). Disaccharides other than sucrose, such as maltose and lactose, are hemiacetals, not dihemiacetals. Therefore, their free energy of hydrolysis is significantly less (Table 4-5), and they cannot serve directly as glycosyl donors in this system. Sucrose, on the other hand, has a free energy of hydrolysis of −6,600 cal/mol, which is in the same range as the nucleoside di-

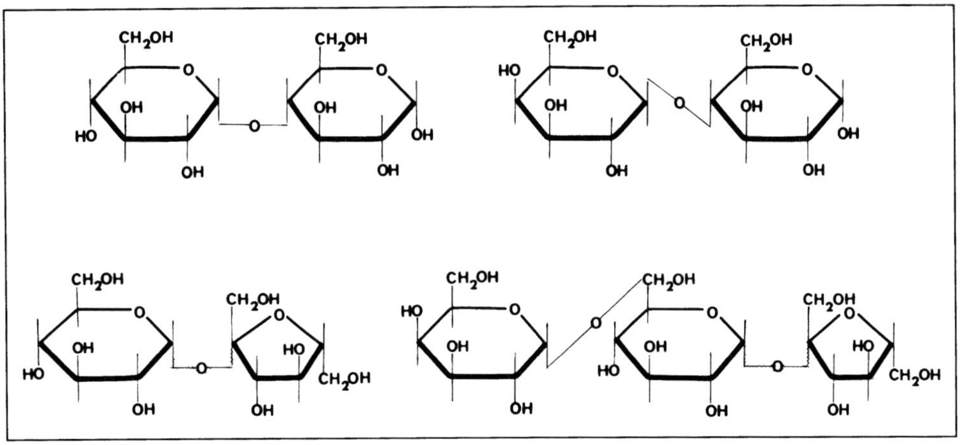

Fig 4-8 Chemical structure of maltose *(upper left)*, lactose *(upper right)*, sucrose *(lower left)*, and raffinose *(lower right)*. The potentially high-energy dihemiacetal linkages between the aldehyde and ketone carbons of glucose and fructose, respectively, in sucrose and raffinose are shown by *stippling*. In maltose, lactose, and between glucose and galactose in raffinose, the glucosidic link is hemiacetal between an aldehyde and an alcohol group and is of much lower energy.

Table 4-5 Free energy of hydrolysis of glucosyl donors, and some polysaccharides

Compound	Standard free energy of hydrolysis ΔG_H(cal-mole)
Glucose 1-phosphate	−5000
UDP-glucose*	−7600
Sucrose	−6600
Maltose	−3000
Lactose	−3000
Glycogen	−4300
Dextran	−2000
Levan	−4600

*UDP, uridine diphosphate.

phosphate sugars, −7,600 cal/mole, and higher than glucose 1-phosphate.[4]

The enzymes involved in the synthesis, glucosyl- and fructosyltransferases, have been isolated and purified from *S sanguis* and *S mutans*.* The properties of these enzymes, which are of considerable clinical relevance, are listed below.

*References 22, 23, 26, 40, 43, 49, 82, 104, 105, 122.

1. They are highly specific for sucrose and will not utilize sugars such as fructose, glucose, maltose, or lactose.
2. They have a broad pH optimum, 5.2 to 7.0, coinciding with the pH range of dental plaque.
3. In the presence of adequate nutrients the enzymes can be made by these organisms and sucrose is not a required inducer. Whenever sucrose is ingested they are ready to synthesize polysaccharides.
4. The equilibrium of the reaction shown below for glucan synthesis is far to the right:

$$\underset{\text{sucrose}}{n\,C_{12}H_{22}O_{11}} \rightarrow \underset{\text{glucan}}{(C_6H_{10}O_5)_n} + \underset{\text{fructose}}{n\,C_6H_{12}O_6}$$

As long as sucrose is present in plaque, the glucosyltransferase enzymes will continue to utilize it to form plaque matrix material and fructose. The latter can readily be fermented by the plaque flora to form organic acids. The glucosyltransferases (GTF) of the mutans-group of streptococci have received considerable attention,[27] and several isozymes have been isolated. There are two types of these enzymes: *(1)* those that synthesize a soluble glucan with predominantly 1,6-α-D-glucose sequences (GTF-S), and *(2)* those that synthesize an insoluble, essentially linear 1,3-α-D glucan (GTF-I). Bifunctional enzymes with 1,6-α-bond and 1,3,6-branch-forming activities have been purified.[150] By cooperative action of these enzymes, a sticky, water-insoluble polysaccharide is synthesized from sucrose that is a major factor in the accumulation of mutans-group streptococci on smooth tooth surfaces.

The pathways by which various ingested carbohydrates are used in plaque are shown schematically in Fig 4-9. Starches are probably prevented from direct entry into plaque because of limited diffusion of such large molecules. The first step in the catabolism of sugars (mono- and disaccharides) is their transport into the cytoplasm of the microorganism. Sugars are generally transported either by a carrier-mediated active transport (permease) system or by group translocation (phosphotransferase system, PTS). Active transport releases the sugar unmodified into the cytoplasm, whereas by group translocation the sugar is chemically modified to a phosphate ester before it appears inside the cell. The uptake of sugars by oral streptococci (*S mutans, Streptococcus sanguis,* and *Streptococcus salivarius*) involves a phosphoenol pyruvate–dependent PTS located in the bacterial cell membrane.[20,97,101,125] The first component in PTS, E_{II}, is induced by and is specific for the particular sugar, whereas the second component, E_I, involved in the transfer of phosphate from phosphoenol pyruvate to a carrier protein, HPr, is constitutive.

Sucrose is utilized directly by *S mutans* mostly via PTS, rather than via prior hydrolysis to glucose and fructose by invertase.[120,132,133] This system *(1)* is inducible by sucrose in the environment, *(2)* is repressed by fructose, and *(3)* has a low Michaelis constant (Km) for sucrose. The Km of extracellular invertase for sucrose is considerably higher; therefore, the sucrose phosphotransferase system is more important because it can

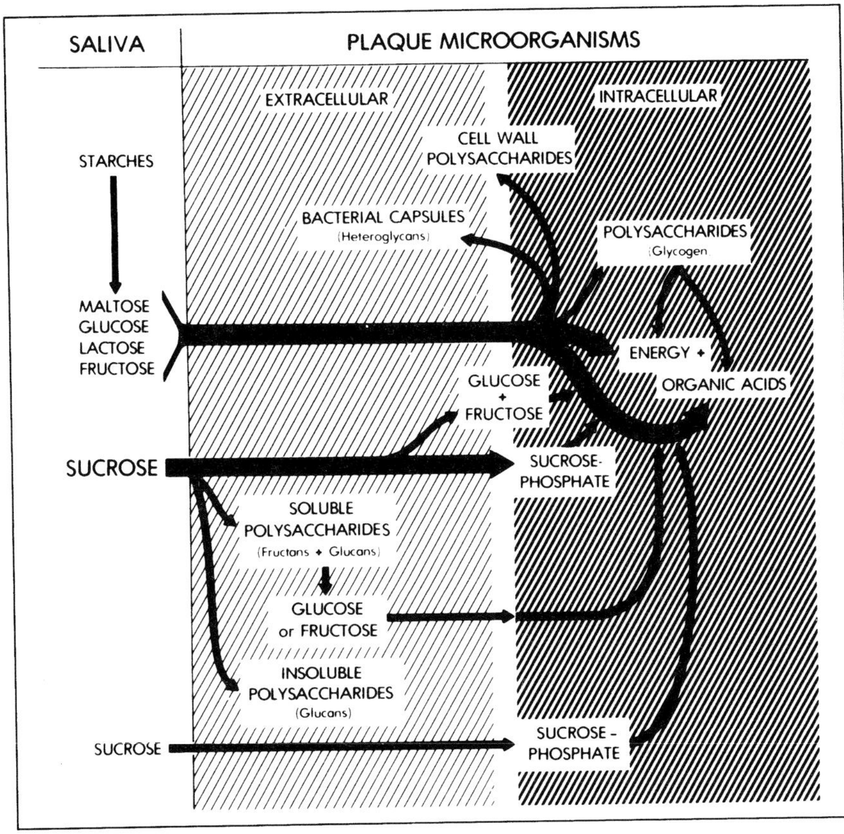

Fig 4-9 Metabolic fate of ingested carbohydrates in the plaque. Heavy arrows indicate major pathways. (Modified after König.[77])

function even at low substrate concentration, scavenging sucrose from the environment. Moreover, it is economical because the energy of only one high-energy bond serves both for translocation and phosphorylation of sucrose. The intracellular product, sucrose 6-phosphate, is then cleaved by a sucrose 6-phosphate hydrolase, yielding glucose 6-phosphate and fructose.[121] The sucrose 6-phosphate hydrolase has dual specificity for both sucrose 6-phosphate and for sucrose; however, the catalytic activity for the latter hydrolysis (invertase) is lower.[25]

The hydrolase enzyme is constitutive and repressed by fructose. The sugar phosphates are subsequently integrated into the catabolic pathways, which, in the case of the oral streptococci, is predominantly the Embden-Meyerhof pathway. When the sugars are abundant, lactate is the major end product, but when the availability of sugar is limited, the major products are ethanol, formate, and acetate (see pages 21 to 23).

Maltose, lactose, fructose, and glucose can be used by the oral flora for the synthesis of bacterial cell walls, capsular and intracellular polysaccharides, and organic acids. The bulk of the glucosyl and fructosyl moieties of sucrose are fermented to organic acid products as shown in Fig 4-9. The ability to ferment sucrose is influenced by the previous exposure of the microorganism to sucrose. A strain (PK-1) of *S mutans* previously grown on sucrose produced much more lactate when given sucrose as a substrate than the same strain of cells previously grown on glucose.[158] Studies suggest that sucrose phosphorylase and invertase are induced in sucrose-grown streptococci.

Sucrose is unique in that it can also serve in the formation of insoluble extracellular polysaccharides and thereby enhance plaque formation and microbial aggregation on the tooth surface. Only small amounts of all glucosyl moieties of sucrose are polymerized,[144,147] and insoluble glucans constitute only a small proportion, on a weight basis, of plaque.[62] The insoluble polysaccharides, though small quantitatively, are important because organisms that have lost this property no longer induce smooth surface lesions.[142,148]

Of considerable ecological significance are some of the properties of these extracellular glucans, which are high molecular weight polymers of glucose. Many are sticky and insoluble, which makes them more resistant to oral bacterial degradation. Glucans cause clumping of specific strains of oral bacteria and can be adsorbed onto hydroxyapatite.

Agglutination or clumping of *S mutans* cells by extracellular glucans involves receptor sites on the bacterial surface that bind the glucan. These receptor sites are distinct from the binding sites for glucosyltransferases.[108] The adhesion of these organisms promoted by the glucan appears to be a crucial determinant of virulence on smooth surfaces. *Actinomyces viscosus* also aggregates rapidly when mixed with high molecular weight glucan. The reaction is specific and does not occur with a variety of other simple and complex carbohydrates.[98] Furthermore, glucans mediate interbacterial aggregation of *A viscosus* with *S sanguis* and with *S mutans*.[11]

Although the adherence of *S mutans* to smooth surfaces is greatly increased by the production of glucans in the presence of sucrose, these organisms can attach to surfaces in the absence of sucrose, albeit at much lower levels. Colonization of tooth surfaces is now seen as a two-step process. The initial attachment is to the acquired pellicle of the tooth and is mediated by cell-surface proteins rather than by glucans. Evidence for the protein-mediated attachment is the reduced adherence of *S mutans* when treated with proteases. The second step involves cellular accumulation mediated by sucrose-derived glucans and cell surface lectins.[137]

Other dietary components and dental caries

Phosphates

Phosphates as possible caries-preventive agents have been tested on experimental animals and in human clinical trials. A significant cariostatic action has been demonstrated by inorganic phosphates when added to cariogenic diets of rats or hamsters. Phosphates increase in cariostatic activity depending on type of anion(cyclic, trimeta-, tripoly-, hexameta-, ortho-, and pyro-, respectively) and type of cation (H, Na, K, Ca, and Mg, respectively). Organic phosphates (phytates, glycerophosphates) also reduce caries.[56] The exact mechanism of action of phosphates in caries reduction is uncertain, but the conclusion of numerous investigations points to a local effect in the mouth rather than a systemic influence through ingestion. There is a striking difference in the cariostatic effect of phosphate when ingested orally compared to when it is administered to rats by stomach intubation.[99] This local effect can be attributed to a number of factors, notably the ability of:

1. Phosphate ions to reduce the rate of dissolution of the hydroxyapatite of the enamel
2. Supersaturated solutions of phosphate ions to redeposit calcium phosphate, particularly in areas of enamel that have been partially demineralized
3. Phosphates to buffer organic acids formed by fermentation of plaque microflora
4. Phosphate ions to desorb proteins from the enamel surface, thereby modifying the acquired pellicle[110]

Although dietary supplementation with phosphates has proven effective in reducing caries in experimental animals, the results of human clinical trials have been disappointing and less than convincing. There are distinct physiological differences between rodents and humans that may explain the low cariostatic response in humans to dietary supplements of phosphate. Rodents have a higher salivary pH and lower salivary phosphate content than humans.[34] Another important difference in animal experiments is that the phosphate supplement is usually homogenized into the entire diet, whereas in human trials the phosphate supplement has usually been incorporated in only one portion of the diet (baked goods, cereals, manioc, chewing gum, sweets).

Within reasonable limits of intake, many dietary phosphate supplements are generally recognized as safe by the Food and Drug Administration. At the present time, however, there is only limited evidence to justify adding phosphates to sugar or other foodstuffs as a means of reducing the incidence and prevalence of dental caries.[157] More testing and more positive demonstration of efficacy in preventing human caries is necessary before commercial implementation can be recommended.

Lipids

It has been known for a long time that adding lipids to a cariogenic diet reduces caries in animals.[3,51,112,129] However, these earlier findings may have been due to substitution of the fat or oil for carbohydrate. Medium chain fatty acids (C_8–C_{12}) and their salts have antibacterial properties at low pH; the mechanism of action is not well defined. They serve as anionic surfactants and uncouple substrate transport and oxidative phosphorylation from electron transport in bacteria. Changes in cell permeability may be involved.[73] Potassium nonanoate, $CH_3(CH_2)_7COOK$, has been studied because, when added to a cariogenic diet fed to rats, it produced a significant reduction in caries score.[57] Human studies with a daily mouthwash containing nonanoate have demonstrated a change in plaque flora, including a reduction in the proportion of acidogenic organisms.[46,58] The potential of lipids as anticariogenic food additives requires further exploration, keeping in mind the dietary goal of limiting consumption of saturated fats.[151]

Trace elements

The widely recognized inverse relationship between the prevalence of dental caries and the ingestion of fluoridated drinking water has prompted investigators to look at other elements. Molybdenum (Mo), selenium (Se), vanadium (V), strontium (Sr), and a variety of other elements (Table 4-6) may have an influence on the prevalence of caries in man.[16,30,53,89] Evidence has accumulated demonstrating that ingestion of selenium actually increased dental caries in man and experimental animals if taken during the period of tooth formation. Cariostatic effects have been claimed, but not proven, for a number of these trace elements.

In any study of the effect of a dietary component on caries, it is important that the amount of that component (trace element, phosphate, etc) in the basic diet as well as the amount of supplement be known. Otherwise, it is quite possible that the amount of supplement is negligible in comparison with its concentration in the basic diet. The addition of a compound to a diet often alters its taste or palatability. To avoid erroneous conclusions, one should ensure that the amount of frequency of eating has not been changed in the test group. Regrettably, most dietary studies have not controlled these variables.

Table 4-6 Relationship of mineral elements to caries

Effect	Mineral
Cariostatic	F, P
Mildly cariostatic	Mo, V, Cu, Sr, B, Li, Au, Fe
Doubtful	Be, Co, Mn, Sn, Zn, Br, I, Y
Caries inert	Ba, Al, Ni, Pd, Ti
Caries-promoting	Se, Mg, Cd, Pt, Pb, Si

Frequency of eating and caries formation

Human studies

The most informative experiment on caries in humans was the classic Vipeholm dental caries study.[52] The main purpose of the investigation was to determine the effects of frequency and quantity of sugar (sucrose) intake on the formation of caries. However, the important point is that the longer sugar remained in the mouth, the greater was the caries activity. Of course, the caries activity also depended on the frequency of sugar intake. The Vipeholm study used institutionalized patients so that the composition of the diet and the eating schedule were well controlled. Baseline data on a standard diet established the initial caries activity to be low. In those groups that consumed sweets in the form of toffee or caramel between meals, caries activity increased tenfold (Fig 4-10).

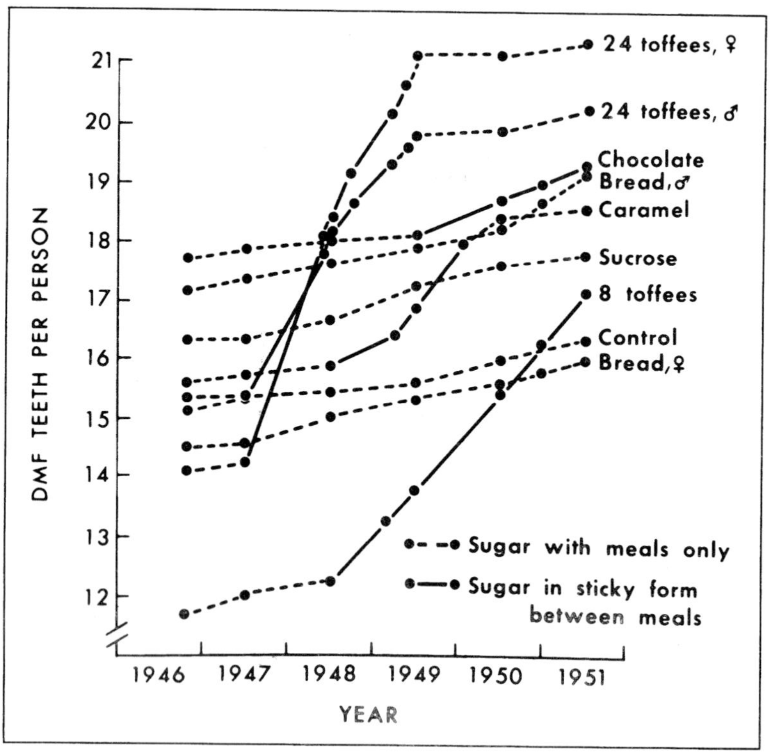

Fig 4-10 Results of the Vipeholm dental caries study. Sugar in various forms was given either between or with meals over several years, and the rate of caries increase was studied. The caries increment was much lower when sugar was given with meals compared with sugar between meals. (Courtesy of B.E. Gustafsson.[52])

A survey of the dietary habits of preschool children (average age 5 years, 9 months) indicated that the typical "between-meal" items such as gum, candy, pastries, soft drinks, and ice cream are also high in sugar content.[154] A direct and consistent relationship has been revealed between the between-meal eating frequency and the caries prevalence in children (Fig 4-11).

Because sugary foods are less adhesive in liquid form they are generally considered less cariogenic than in solid form. However, if the

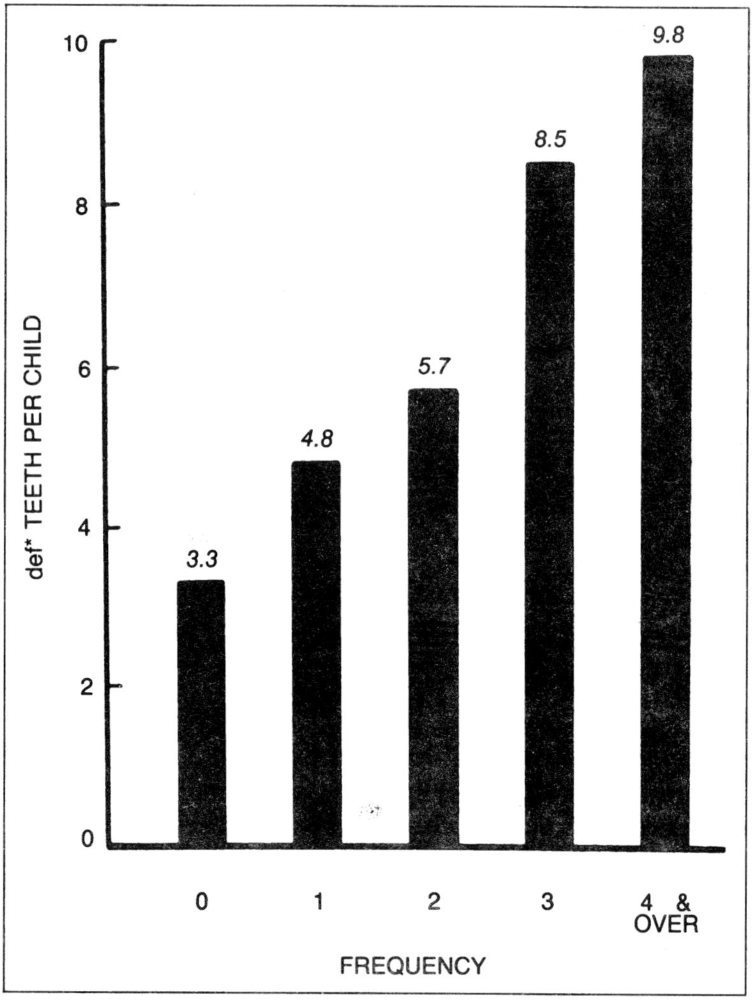

Fig 4-11 The effect of between-meal eating on caries activity in 5- to 6-year-old children. The more snacks children eat, the higher is the caries increment. *(def)* Decayed, extracted, filled (teeth). (Courtesy of Weiss and Trithart.[154])

sugary beverage is consumed with high frequency, then it is certainly cariogenic. In the United States the per capita consumption of soft drinks has increased steadily; the average American now consumes the equivalent of 420 twelve-ounce cans annually. A significant positive association between the frequency of at- and between-meal consumption of soft drinks and high DMFT scores has been demonstrated.[72] Habitual "sippers" of carbonated beverages also run the risk of dental erosion.

A survey of the menus of 4,000 households during 1962 to 1963 and 1967 to 1968 indicated a change in dietary habits (Table 4-7). Market research found that desserts no longer occupied the same place and status in the American diet as formerly; they were considered somewhat of an indulgence. Between surveys, the total number of servings of these food products as desserts decreased 30%. During the same time interval, servings of these food products as snack items increased by 40%. Snack foods accounted for about 15% of total caloric intake. This represents a substantial growth in the snack food area and, as a corollary, an increased rate in the incidence of caries.

There may be beneficial metabolic effects from a more frequent eating ("nibbling") pattern. A more constant energy supply is provided by the diet, which reduces the stress caused by the variable flux of energy associated with a gorging pattern.[152] An inverse relationship between meal frequency and rate of occurrence of ischemic heart disease has been observed. In view of such data, dentists might modify the traditional advice against between-meal eating. Instead, patients should be encouraged to eat noncariogenic, "safe" snack items.[107]

Table 4-7 Percent change in household servings of selected food products*

Type of food	Dessert servings, change (%)	Snack servings, change (%)
Soft drinks	+114	+26
Cakes	−33	+70
Cookies	−43	+40
Pies	−20	+24
Other baked desserts	−24	+75
Gelatin	+5	+54
Pudding desserts	−8	+43
Ice cream and related products	−17	+3
Fruit	−38	+56
Quick breads, toasted products	−16	+36
Coffee cake	−24	+13
Donuts	−42	+4
Snacks, curls, chips, nuts	+1	+63
Candy (chocolate)	−37	+46
Other candy	−8	+48

*− = decrease, + = increase; from national household menu census of the Marketing Research Corporation of America, 1962–1963 and 1967–1968.

Animal studies

It is much easier to regulate time factors in the diet when experimental animals are used. For example, Stephan[139] compared the caries score of rats fed a high-sugar diet twice a day for 1 hour to the score of rats feeding ad libitum (Table 4-8). The differences in caries score are convincing. More elegantly controlled feeding techniques, such as a programmed feeding machine, are available.[79] This device consists of a circular tray with 18 food cups. A plastic tube leads from each cage to the tray, one cup at a time being accessible. An endless computer punch card controls the stepwise movement of the tray and a synchronous motor keeps the 24-hour feeding program in motion. This machine imposes eating patterns of widely different frequencies on the rats. There is a consistent increase in the average incidence of caries with increased frequency of the programmed meals when tested on a particular stock of rats (see Table 4-8). Moreover, the highly significant positive correlation between frequency of eating and caries incidence is found not only on a sucrose diet but also on a bread (from wheat flour) diet. However, the incidence of caries is much lower on the bread diet.[76] When rats fed a cariogenic diet receive the same numbers of meals but at different intervals, the longer the interval between each feeding the more caries results. "What, when and how often we eat, how we eat, what else we have been eating and even what we do when we are not eating, all play a role in dental caries . . . it is clear that there is more to caries than what meets the teeth."[36]

Table 4-8 Relationship of caries incidence to frequency of eating in rats fed a cariogenic diet

Feeding frequency (times/day)	Availability of food (hr)	Mean caries score	SE	Reference
2	2	11.3	2.03	Stephan[139]
Ad libitum	24	63.0	12.37	
	Mean duration of eating (hr)	**Mean fissure lesions**	**SD**	
12	1	0.7	0.8	König et al[79]
18	1.5	2.2	0.8	
24	2	4.0	2.4	
30	2.5	4.7	2.3	
Ad libitum	6.25	4.2	4.3	

Chapter review

- Indicate how the caries-producing potential of different foods can be measured.
- List the major conclusions of the Vipeholm dental caries study.
- Given a list of foods, identify them as *(1)* highly cariogenic or *(2)* relatively noncariogenic.
- Indicate what highly cariogenic foods have in common.
- Diagram the possible fate of a sucrose molecule in dental plaque. Indicate how it differs from other carbohydrates.
- List what types of carbohydrate food can and cannot be eaten by a patient with hereditary fructose intolerance. State the clinical significance of these dietary habits as far as caries is concerned.
- Indicate how sucrose differs from other disaccharides such as maltose and lactose.
- List the properties of the glucosyltransferases isolated from oral streptococci. State the clinical significance of these properties.
- State the mechanisms whereby phosphates reduce animal caries.
- Draw the relationship of caries prevalence to eating frequency; indicate the coordinates.

Selected readings

Andlaw, R.J. 1977. Diet and dental caries—review. *J Hum Nutr* 31:45–52.

Brown, A.T. 1975. The role of dietary carbohydrates in plaque formation and oral disease. *Nutr Rev* 33:353–361.

Burt, B.A., and Ismail, A.I. 1986. Diet, nutrition, and food cariogenicity. *J Dent Res* 65:1475–1484.

Curzon, M.E.J., and Cutress, T.W. (eds) 1983. *Trace elements and dental disease.* Boston: John Wright PSG Inc.

Gould, R.F. (ed) 1970. *Dietary Chemicals vs. Dental Caries.* Advances in Chemistry Series 94. Washington, D.C.: American Chemical Society.

Hartles, R.L., and Leach, S.A. 1975. Effect of diet on dental caries. *Br Med Bull* 31:137–141.

Hefferren, J.J., and Koehler, H.M. (ed) 1981. *Foods, Nutrition and Dental Health.* Park Forest South, Ill.: Pathotox Publisher.

Imfeld, T.N. 1983. Identification of low caries risk dietary components. In *Monographs in Oral Science,* vol. 11, H. Myers (ed), Basel: S. Karger.

Lilienthal, B. 1977. Phosphates and dental caries. In *Monographs in Oral Science,* vol. 6, H. Myers (ed), Basel: S. Karger.

Newbrun, E. 1974. Diet and dental caries relationships. *Adv Caries Res* 2:xv–xxiv.

Newbrun, E. 1979. Dietary carbohydrates. Their role in cariogenicity. *Med Clin North Am* 63:1069–1086.

Newbrun, E. 1982. Sugar and dental caries. A review of human studies. *Science* 217:418–423.

Nizel, A.E. 1981. *Nutrition in Preventive Dentistry: Science and Practice.* 2nd ed. Philadelphia: W.B. Saunders.

Rowe, N.H. (ed) 1978. *Diet, Nutrition and Dental Caries.* Proceedings of Symposium. Ann

Arbor: University of Michigan.
Rugg-Gunn, A.J. 1981. Diet and dental caries. *Front Oral Physiol* 3:53–65.
Sreebny, L.M. 1982. Sugar and human dental caries. *World Rev Nutr Diet* 40:19–65.
Tanzer, J.M. (ed) 1981. *Animal Models in Cariology*. Sp. Suppl. Microbiol. Abstr. Washington, D.C.: Information Retrieval, Inc.
Wei, S.H.Y. (ed) 1979. *National Symposium on Dental Nutrition*. Iowa City: University of Iowa.

References

1. Anaise, J.Z. 1978. Prevalence of dental caries among workers in the sweets industry in Israel. *Community Dent Oral Epidemiol* 6:286–289.
2. Auerswald, W., and Kupetz, G.W. 1969. Beitrag zur Klinik der hereditären Fruktose-Intoleranz. *Dtsch Gesundheitsw* 24:875–877.
3. Bavetta, L.P., Alfin-Slater, R.L., Bernick, S., and Ershoff, B.H. 1959. Effect of fat-free diet on bone, periodontium and the evidence and severity of caries in the immature rat. *J Dent Res* 38:686–687.
4. Bernfeld, P. (ed) 1963. The biogenesis of carbohydrates. In *Biogenesis of Natural Compounds*, Oxford: Pergamon Press, p. 278.
5. Bibby, B.G. 1975. The cariogenicity of snack foods and confections. *J Am Dent Assoc* 90:121–132.
6. Bibby, B.G., Goldberg, H.J.V., and Chen, E. 1951. Evaluation of caries-producing potentialities of various food stuffs. *J Am Dent Assoc* 42:491–509.
7. Bibby, B.G., and Mundorff, S.A. 1975. Enamel demineralization by snack foods. *J Dent Res* 54:461–470.
8. Bibby, B.G., and Shern, R.J. (eds) 1978. *Methods of Caries Prediction*. Sp. Suppl. Microbiol. Abstr. Washington, D.C.: Information Retrieval, Inc.
9. Birkhed, D. 1984. Sugar content, acidity and effect on plaque pH of fruit juices, fruit drinks, carbonated beverages and sports drinks. *Caries Res* 18:120–127.
10. Birkhed, D., Frostell, G., and Lamm, C.J. 1980. Cariogenicity of glucose, sucrose and amylopectin in rats and hamsters infected and non-infected with *Streptococcus mutans*. *Caries Res* 14:441–447.
11. Bourgeau, G., and McBride, B.C. 1976. Dextran-mediated interbacterial aggregation between dextran-synthesizing streptococci and *Actinomyces viscosus*. *Infect Immun* 13:1228–1234.
12. Bradford, E.W., and Crabb, H.S.M. 1961. Carbohydrate restriction and caries incidence. *Br Dent J* 111:273–279.
13. Brauman, J., Kentos, P., Frisque, P., Gepts, W., and Verbanck, M. 1971. Intolerance hereditaire au fructose chez une femme de 83 ans. *Acta Clin Belg* 26:65–77.
14. Brudevold, F., Attarzadeh, F., Tehrani, A., van Houte, J., and Russo, J. 1984. Development of a new intraoral demineralization test. *Caries Res* 18:421–429.
15. Burt, B.A., Eklund, S.A., Morgan, K.J., Larkin, F.E., Guire, K.E., Brown, L.O., and Weintraub, J.A. 1988. The effects of sugar intake and frequency of ingestion on dental caries increment in a three-year longitudinal study. *J Dent Res* 67:1422–1429.
16. Bütner, W. 1969. Trace elements and dental caries in experiments on animals. *Caries Res* 3:1–13.
17. Caldwell, R.C. 1962. Adhesion of food to teeth. *J Dent Res* 41:821–832.
18. Caldwell, R.C. 1968. The retention and clearance of food from the mouth. *Ann NY Acad Sci* 153:64–70.
19. Caldwell, R.C. 1970. Physical properties of foods and their caries-producing potential. *J Dent Res* 49:1293–1298.
20. Calmes, R. 1978. Involvement of phosphoenolpyruvate in the catabolism of caries-conducive disaccharides by *Streptococcus mutans:* lactose transport. *Infect Immun* 19:934–942.
21. Campbell, R.G., and Zinner, D.D. 1979. Effect of certain dietary sugars on hamster caries. *J Nutr* 100:11–20.
22. Carlsson, J. 1970. A levansucrase isolated from *Streptococcus mutans*. *Caries Res* 4:97–113.
23. Carlsson, J., Newbrun, E., and Krasse, B. 1969. Purification and properties of dextran-sucrase from *Streptococcus sanguis*. *Arch Oral Biol* 14:469–478.

24. Chambers, R.A., and Pratt, R.T.C. 1956. Idiosyncrasy to fructose. *Lancet* 2:340.
25. Chassy, B.M., and Porter, E.V. 1979. Initial characterization of sucrose-6-phosphate hydrolase from *Streptococcus mutans* and its apparent identity with intracellular invertase. *Biochem Biophys Res Comm* 89:307–314.
26. Chludzinski, A.M., Germaine, G.R., and Schachtele, C.F. 1974. Purification and properties of dextransucrase and invertase from *Streptococcus mutans. J Bacteriol* 118:1–7.
27. Ciardi, J.E. 1983. Purification and properties of glucosyltransferases from *Streptococcus mutans:* a review. In *Glucosyltransferases, glucans, sucrose and dental caries,* R.J. Doyle and J.E. Ciardi (eds), Sp. Suppl. Chemical Senses, pp. 51–64.
28. Cornblath, M., Rosenthal, I.M., Reisner, S.H., Wybregt, S.H., and Crane, R.K. 1963. Hereditary fructose intolerance. *N Engl J Med* 269:1271–1278.
29. Curzon, M.E.J. 1986. Integration of methods of determining the cariogenic potential of foods: is this possible with present technologies? *J Dent Res* 65:1520–1524.
30. Curzon, M.E.J., and Losee, F.L. 1977. Dental caries and trace element composition of whole human enamel. Eastern United States. *J Am Dent Assoc* 94:1146–1150.
31. Dako, D.Y., Trautner, K., and Somogyi, J.C. 1970. Der Glukose-, Fructose- une Saccharosegehalt verschiedener Früchte. *Schweiz Med Wochenschr* 100:897–903.
32. Dreizen, S., and Spies, T.D. 1952. The incidence of dental caries in habitual sugar cane chewers. *J Am Dent Assoc* 45:193–200.
33. Edwardsson, S., and Krasse, B. 1967. Human streptococci and caries in hamsters fed diets with sucrose or glucose. *Arch Oral Biol* 12:1015–1016.
34. Ericsson, Y. 1965. Phosphates in relation to dental caries. *Int Dent J* 15:311.
35. Firestone, A.R. 1982. Human interdental plaque-pH data and rat caries tests. Results with the same substances. *J Dent Res* 61:1130–1136.
36. Firestone, A.R., Schmid, R., and Muhlemann, H.R. 1984. Effect of the length and number of intervals between meals on caries in rats. *Caries Res* 18:128–133.
37. Food and Agriculture Organization of the United Nations. 1977. *Food Consumption Surveys.* vol. 1. Rome.
38. Froesch, E.R. 1978. Essential fructose urea and hereditary fructose intolerance. In *The Metabolic Basis of Inherited Disease,* 4th ed, J.B. Standbury, J.B. Wyngaarden, and D.C. Fredrickson (eds), New York: McGraw-Hill, pp. 126–132.
39. Froesch, E.R., Wolf, H.P., and Baitsch, H. 1963. Hereditary fructose intolerance. *Am J Med* 34:151–167.
40. Fukui, K., Fukui, Y., and Mariyama, T. 1974. Purification and properties of dextransucrase and invertase from *Streptococcus mutans. J Bacteriol* 118:796–804.
41. Fukui, K., Moriyama, T., Miyake, Y., Mizutani, K., and Tanaka, O. 1982. Purification and properties of glucosyltransferase responsible for water-insoluble glucan synthesis from *Streptococcus mutans. Infect Immun* 37:1–9.
42. Geddes, D.A.M., Edgar, W.M., Jenkins, G.N., and Rugg-Gunn, A.J. 1977. Apples, salted peanuts and plaque pH. *Br Dent J* 142:317–319.
43. Germaine, G.R., Chludzenski, A.M., and Schachtele, C.F. 1974. *Streptococcus mutans* dextransucrase. Requirement for primer dextran. *J Bacteriol* 120:287–294.
44. Glass, R.L., and Fleisch, S. 1974. Diet and dental caries. Dental caries incidence in the consumption of ready-to-eat cereals. *J Am Dent Assoc* 88:807–813.
45. Grenby, T.H. 1963. The effects of some carbohydrates on experimental dental caries in the rat. *Arch Oral Biol* 8:27–30.
46. Griffiths, S.J. 1979. The acidogenic potential of plaque from caries-free and caries-prone subjects and the effects of nonanoate-glucose mouthrinse. *Br Dent J* 147:329–331.
47. Guggenheim, B. 1970. Extracellular polysaccharides and microbial plaque. *Int Dent J* 20:657–678.
48. Guggenheim, B., König, K.G., Herzog, E., and Mühlemann, H.R. 1966. The cariogenicity of different carbohydrates tested on rats in relative gnotobiosis with a streptococcus producing extracellular polysaccharide. *Helv Odontol Acta* 10:101–113.
49. Guggenheim, B., and Newbrun, E. 1969. Extracellular glucosyltransferase activity of an HS strain of *Streptococcus mutans. Helv Odontol Acta* 13:84–97.
50. Gustafson, G., Stelling, M., Abramson, E., and Brunius, E. 1955. The cariogenic effects of some carbohydrates in dry and moist diets. Experimental dental caries in golden hamsters. *V Odont Tidsk* 63:506–523.
51. Gustafson, G., Stelling, E., and Brunius, E. 1953. Experimental dental caries in golden hamsters. Experiments with dietary fats having different contents of unsaturated fatty acids. *Br Dent J* 95:124–125.
52. Gustafsson, B.E., Quensel, C.E., Lanke, L.S., Lundqvist, C., Grahnén, H., Bonow, B.E., and Krasse, B. 1954. The Vipeholm dental caries study. The effect of different

levels of carbohydrate intake on caries activity in 436 individuals observed for five years. *Acta Odontol Scand* 11:232–364.

53. Hadjimarkos, D.M. 1968. Effect of trace elements on dental caries. In *Advances in Oral Biology*, P.H. Staple (ed), New York: Academic Press, pp. 253–292.
54. Hardwick, J.L. 1960. The incidence and distribution of caries throughout the ages in relation to the Englishman's diet. *Br Dent J* 108:9–17.
55. Harris, R. 1963. Biology of the children of Hopewood House, Bowral, Australia. IV. Observations of dental caries experience extending over five years (1957–1961). *J Dent Res* 42:1387–1398.
56. Harris, R.S. 1970. Minerals: calcium and phosphates. In *Dietary Chemicals vs. Dental Caries*, R.F. Gould (ed), Advances in Chemistry Services 94, Washington, D.C.: American Chemical Society, pp. 116–122.
57. Hayes, M.L., and Berkovitz, B.K.B. 1979. The reduction of fissure caries in Wistar rats by a soluble salt of nonanoic acid. *Arch Oral Biol* 24:663–666.
58. Hayes, M.L., and Carter, E.C. 1980. Effects of nonanoate glucose mouthrinses on acidogenic plaque organisms. *J Dent Res* 59:(Sp. Issue A, Abstr. 526)399.
59. Hefti, A., and Schmid, R. 1979. Effect on caries incidence in rats of increasing dietary sucrose levels. *Caries Res* 13:298–300.
60. Hess, J., and Graf, H. 1975. Zahnplaque-pH bei Patienten mit hereditären Fruktose-Intoleranz. *Schweiz Monatsschr Zahnheilkd* 85:141–153.
61. Hoover, C.I., Newbrun, E., Mettraux, G., and Graf, H. 1980. Microflora and chemical composition of dental plaque from subjects with hereditary fructose intolerance. *Infect Immun* 28:853–859.
62. Holtz, P., Guggenheim, B., and Schmid, R. 1972. Carbohydrates in pooled dental plaque. *Caries Res* 6:103–121.
63. Houte, J. van. 1964. Relationship between carbohydrate intake and polysaccharide-storing micro-organisms in dental plaque. *Arch Oral Biol* 9:91–93.
64. Hubschmann, K., and Cobet, G. 1964. Contribution to hereditary fructose intolerance. *Dtsch Med Wochenschr* 89:938.
65. Huxley, H.G. 1971. The cariogenicity of various percentages of dietary sucrose and glucose in experimental animals. *N Z Dent J* 67:85–98.
66. Igarishi, K., Kamiyama, K., and Yamada, T. 1981. Measurement of pH in human dental plaque in vivo with an ion-sensitive transistor electrode. *Arch Oral Biol* 26:203–207.
67. Imfeld, T. 1977. Evaluation of the cariogenicity of confectionery by intra-oral wire telemetry. *Helv Odontol Acta* 21:437–464.
68. Imfeld, T.N. 1983. Identification of low caries risk dietary components. In *Monographs in Oral Science*, vol. 11, H. Myers (ed), Basel: S. Karger.
69. Imfeld, T., Hirsch, R.S., and Mühlemann, H.R. 1978. Telemetric recordings of interdental plaque pH during different meal patterns. *Br Dent J* 144:40–45.
70. Imfeld, T., and Mühlemann, H.R. 1977. Evaluation of sugar substitutes in preventive cariology. *J Prev Dent* 4:8–14.
71. Ishii, T., König, K.G., and Mühlemann, H.R. 1968. The cariogenicity of different between-meal snacks in Osborne-Mendel rats. *Helv Odontol Acta* 12:41–47.
72. Ismail, A.I., Burt, B.A., and Eklund, S.A. 1984. The cariogenicity of soft drinks in the United States. *J Am Dent Assoc* 199:241–245.
73. Kabara, J.J., Swieczkowski, D.M., Conley, A.J., and Truant, J.P. 1972. Fatty acids and derivatives as antimicrobial agents. *Antimicrobial Agents Chemother* 2:23–28.
74. Kaufmann, U., and Froesch, E.R. 1973. Inhibition of phosphorylase-a by fructose-1-,α-glycerophosphate and fructose-1, 6-diphosphate. Explanation for fructose-induced hypoglycaemia in hereditary fructose intolerance and fructose-1, 6-diphosphatase deficiency. *Eur J Clin Invest* 3:407–413.
75. Knowles, E.M. 1946. The effect of enemy occupation on the dental condition of children in the Channel Islands. *Monthly Bull Minn Hlth Energy Pub Hlth Serv*, pp. 162–172.
76. König, K.G. 1969. Caries activity induced by frequency-controlled feeding of diets containing sucrose or bread to Osborne-Mendel rats. *Arch Oral Biol* 14:991–993.
77. König, K.G. 1971. *Karies and Kariesprophylaxe*. Munich: W. Goldman Verlag.
78. König, K.G., Larson, R.H., and Guggenheim, B. 1969. A strain-specific eating pattern as a factor limiting the transmissibility of caries activity in rats. *Arch Oral Biol* 14:91–103.
79. König, K.G., Schmid, P., and Schmid, R. 1968. An apparatus for frequency-controlled feeding of small rodents and its use in dental caries experiments. *Arch Oral Biol* 13:13–26.

80. Koulourides, T., Phantumvanit, P., Munksgaard, E.C., and Housch, T. 1974. An intraoral model used for studies of fluoride incorporation in enamel. *J Oral Pathol* 3:185–195.
81. Kunzel, W., Borroto, R.C., Lanier, S., and Soto, F. 1973. Auswirkungen habituellen Zuckerrohrkauens auf Kariesbefall und Parodontalzustand Kubanischer Zuckerrohrarbeiter. *Dtsch Stomatol* 23:554–561.
82. Kuramitsu, H.K. 1975. Characterization of extracellular glucosyltransferase activity of *Streptococcus mutans*. *Infect Immun* 12:738–749.
83. Leach, S.A., Green, R.M., Hayes, M.L., and Dada, O.A. 1969. Biochemical studies on the formation and composition of dental plaque in relationship to dental caries. Extracellular polysaccharides. *J Dent Res* 48:811–817.
84. Lee, C.Y., Shallenberger, R.S., and Vittum, M.T. 1970. Free sugars in fruits and vegetables. *N Y Food Life Sci Bull* 1:1–12.
85. Lehner, T. 1980. Future possibilities for the prevention of caries and periodontal disease. *Br Dent J* 149:318.
86. Lenke, J., Enright, C.A., Harper, D.S., and Hefferren, J.J. 1982. A simple indwelling electrode for measurement of oral pH. *J Dent Res* 61:(Program and Abstracts, Abstr. 785)266.
87. Levin, B., Snodgrass, G.J.A.I., Oberholzer, V.G., Burgess, E.A., and Dobbs, R.H. 1968. Fructosaemia observations on seven cases. *Am J Med* 45:826–838.
88. Linden, L., and Nissell, J. 1964. Hereditary intolerance to fructose. *Svensk Läkartidn* 61:3185.
89. Losee, F.L., and Ludwig, T.G. 1970. Trace elements and caries. *J Dent Res* 49:1229–1235.
90. Lundqvist, C. 1952. Oral sugar clearance. *Odontol Revy* 3(Suppl. 1):1–121.
91. Mansbridge, J.N. 1960. The effect of oral hygiene and sweet consumption on the prevalence of dental caries. *Br Dent J* 109:343–354.
92. Marthaler, T. 1967. Epidemiological and clinical dental findings in relation to intake of carbohydrates. *Caries Res* 1:222–238.
93. Marthaler, T. 1968. Apfel, Gesundheit und Kauorgan, Schweiz. *Monatsschr Zahnheilkd* 78:823–836.
94. Marthaler, T.M. 1979. Sugar and oral health. Epidemiology in humans. In *Health and Sugar Substitutes,* Proceedings of ERGOB Conference on Sugar Substitutes, B. Guggenheim (ed), Basel: S. Karger, pp. 27–34.
95. Marthaler, T.M., and Froesch, E.R. 1967. Hereditary fructose intolerance—dental status of 8 patients. *Br Dent J* 123:597–599.
96. Matsukubo, T., Maki, Y., Miyake, S., and Takaesu, Y. 1982. Cariogenic potential index and classification of foodstuffs using in vitro assessment. *J Dent Res* 61:(Program and Abstracts, Abstr. 1079)298.
97. Mayo, J.A., Feary, T.W., and Doerr, P.L. 1978. Transport of sucrose by *Streptococcus sanguis*. *J Dent Res* 57:(Sp. Issue A, Abstr. 644)235.
98. McBride, B.C., and Bourgeau, G. 1975. Dextran-induced aggregation of *Actinomyces viscosus*. *Arch Oral Biol* 20:837–842.
99. McClure, F.J. 1965. Cariostatic effect of dietary vs. intubated phosphate. *Arch Oral Biol* 10:1011–1013.
100. McDonald, J.L., and Stookey, G.K. 1977. Animal studies concerning the cariogenicity of dry breakfast cereals. *J Dent Res* 56:1001–1006.
101. Mimura, C.S., Eisenberg, L.B., and Jacobson, G.R. 1984. Resolution of the phosphotransferase enzymes of *Streptococcus mutans:* purification and preliminary characterization of a heat-stable phosphocarrier protein. *Infect Immun* 44:708–715.
102. Moore, W.J., and Corbett, M.E. 1978. Dental caries experience in man. In *Diet, Nutrition, and Dental Caries,* N.H. Rowe (ed), Ann Arbor: University of Michigan, pp. 3–19.
103. Newbrun, E. 1967. Sucrose, the arch criminal of dental caries. *Odontol Revy* 18:373–386.
104. Newbrun, E. 1971. Dextransucrase from *Streptococcus sanguis*. Further characterization. *Caries Res* 5:124–134.
105. Newbrun, E. 1976. Polysaccharide synthesis in plaque. In *Microbial Aspects of Dental Caries,* H.M. Stiles, W.W. Loesche, and T.C. O'Brien (eds), Sp. Suppl. Microbiol. Abstr. 3:649–664.
106. Newbrun, E., Hoover, C., Mettraux, G., and Graf, H. 1980. Comparison of dietary habits and dental health of subjects with hereditary fructose intolerance and control subjects. *J Am Dent Assoc* 101:619–626.
107. Nizel, A.E. 1981. *Nutrition in Preventive Dentistry: Science and Practice.* 2nd ed. Phila-

delphia: W.B. Saunders, pp. 417–452.

108. Olson, G.A., Guggenheim, B., and Small, P.A. 1974. Antibody-mediated inhibition of dextran/sucrose-induced agglutination of *Streptococcus mutans*. *Infect Immun* 9:273–378.
109. Petersen, P.E. 1983. Dental health among workers at a Danish chocolate factory. *Community Dent Oral Epidemiol* 11:337–341.
110. Pruitt, K.M., Jamieson, A.D., and Caldwell, R.C. 1970. Possible basis for the cariostatic effect of inorganic phosphates. *Nature* 225:1249.
111. Retief, D.H., Cleaton-Jones, P.E., and Walker, A.R. 1975. Dental caries and sugar intake in South African pupils of 16 to 17 years in four ethnic groups. *Br Dent J* 138:463–469.
112. Rosebury, T., and Karshan, M. 1939. Susceptibility of dental caries in the rat. VIII. Further studies on the influence of vitamin D and of fats and fatty oils. *J Dent Res* 18:189–202.
113. Rosen, S. 1969. Comparison of sucrose and glucose in the causation of dental caries in gnotobiotic rats. *Arch Oral Biol* 14:445–450.
114. Rosen, S., Min, D.B., Harper, D.S., Harper, W.J., Beck, E.X., and Beck, F.M. 1984. Effect of cheese, with and without sucrose, on dental caries and recovery of *Streptococcus mutans* in rats. *J Dent Res* 63:894–896.
115. Rowe, N.H., Anderson, R.H., and Wanninger, L.A. 1974. Effects of ready-to-eat breakfast cereals on dental caries experience in adolescent children. A three-year study. *J Dent Res* 53:33–36.
116. Rugg-Gunn, A.J., Edgar, W.M., Geddes, D.A.M., and Jenkins, G.N. 1975. The effect of different meal patterns upon plaque pH in human subjects. *Br Dent J* 139:351–356.
117. Rugg-Gunn, A.J., Edgar, W.M., and Jenkins, G.N. 1978. The effect of eating some British snacks upon the pH of human plaque. *Br Dent J* 145:95–100.
118. Rugg-Gunn, A.J., Edgar, W.M., and Jenkins, G.N. 1981. The effect of altering the position of a sugary food in a meal upon plaque pH in human subjects. *J Dent Res* 60:867–872.
119. Rugg-Gunn, A.J., Hackett, A.F., Appleton, D.R., Jenkins, G.N., and Eastoe, J.E. 1984. Relationship between dietary habits and caries increments assessed over two years in 405 English adolescent schoolchildren. *Arch Oral Biol* 29:983–992.
120. St. Martin, E.J., and Wittenberger, C.L. 1979. Characterization of a phosphoenolpyruvate-dependent sucrose phosphotransferase system in *Streptococcus mutans*. *Infect Immun* 24:865–868.
121. St. Martin, E.J., and Wittenberger, C.L. 1979. Regulation and function of sucrose 6-phosphate hydrolase in *Streptococcus mutans*. *Infect Immun* 26:487–491.
122. Scales, W.R., Long, L.W., and Edwards, J.R. 1975. Purification and characterization of a glucosyltransferase complex from the culture broth of *Streptococcus mutans* FA1. *Carbohydr Res* 42:325–338.
123. Schachtele, C.F., and Jensen, M.B. 1981. Human plaque pH studies. Estimating the cariogenic potential of foods. *Cereal Foods World* 26:14–17.
124. Schachtele, C.F., Loken, A.E., and Schmitt, M.K. 1972. Use of specifically labeled sucrose for comparison of extracellular glucan and fructan metabolism by oral streptococci. *Infect Immun* 5:263–266.
125. Schachtele, C.F., and Mayo, J.A. 1973. Phosphoenolpyruvate-dependent glucose transport in oral streptococci. *J Dent Res* 52:1209–1215.
126. Schafer, W.G. 1949. The caries-producing capacity of starch, glucose and sucrose diets in the Syrian hamster. *Science* 110:143–144.
127. Schulerud, A. 1950. *Dental caries and nutrition during wartime in Norway*. Oslo: Fabritius & Sonners.
128. Shannon, I.L. 1977. *Brand Name Guide to Sugar*. Chicago: Nelson-Hall.
129. Shaw, J.H. 1950. Effects of dietary composition on tooth decay in the albino rat. *J Nutr* 41:13–24.
130. Shaw, J.H., Krumins, F., and Gibbons, R.J. 1967. Comparison of sucrose, lactose, maltose and glucose in causation of experimental oral diseases. *Arch Oral Biol* 12:755–768.
131. Shimamura, A., Tsumori, H., and Mukasa, H. 1982. Purification and properties of *Streptococcus mutans* extracellular glycosyltransferase. *Biochem Biophys Acta* 702:72–80.
132. Slee, A.M., and Tanzer, J.M. 1979. Phosphoenolpyruvate-dependent sucrose phosphotransferase activity in *Streptococcus mutans*. NCTC 10449. *Infect Immun* 24:821–828.
133. Slee, A.M., and Tanzer, J.M. 1979. Phosphoenolpyruvate-dependent sucrose phos-

photransferase activity in 5 serotypes of *Streptococcus mutans*. *Infect Immun* 26:783–786.

134. Sognnaes, R.F. 1948. Analysis of wartime reduction of dental caries in European children. *Am J Dis Child* 75:792–821.
135. Somogyi, J.C., and Trautner, K. 1974. Der Glukose-, Fruktose- und Saccharosegehalt verschiedener Gemüsearten. *Schweiz Med Wochenschr* 140:177–182.
136. Sreebny, L.M. 1982. Sugar availability, sugar consumption and dental caries. *Community Dent Oral Epidemiol* 10:1–7.
137. Staat, R.H., Langley, S.D., and Doyle, R.J. 1980. *Streptococcus mutans* and adherence. Presumptive evidence for protein-mediated attachment followed by glucan-dependent cellular accumulation. *Infect Immun* 27:675–681.
138. Steinberg, A.D., Zimmerman, S.O., and Bramer, M.L. 1972. The Lincoln dental caries study II. The effect of acidulated carbonated beverages on the incidence of dental caries. *J Am Dent Assoc* 85:81–89.
139. Stephan, R.M. 1966. Effect of different types of human foods on dental health in experimental animals. *J Dent Res* 45:1551–1561.
140. Stookey, G.K. 1986. Considerations in determining the cariogenic potential of foods: how should existing knowledge be combined? *J Dent Res* 65:1525–1527.
141. Stoppelaar, J.D. de, Houte, J. van, and Backer Dirks, O. 1970. The effect of carbohydrate restriction on the presence of *Streptococcus mutans, Streptococcus sanguis*, and iodophilic polysaccharide-producing bacteria in human dental plaque. *Caries Res* 4:114–123.
142. Stoppelaar, J.D. de, König, K.G., Plasschaert, A.J.M., and Hoeven, J.S. van der. 1971. Decreased cariogenicity of a mutant of *Streptococcus mutans*. *Arch Oral Biol* 16:971–875.
143. Takeuchi, M. 1961. Epidemiological study on dental caries in Japanese children before, during and after World War II. *Int Dent J* 11:443–457.
144. Tanzer, J.M. 1972. Studies on the fate of glucosyl moiety of sucrose metabolized by *Streptococcus mutans*. *J Dent Res* 51:415–423.
145. Tanzer, J.M. 1979. Essential dependence of smooth surface caries on, and augmentation of fissure caries by, sucrose and *Streptococcus mutans* infection. *Infect Immun* 25:526–531.
146. Tanzer, J.M. (ed) 1981. *Animal Models in Cariology*. Sp. Suppl. Microbiol. Abstr. Washington, D.C.: Information Retrieval, Inc.
147. Tanzer, J.M., Chassy, B.M., and Krichevsky, M.I. 1972. Sucrose metabolism by *Streptococcus mutans*, SL-1. *Biochim Biophys Acta* 261:379–387.
148. Tanzer, J.M., Freedman, M.L., Fitzgerald, R.J., and Larson, R.H. 1974. Diminished virulence of glucan synthesis-defective mutants of *Streptococcus mutans*. *Infect Immun* 10:197–203.
149. Toverud. G. 1964. Child dental health. *Br Dent J* 116:299–304.
150. Tsumori, H., Shimamura, A., and Mukasa, H. 1983. Purification and properties of extracellular glucosyltransferases from *Streptococcus mutans* serotype a. *J Gen Microbiol* 129:3251–3259.
151. U.S. Senate Select Committee on Nutrition and Human Needs. 1977. *Dietary Goals for the United States*. Washington, D.C.: U.S. Government Printing Office, p. 12.
152. Wadhwa, P.S., Young, E.A., Schmidt, K., Elson, C.E., and Pringle, D.J. 1973. Metabolic consequences of feeding frequency in man. *Am J Clin Nutr* 26:823–830.
153. Walker, A.R.P., Dison, E., Duvenhage, A., Walker, B.F., Friedlander, I., and Aucomp, V. 1981. Dental caries in South African black and white school pupils in relation to sugar intake and snack habits. *Community Dent Oral Epidemiol* 9:37–43.
154. Weiss, R.L., and Trithart, A.H. 1960. Between-meal eating habits and dental caries experience in preschool children. *Am J Public Health* 50:1097–1104.
155. Wilson, C.J. 1979. Ready-to-eat cereals and dental caries in children. A three-year study. *J Dent Res* 58:1853–1858.
156. Winter, G.B., Hamilton, M.C., and James, P.M.C. 1966. Role of the comforter as an aetiological factor in rampant caries of the deciduous dentition. *Arch Dis Child* 41:207–212.
157. World Health Organization. 1972. *The etiology and prevention of dental caries*. Techn. Rep. Ser. No. 494. Geneva, Switzerland, p. 12.
158. Yamada, T., Hojo, S., Kobyashi, K., Asano, Y., and Araya, S. 1970. Studies on the carbohydrate metabolism of cariogenic *Streptococcus mutans* Strain PK-1. *Arch Oral Biol* 15:1205–1217.
159. Zita, A.C., McDonald, R.E., and Andrews, A.L. 1959. Dietary habits and dental caries. *J Dent Res* 38:860–865.

Chapter 5

Sugar, Sugar Substitutes, and Noncaloric Sweetening Agents

Just a spoonful of sugar makes the medicine [soft drink, cereal, pastry, cookie, candy, chocolate, etc] *go down, In a most delightful way.*

–Mary Poppins

Most of us enjoy eating sweet-tasting foods, and some might almost have a psychological need for them. Sweetness is the taste that is strongly identified with affection and reward. Indulgence in sweets has been described as a "universal human weakness," as evidenced by the ubiquity of sugar bowls, candy counters, automatic candy machines, bakery and pastry shops, and the soda fountain.[128] Fruits, berries, and honey were the earliest sweet foods known; a famous Stone Age painting in southern Spain depicts the theft of honey from a bee's nest; dates were cultivated in Mesopotamia and the Nile Valley as early as 3500 BC. Since about the seventeenth century, sugar (sucrose) has been the primary sweetening agent. The search for a suitable sugar substitute, or nonnutritive sweetening agent, was originally prompted by the requirement of diabetic patients for a tasty diet. But because obesity is a major nutritional problem in affluent countries today (about 40% of adults in the United States are overweight or obese[167]), the concern of many consumers about their caloric intake has further stimulated the production of foods and beverages containing noncaloric sweetening agents.

The dental profession shares an interest in the search for safe, palatable sugar substitutes. The association between the frequency of sugar consumption and dental caries has been well documented.[88,100,128,172] Many dentists, anxious to prevent dental caries, have attempted to persuade their patients to adopt special dietary programs to limit the frequency with which sugar-containing foods are ingested.[127] Unfortunately, such controlled diets are not a practicable means of caries prevention on a public health scale. Jenkins[83] has written: "It is quite unrealistic to suppose that significant numbers of people would change their dietary habits." It is indeed difficult to change dietary habits, especially if the change requires the elimination of palatable, conveniently available foods. Dentists are placed in a difficult situation, because they must educate patients and somehow motivate them to alter their customary dietary behavior. Furthermore, health education must compete with the food manufacturers' marketing techniques, such as advertisements that sugar-containing food is "rich in energy."[177] It will require the active collaboration of the food industry if dietary control methods are to have a significant effect on dental caries in the population at large. This chapter provides information on the characteristics and the limitations of currently available sugar substitutes and nonnutritive sweetening agents.

Taste and sweetening agents

There are four basic taste modalities, namely:

1. Sour	A property common to protonic acids, $[H^+]$-dependent.
2. Salt	A taste found with many salts of the group I metals, dependent on both anion and cation of the salt.
3. Bitter } 4. Sweet }	Not confined to such well-known classes of substances; bitter and sweet tastes are found in nearly every chemical class.

The ability to differentiate between sweet and bitter substances may have had survival value for early man, since nutritious plants are usually sweet whereas poisonous plants are often bitter. Of the four primary tastes, sweetness is the only one that is pleasant at most concentrations, especially if one is hungry and often even if one is not.[26,27] The sweetness (discriminative) and pleasantness (hedonic) aspects of taste can be separated.[114] There exists a break point at a fixed sweetness (0.21 M sucrose or 7.1% wt/vol) beyond which pleasantness decreases although the sweetness increases.

We usually associate sweetness with sugar, but D-isomers of amino acids also are sweet. Sweet taste is often associated with bitter taste, and sometimes as one ascends a homologous series, taste will change from sweet to bitter. That sweetness should be common to substances with such diverse chemical structures as sugar, saccharin, dulcin, and cyclamate has always seemed inexplicable to the student of the relationship between taste and structure.[109] Several theories have been proposed to explain the mechanism of action of sweet substances on the taste receptor, but it is still not well understood.[143] These theories include:

1. Hydrophobic and hydrogen bonding
2. Complex formation with a "sweet-sensitive protein"
3. Bifunctional molecular theory

They will be reviewed briefly.

Hydrogen and hydrophobic bonding

An important prerequisite for sweetness is high anionic character or ability to form hydrogen bonds with water, that is, to dissolve.[43] The receptor site on the tongue consists of an area for hydrophobic bonding coupled with a site for electronic bonding. Sugars are very soluble in water but are rather low on the relative sweetness scale, so that their attachment to the receptor site is weak and critically dependent on their stereochemistry.

Note that the very sweet compounds dulcin, saccharin, and ultrasüss (1-propoxy-2-amino-4-nitrobenzene) all have a benzene ring that presumably plays a part in the hydrophobic bonding to the receptor site. The sweetness of the 2-amino-4-nitrobenzenes is dependent on the position of the substituent and its effect on the electrons of the ring.

Complex formation with a sweet-sensitive protein

In higher animals, a chemoreceptor is responsible for gustation. Understanding of the biochemistry of taste is rudimentary. It was suggested that in the initial interaction, weak complexes form between the stimulus compound and some receptor molecule at or near the surface of the taste bud.[41] However, the "sweet-sensitive protein" has since been found in large amounts throughout the epithelium of the tongue, whether or not taste buds were present; it is, therefore, not unique to taste buds.[29]

Bifunctional molecular theory

The sweet unit of the sweet compound is viewed as a bifunctional entity with an AH and B component. The taste receptor site is also a bifunctional unit similar in nature to the AH-B system of a sweet compound, as follows:

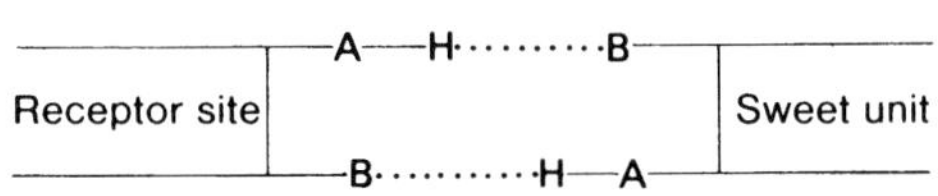

Sweet taste results from an interaction that is probably the result of hydrogen bonding. The interatomic distance of AH-B systems in representative sweet compounds is about 0.3 nm.[142]

Taste receptor response

The primary event involves the interaction of a stimulant molecule with a receptor located at the taste cell plasma membrane. The taste cells, located in the circumvallate and fungiform papillae, contain microvilli (fingerlike projections) at their apical ends that are in constant contact with saliva. The interaction between tastant molecule and receptor occurs on the membrane of the microvilli.

The taste substance interacting with the taste receptor alters the phys-

Table 5-1 Relative sweetnesses of various sweeteners*

Sweetener	Sweetness†
Sucrose	1
Raffinose	0.2
Rhamnose	0.3
Lactose	0.4
Dulcitol	0.4
Palatinose	0.4
Maltose	0.5
Sorbitol	0.5
Galactose	0.6
D-Glucose	0.7
D-Xylose	0.7
Mannitol	0.7
Glycine	0.7
Invert sugar	0.7–0.9
Glycerol	0.8
Xylitol	1
D-Fructose	1.1
Ethylene glycol	1.3
Sodium 3-methylcyclopentylsulfamate	15
p-Anisylurea	18
Sodium cyclohexylsulfamate (cyclamate)	30–80
Chloroform	40
Glycyrrhizin	50

*Adapted from Inglett, G.E. Sweeteners: an overall perspective. In *Aspartame*, L.D. Stegink and L.J. Filer (eds), New York: Dekker, 1984.

†Sucrose is assigned a value of 1 for comparison. Sweet taste depends upon concentration of sweetener, temperature, pH, type of medium used, and sensitivity of the taster.

icochemical properties of the membrane and changes the membrane potential. The magnitude of the potential across the taste cell membrane changes with stimulation. Presumably the adsorption of the chemical stimulus molecules to specific receptor sites on the membrane of the taste cell leads to conformational changes in certain membrane molecules and a resultant depolarization of the taste cell membrane.[13]

Relative sweetness—organoleptic evaluation

The intensity of a compound's sweetness cannot be measured quantitatively in absolute physical or chemical terms but requires the use of subjective sensory methods with trained taste panels. Sucrose is the usual standard, and the sweetening power of other sweeteners is then compared on a relative weight basis.

These ratios are only approximate at best and hold true only up to a certain concentration. At higher concentrations, especially of saccharin, there is an increasing level of bitterness and aftertaste.

Sucrose has a relative quick sweetness impact followed by a fairly sharp, clean cutoff. Nonnutritive sweeteners build up to their maximum sweet-

Table 5-1 Relative sweetnesses of various sweeteners—cont'd

Sweetener	Sweetness†
Acesulfame-K	130
Aspartylphenylalanine methyl ester	100–200
5-Nitro-2-methoxyaniline	167
5-Methylsaccharin	200
Perillartine 200	200
p-Ethoxyphenylurea (dulcin)	70–350
6-Chlorosaccharin	100–350
n-Hexylchloromalonamide	300
Sodium saccharin	200–700
Stevioside	300
2-Amino-4-nitrotoluene	300
Naringin dihydrochalcone	300
p-Nitrosuccinanilide	350
Suosan	350
Phyllodulcin	400
1-Bromo-5-nitroaniline	700
5-Nitro-2-ethoxyaniline	950
Perillaldehyde anti-aldoxime	2,000
Neohesperidin dihydrochalcone	2,000
Talin	2,500
Thaumatin	3,000
Monellin	3,000
5-Nitropropoxyaniline (P-4000)	4,000

ness intensity at a slower rate, and the sensation persists for a longer period.

Different individuals exhibit different reactions to taste stimuli.[30] For example, sensitivity to the taste of phenylthiocarbamide is inherited as a Mendelian recessive trait. Therefore, tables of relative sweetness depend on the average opinion of a number of people and are only approximate.

The sucrose-recognition taste threshold has been compared for caries-resistant adults and caries-susceptible subjects matched with respect to age, sex, and race.[180] Surprisingly, the caries-resistant persons had an elevated sucrose taste threshold that could not be explained as being responsible for caries resistance. Presumably the sucrose taste threshold is a reflection of a physiological or genetic characteristic of this group.

Of considerable interest is the observation that for adults, as the sugar concentration (and, therefore, also the sweetness) increases, so does liking (hedonic preference), until a certain level, called the "bliss point," is reached. Thereafter, further increase in the sugar concentration or sweetness reduces the liking. The bliss point concentration is 9% sucrose (wt/vol) or 18% (1.0 M) glucose. In children, however, the liking pattern does not follow the same inverted-U curve of arousal. Rather, the children exhibited no bliss point and rated beverages in preference directly according to their sweetness and sugar concentration.[115] This may, in part, account for the greater caries susceptibility of children than adults. However, in a study of 15-year-old children, groups with high and low caries prevalence showed no significant differences in sucrose taste threshold or in preference for sweet taste.[126]

The sweetness of a variety of substances is shown in Table 5-1. Most of the naturally occurring sugars are less sweet than sucrose. Fructose is an exception and is appreciably sweeter than sucrose. There are a few natural products or their derivatives, such as ammoniated glycerrhizin, stevioside, the dihydrochalcones, and monellin, which are intensely sweet. However, most of the intensely sweet compounds are chemically synthesized and are called noncaloric or nonnutritive sweeteners. The terms "synthetic" and "artificial" sweeteners are no longer used by food technologists because the important difference between sugars and related polyols and the noncaloric sweeteners is a nutritional one.[11]

Sucrose

The etymology of the word "sugar" has been traced to the Chinese term *shache,* literally, "sand-sugar plant," then to the Sanskrit, *Rarkara,* meaning sand or gravel, and more directly from the Arabic, *sukkar.*[97]

Sucrose is found in all green plants, where it is an early product of photosynthesis and is the main agent for translocating carbon to the rest of the plant. The maple tree, certain palm trees, and sweet sorghum contain appreciable amounts of sucrose but are unimportant commercially. Sugar cane and sugar beet are the major industrial sources of sugar.

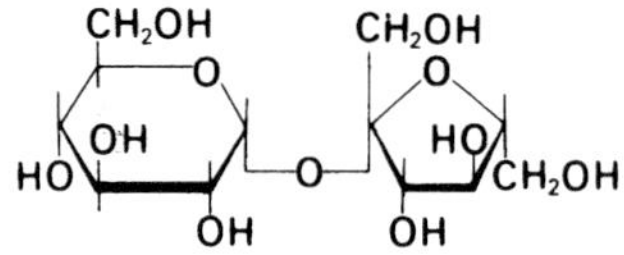

SUCROSE

Sucrose is a nonreducing disaccharide, β-D-fructofuranosyl-α-D-glucopyranoside. It has a positive optical rotation, $[\alpha]_D = +66.5°$, and can be readily hydrolyzed. The resulting mixture of glucose and fructose has a negative optical rotation and is known as "invert sugar," which is slightly sweeter than sucrose. Sucrose is fermentable but resists bacterial decomposition when in high concentration (65% or more).

History

Sugar cane, *Saccharum officinarum,* is a giant grass resembling bamboo, growing to a height of 4 to 5 m and requiring a moist soil and a sunny tropical climate. It contains about 13% sucrose. The plant originated in the South Pacific, probably in New Guinea, and moved northward to Southeast Asia and India. Sugar was specifically mentioned for the first time in the West in 325 BC by Nearchus, an officer in Alexander's invading army in India. Sugar cane cultivation and refining spread to China about 100 BC and was a flourishing industry there at the time of Marco Polo (1254–1324). It did not reach the Mediterranean until relatively late, probably as a result of the Arab conquest after AD 635.

Sugar was introduced into Europe in the thirteenth century by Venetian traders. The Portuguese started sugar cane cultivation on the island of Madeira and subsequently on the west coast of Africa and Brazil in the fifteenth century. Spaniards introduced sugar cane to the Canary Islands, whence Columbus brought cane to the Caribbean. The sugar plantations in the New World were very much dependent upon the slave trade because of their need for abundant labor for culturing and harvesting the sugar cane.[5]

Until about the middle of the fifteenth century, sugar in its various forms was a scarce luxury enjoyed only by the court and nobility. Queen Elizabeth was overfond of sugar and sugared dishes and confections, and her teeth suffered as a consequence. Hentzer, a German traveler who visited England in 1598, noted the blackness of her teeth and ascribed this to her excessive consumption of sugar—one of the earliest references to the connection between sugar and dental caries.

There was also a steady demand for sugar in small quantities for medical prescriptions. "An apothecary without sugar" is an old proverbial expression denoting the lack of something essential for a specific trade. Regrettably, many pharmaceutical preparations even today contain large amounts of sucrose, especially in troches and syrups.[18] For example, the sucrose content of several antacid tablets or gums is as follows: Bisodol 13%, Chooz Gum 48%, Rolaids 56%, Tums 41%, and Walgreen Antacid 32%. Most vitamin, cough, and antibiotic syrups contain from 10% to 80% sucrose, usually about 55%. Similarly, many chewable vitamin tablets and especially cough lozenges have a high sucrose content (eg, Chew-Tabs 50%, Tri-Vi-Sol 30%, Flintstones 75%, Vicks Medicating Throat Lozenges 66%, Parke Davis Throat Disc 58%, Cepacol 51%, Chloraseptic 53%, and Silence is Golden 58%).[144]

Many of these products are prepared for pediatric use; they cause an extended drop in pH and their long-term use has been correlated with rampant decay.[52,53] Children with chronic medical disorders often require a long-term medication. To improve palatability and, perhaps, patient compliance, pharmaceutical companies prepare many drugs in syrup form. Children who had been taking sucrose-based medicines for at least 6 months had significantly more caries than a suitable control group (Table 5-2).[133] Comprehensive lists of medications that are virtually sugar-free have been published.[2,3] Conversely, a listing of the sugar content of selected pharmaceuticals is also available.[146]

The sugar beet, *Beta vulgaris,* which contains about 16% sucrose, is

Table 5-2 Comparison of caries score, plaque index, and gingival index in children taking syrup medicines* and control subjects†

Indices of dental disease	Mean score: Syrup group (n = 44)	Mean score: Control (n = 47)	Significance (*P*)
Caries score (defs)	5.55	1.26	0.02
Plaque index	0.87	0.55	0.06 NS
Gingival index	0.91	0.51	0.03

*Children between 9 months and 6 years old with chronic medical disorders taking syrup medicines for ≥6 months.
†From Roberts and Roberts.[131]
(defs) = Decayed, extracted, and filled surfaces; *(NS)* = not significant.

now the second major source of sucrose. It was known as a sweetish vegetable during the Middle Ages. In 1744, Andreas Marggraf, a German chemist, established the identity of beet and cane sugar. Practical methods of extracting sugar from the beet were developed. Sugar beet cultivation and processing have become a major agricultural activity of most European countries, particularly Russia, Germany, the United Kingdom, and Italy. The United States produces about 10% of the world's cane and beet sugar.

Manufacture

Prompt harvesting and processing of the ripened cane are essential to avoid spoilage. The cut cane is shredded and crushed between rollers to extract the juice. The juice is heated and lime is added, enabling some impurities to be skimmed off as scum. Evaporation and boiling are used to concentrate the juice, yielding a mixture of crystals and syrup called *massecuite.* The crystals, known as raw sugar, can be separated (eg, by centrifugation) and are about 96% sucrose, the remaining 4% consisting of water, invert sugar, dirt, and impurities.

The syrup, or molasses, is prevented from crystallization by interfering substances, and contains about 70% sucrose. It provides the raw material for the manufacture of rum or is sold for livestock feed. Molasses is usually rich in iron and also contains some calcium, but otherwise is no more nutritious than sugar. Treacle is essentially a superior form of molasses, containing more sucrose and less impurities.

Raw sugar is transported to refineries, usually distant from the plantations, for further purification. This involves melting, carbonation, filtration, charring, crystallization, and granulation. A detailed description of these various steps and the quality control factors can be found elsewhere.[121] The final product, white sugar, is one of the purest chemical substances manufactured on a large scale. Minor modifications of the process can produce granulated sugar, cube sugar, castor sugar, icing sugar, coffee crystals, and other products. Powdered (icing) sugars are produced from granulated sugar by milling and adding small amounts of anticaking agents such as starch and tricalcium phosphate. Table syrups are specially refined, partially inverted sugar solutions containing about 83% solids, of which about 3% are nonsugars that give the characteristic color and flavor.

Some of the advertising claims of sugar manufacturers are rather dubious to say the least. For example, the following statement was made by the public relations department of one firm:

> Sugar helps you eat less of all foods if you are on a weight control diet. A few bites of food containing sugar before or with meals satisfies your hunger with less food.

There is no evidence to indicate that intake of sucrose (at four calories/g) is desirable in weight control diets. Another product, Sugar in the Raw, was advertised as "organically" grown sugar, containing "its natural vitamins and minerals" with no chemicals or preservatives added. The Federal Trade Commission has prohibited such false advertising (no refined sugar contains nutritionally significant amounts of vitamins or minerals).[72]

Consumption

The so-called sugar consumption figures widely cited in the literature are really average utilization or disappearance values, derived by dividing the amount available in the market to consume (that is, what disappears) by the total population.[32] This does not include industrial and household waste such as spillage and discarded leftovers. When actual consumption of sucrose per capita has been calculated from dietary recall questionnaires or interviews, it has been found to be less than the per capita disappearance values.[102,124,147] Because information on actual sucrose consumption is more difficult to obtain, the disappearance values are most widely used. It should be recognized, however, that these values exceed actual consumption.

As the sugar industry flourished in the Caribbean and South America, the consumption of sugar rose steadily in Europe and North America. In England, for example, it increased from 4 lbs/person/year in 1700 to 12 lbs/person/year in 1780. Sucrose did not become a major carbohydrate food until the nineteenth century. The demand for sugar was further stimulated by the growing use of two other tropical products: coffee and tea. In Germany, annual per capita consumption of sugar rose from 3 kg in 1850 to 30 kg in 1967.

World sugar production from 1900 to 1970 rose from 8 million metric tons to 73 million tons (ie, about ninefold). Between 1950 and 1964, production almost doubled. No other human food or agricultural product has shown an increase of the same order. In high sugar-consuming countries, sucrose accounts for one sixth or more of total caloric intake. In the United States and the United Kingdom, annual per capita utilization was about 50 kg, or 1 kg/week/person, in 1965.[73,156] Based on US Department of Agriculture disappearance data, per capita utilization of total sugars was 50 kg in 1960, 56 kg in 1970, and 58 kg in 1984.[60] Utilization of sucrose has decreased (Fig 5-1), but the total sugar (sucrose, fructose, corn syrups, honey) utilization has remained fairly stable. This change in consumption pattern is in part explained by the rising cost of sucrose and, therefore, the increasing use of high-fructose corn syrup (HFCS) as a sweetener. In January 1980, one of the major soft drink companies began using HFCS in its cola, and other soft drink manufacturers quickly followed suit.[159]

Less than 30% of the annual per capita intake is packaged for household use.[158] Most sugar is delivered to industrial users, beverage makers taking one third of this allocation. Producers of bakery goods, cereal, and allied products rank second as industrial users of sucrose. Next come candy makers, then canners, frozen food packers, and the dairy industry. The products of these manufacturers are eventually consumed and are said to contain the "hidden sugars" of the diet. The proportion of total

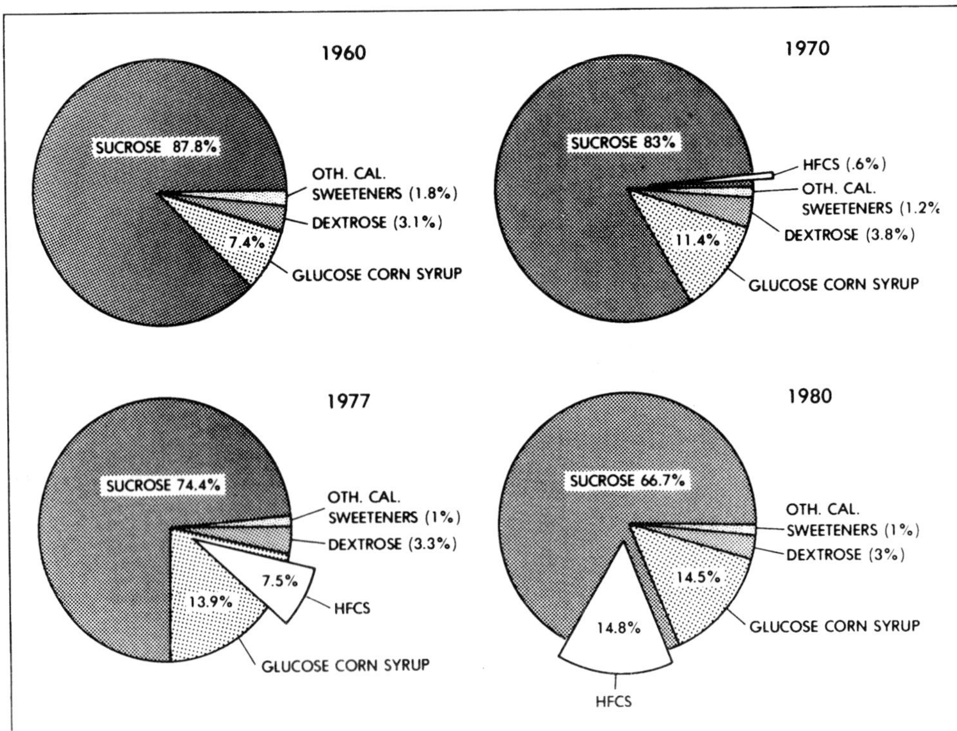

Fig 5-1 Utilization of caloric sweeteners in the United States from 1960 to 1980. Use of high-fructose corn syrup (HFCS) has increased markedly in recent years.

sugar intake consumed in the form of commercially processed foods has increased. This increase is traceable in large part to the desire of food manufacturers to gain a competitive edge.[168] The profusion of varieties of presweetened cereals and soft drinks is a striking example. According to a Swedish survey, more than 50% of the sucrose intake by children was consumed between regular meals.[103] Sucrose is undoubtedly one of the cheapest sources of assimilable energy currently available. It is well established as an important food ingredient that will not easily be replaced[54]; however, reduction of sugar consumption is clearly recognized as a dietary goal for the United States.[168]

Long-term feeding of a high-sucrose diet causes renal glomerulosclerosis, impairment of glucose tolerance, and marked proteinuria in rats[135]; it also shortens their lifespan.[40] It has been proposed that high consumption of sucrose elevates serum triglycerides and may be an important factor in the etiology of atherosclerosis, myocardial infarction, and non-insulin-dependent diabetes.[176,178,179] Other surveys have also reported some correlation between high sucrose intake and coronary heart disease but have not found it to be statistically significant.[48,130] In experimental animals, atherosclerosis comparable to the disease in man has not been produced by sucrose feeding.[181] As yet there is no clear-cut evidence of sucrose as a causative factor in coronary heart disease. Excessive sugar intake does not adversely affect mood.[20,60]

There are dangers inherent in excessive consumption of sucrose-containing foods. Not only does such a practice promote dental caries, but it also clearly causes a high caloric intake, which may be serious for diabetics and undesirable for overweight people.

Sugar substitutes

Sorbitol (D-glucitol)

Sorbitol occurs naturally in cherries, plums, pears, apples, many berries, seaweeds, and algae. It is prepared industrially from glucose by high-

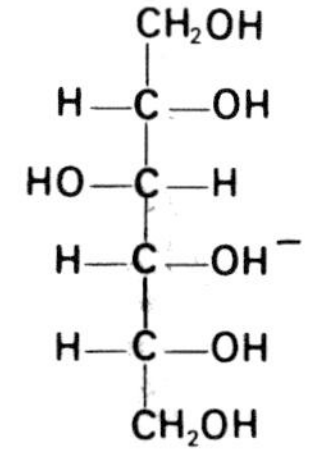

SORBITOL

pressure hydrogenation or by electrolytic reduction. It is moderately sweet (about half that of sucrose) and relatively inexpensive. Commercially it is sold as a sweetener in aqueous solution because of its hygroscopic properties. Sweets containing only sorbitol cannot be stored for very long. The hygroscopic effect can be reduced by adding gum arabic (eg, in throat lozenges). Sorbitol is slowly absorbed through the small bowel by passive transport mechanisms and is converted to glycogen in the liver through the intermediary formation of fructose:

$$\text{Sorbitol} \xrightarrow[\text{Oxidoreductase}]{} \text{Fructose}$$

As with carbohydrates, 1 g of sorbitol yields four calories; however, only about 70% of orally ingested sorbitol is absorbed. Sorbitol may cause gastric upset in large doses. It acts as a laxative because of osmotic transfer of water into the bowel. A number of cases of diarrhea in very young children after ingestion of sorbitol candies have been reported.[63] The Food and Agricultural Organization–World Health Organization Commission's report on food additives recommends that the intake of sorbitol be limited to 150 mg/kg/day.

Dental aspects

Fermentation by oral microorganisms. Practically all strains isolated (96%) of caries-inducing mutans group of streptococci will ferment sorbitol (and mannitol) in vitro to give a final pH of below 5.0.[31,47,64] Most other oral microorganisms will not ferment sorbitol. Sorbitol, if suspended in and incubated with mixed oral flora from saliva or plaque, will be fermented, but only slowly and after extended periods of time.[66] Numerous studies have shown that when sorbitol is applied to dental plaque in situ or in vitro, very little alteration of the pH of the plaque takes place, whereas most sugars (sucrose, glucose, galactose) cause a dramatic and rapid drop of the pH in plaque.* The failure of sorbitol to appreciably lower pH in plaque can be explained by the fact that, although *Streptococcus mutans* ferments sorbitol, the rate of acid production is much slower compared to other fermentable hexoses and disaccharides. This permits salivary buffers to neutralize acid end products as they are formed. Fermentation of sorbitol or mannitol by *S mutans* involves an initial phosphorylation of the hexitol to sorbitol 6-phosphate or mannitol 1-phosphate, respectively, with subsequent oxidation of the hexitol phosphates to fructose 6-phosphate (Fig 5-2). The sorbitol 6-phosphate:NAD oxidoreductase (dehydrogenase) and mannitol 1-phosphate:NAD oxidoreductase are distinct, inducible enzymes[24] that can be repressed by glucose. In vivo it is doubtful that hexitol is the sole carbohydrate available to plaque streptococci; therefore, oxidation of the hexitol phosphates would be repressed.

*References 17, 19, 33, 51, 55, 56, 118.

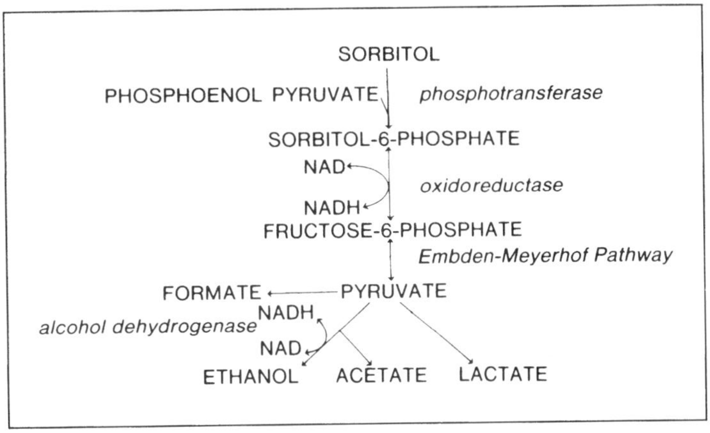

Fig 5-2 Sorbitol metabolism by *Streptococcus mutans*. *(NAD)* Nicotinamide adenine dinucleotide; *(NADH)* reduced nicotinamide adenine dinucleotide.

The reactions catalyzed by these oxidoreductases are reversible, permitting the removal of free fructose other than by glycolysis.[23] The stored polyol may subsequently be used as an energy source, giving *S mutans* an ecological advantage.

Cariogenicity. Sorbitol and partially hydrolyzed hydrogenated starches containing about 28% sorbitol have been tested for their cariogenicity in rodents by several independent investigators.* Usually sorbitol was compared with sucrose or other carbohydrates. Sorbitol ingestion under such conditions caused much less caries and a reduction in plaque accumulation. However, some low-grade caries activity in sulci remained. The reported caries reduction of sorbitol diets should be interpreted with caution, because when sorbitol is added to the diet, there is a measurable decrease in food intake, frequently accompanied by a decreased weight gain.[70]

No adequate human clinical caries studies have been done on the effect of ingestion of sorbitol, although candies and chewing gum sweetened with sorbitol are available commercially both in the United States and in Europe. Some manufacturers have advertised their products as "tooth protective" or "safe for teeth." These claims may be premature, although the Swiss government permits such labeling providing human tests show that ingestion of the sweets will not cause a drop of plaque pH below 5.7.[78,117]

In Roslagen, Sweden, investigators attempted to compare the cariogenicity of candies containing sucrose with candies containing Lycasin, a hydrogenated starch hydrolysate.[58] Children 3 to 6 years old were observed for 18 to 30 months. Almost all the children in the Lycasin group also ate sucrose-containing candies, and some drank sucrose-containing lemonades. Since replacement of sucrose was far from com-

*References 49, 57, 59, 86, 119, 145.

plete, the differences in caries increments were not statistically significant. This study emphasizes the futility of attempting to reduce caries by substituting for sucrose in only one type of food (candies) while maintaining an otherwise high-sucrose diet.

Bacterial adaptation. The question has been raised whether long-term ingestion of sorbitol permits the establishment of caries-inducing organisms capable of fermenting sorbitol. In vitro cultures of *S mutans* (strain Ingbritt) adapt themselves to grow more rapidly in media containing sorbitol and xylitol if maintained in the presence of these polyols for about 5 months.[99] Some adaptation of human oral flora to daily feeding of or rinsing with sorbitol for 2 to 6 months has been reported.[17,56] Other investigators[16,34,39,65] have not found any significant alterations in the oral flora or increased numbers of sorbitol-fermenting organisms following prolonged sorbitol intake. These findings are to be expected, first of all, because the population in general has already been exposed to appreciable amounts of sorbitol for quite some time without major alterations in the oral flora. Many dentifrices contain 6% to 20% sorbitol not only because of its sweetening properties but also because it is a humectant (moistener). Secondly, in order for selective overgrowth of sorbitol fermenters to occur, other carbohydrates would have to be excluded. Indeed, in an experimental carbohydrate-free diet, subjects who ate two sorbitol candies six times daily for 4 days had a significant increase in the proportion of sorbitol-fermenting bacteria in their plaque.[132] However, such exclusion of carbohydrates is most unlikely in a human population.

Xylitol

Xylitol is a pentose alcohol found naturally in a variety of fruits and vegetables (raspberries, strawberries, plums, lettuce, cauliflower, mushrooms, chestnuts)[171] and obtained commercially from birch trees, cottonseed hulls, and coconut shells. It has a sweetness similar to sucrose and a cooling effect in the mouth.[69] It has been proposed as a possible

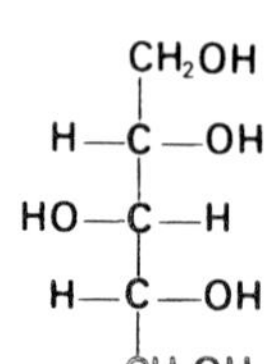

XYLITOL

sugar substitute for diabetes, although in high dosage it may cause diarrhea in both humans[107] and rats.[89,119] Like sorbitol, it is only slowly absorbed from the gastrointestinal tract and, therefore, draws water into the bowel by osmotic effects. It is a metabolic intermediate in the glucuronate pathway in humans.

Xylitol has been tested for its effect on the pH of interdental plaque using biotelemetry.[78,79,118] A rinse with 10% xylitol did not change plaque pH over a 30-minute test period. Xylitol administered to rats is of very low cariogenicity, even less than sorbitol.[62,119,120] However, these observations are not definitive because of lower growth rates or poor survival, or both, of the rats fed xylitol. This reduction in caries could be a nonspecific effect due to less dietary intake and decreased eating frequency. Students had a lower plaque index when consuming xylitol than with most other sugars.[99,116,138]

In Turku, Finland, the caries increment, plaque formation, and plaque flora were compared in adults, average age 27.5 years, on diets using either sucrose, fructose, or xylitol as the sweetening agent. In this clinical trial, the specific sugars were used as sweeteners in about 100 products, such as tea, soft drinks, juices, porridges, jams, marmalade, pastries (about 30 varieties), sweets, chocolates, bonbons, chewing gum, marinated herring, pickles, mustard, and cough mixture. After only 1 year, a dramatic reduction in caries increments was found in the group consuming xylitol-containing products (about 90% less caries than the sucrose group). Patients in the xylitol group had less plaque and lower colony counts of *S mutans* in their plaque. Large intake of xylitol-containing soft drinks did produce transitory loose stools, usually not a problem with the solid products. Only one of the more than 50 persons using xylitol products dropped out of the study because of diarrhea.[139]

The caries index used measures very early caries (chalky or discolored enamel) as well as lesions with visible loss of substance or cavitation, differing from the more commonly used caries-scoring system. Very early carious lesions present at the time of the initial examination would be related to sucrose intake before the start of the study. Once dietary sucrose is eliminated and xylitol is used as a sugar substitute, these early lesions would have a chance to remineralize. Incipient lesions, seen microscopically in vivo, can be reversed upon stopping frequent sucrose use, instituting good oral hygiene practice, and regularly applying fluoride. In the Turku study one would, therefore, anticipate a greater reversal (by remineralization) in the xylitol group because of the scoring system employed. If incipient lesions are disregarded and the usual diagnostic criteria for caries are employed, the reduction in DMFS was 56% after 1 year and 60% after 2 years. The Turku study, involving virtually complete sucrose substitution, clearly demonstrated that xylitol is noncariogenic in humans.

Several studies have provided dietary xylitol, in the form of xylitol-sweetened chewing gum, as an "add-on" (1 to 10 g/day) without attempting to restrict sucrose intake.[82,85,139] Alternatively, partial substitution of xylitol for dietary sucrose (maximum 20 g/day) in candy, chewing gum, ice lolly, chocolate, gumdrop, and wafer has been tested in institutionalized Hungarian and noninstitutionalized Polynesian children.[84,137] Although the design of these field studies does not conform to the requirements of standardized clinical trials (nonrandomized populations with differing baseline caries prevalence, examiners were not blinded), the results have consistently shown that even relatively small amounts of xylitol reduce formation of new caries.[6]

The mechanism whereby xylitol reduces caries is as yet not clearly understood.[101] Short-term chewing of xylitol gum (two packages per day for 4 weeks) significantly reduced salivary levels and plaque proportions of *S mutans*, whereas sorbitol- or fructose-sweetened gum had no such effect.[97] Xylitol, due to its organoleptic properties, stimulates salivation, thereby increasing plaque pH, and thus promotes remineralization.

During toxicity studies of xylitol by the Huntington Research Centre in England, it was found that mice ingesting diets with the highest xylitol content (10% and 20%) showed an increase in urinary bladder calculi, epithelial hyperplasia, and neoplasia of the bladder. Xylitol can be converted, via glycollate, to oxalate, which appears in the urine and can accumulate to form calcium oxalate crystals. The adverse effects observed in animal studies, such as pelvic nephrocalcinosis and bladder calculi, were induced by gross physiological and/or nutritional disturbance related to very high dose levels of the test compound.[7] Therefore, xylitol at a dose high enough to form bladder stones may serve as a tumor promoter rather than a true carcinogen. This dose (20% in the diet) is equivalent to a 70-kg man consuming over half a kilogram of xylitol daily. Unlike rodents, humans do not produce biologically significant amounts of oxalate from xylitol. Humans exposed to "normal" levels of xylitol would not be at risk of developing bladder tumors.[134] Xylitol exhibits no mutagenic activity by the Ames test, in direct microbial assay, or in a host-mediated assay test system.[9]

Xylitol is approved for foods, cosmetics, and pharmaceuticals in about 40 countries. In the United States, xylitol has been approved for special dietary use since 1963. It is used as a sweetener mainly in noncariogenic confectionery (chewing gum, candies, gum drops) and less frequently in dietetic food (for diabetics), in pharmaceutical products (tablets, throat lozenges, vitamin tablets, cough syrup), and occasionally in dentifrices. Use in soft drinks is limited because the intake of excessive quantities of polyol-sweetened liquids would tend to exceed the threshold dose, causing gastrointestinal side effects (laxation). A significant deterrent to the widespread use of xylitol as a sweetener is its cost, currently ten times that of sucrose.

Starch hydrolysates

Dextrin-based sucrose substitutes have been developed using starches from cereals (maize, wheat) or potatoes. The starches are hydrolyzed using acid and/or microbial enzymes to produce the desired degree of depolymerization.[141] The final products are normally sold as syrups containing dextrins, maltose, and glucose. Future developments in this field include partial hydrogenation converting glucose to sorbitol and the use of glucose isomerase to convert glucose to fructose. Corn sweeteners must be considered cariogenic, certainly with respect to fissure caries.

High-fructose corn syrups (HFCS)

High-fructose corn syrups, developed in the early 1970s, are produced from hydrolyzed corn starch by the use of the enzyme glucose-isomerase, which converts some of the glucose to fructose. Because fructose is about three times as sweet as glucose, the overall product is considerably sweeter than corn syrup or sucrose solutions. More and more HFCSs, particularly one containing 55% fructose, are being substituted for sucrose, invert sugar, and glucose syrups for use in processed foods and as a liquid table-top sweetener. Estimated use of HFCS for 1980 was 19 pounds per capita per year (8.6 kg). Soft drink manufacturers are the main users of HFCS, but HFCS use is increasing at a dramatic rate in other food industries such as baking, canning, processed foods, and dairy products (see Fig 5-1). HFCS's gains have adversely affected the United States cane and beet sugar industries. HFCS has become dominant because of the industry's modern, automated, and efficient plant facilities and highly advanced technology. Furthermore, HFCS facilities can be operated year-round, as compared with the 3 to 5 months beet factories and cane mills are operated. HFCS supplies are more reliable and pre-

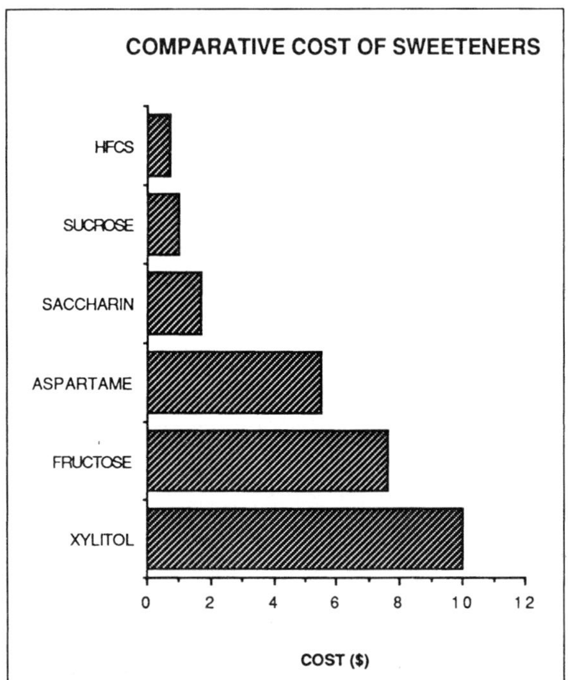

Fig 5-3 Price comparison of commercially available sweeteners with adjustment for cost of sweetener equal in sweetening power to sucrose.

dictable and its price is less volatile than that of sucrose[6]; it is also slightly cheaper when costs are adjusted for equal sweetening power (Fig 5-3). This cost advantage exists only in the United States, where corn prices are artificially low because of government subsidies and where domestic sucrose prices are higher than world prices because of import quotas.

Coupling sugar: glycosylsucrose

Glycosylsucrose is the general term for oligosaccharide derivatives of sucrose. When the enzyme cyclodextrin glucosyltransferase, isolated from *Bacillus megaterium*, acts on a mixture of starch and sucrose, a mixture of monosaccharides, glucosylsucrose, maltosylsucrose, oligosaccharides, and oligosaccharides terminated at the reducing end by sucrose are formed (Fig 5-4).[90] This mixture, called "coupling sugar," is presently used in Japan in a variety of foods, including candies, chocolate, cookies, jam, and jelly. Its sweetness is about 50% to 60% that of sucrose, it is relatively cheap, is resistant to heat and, therefore, suitable for baking and cooking. Also, it is pH stable and does not cause diarrhea. Although coupling sugar is fermented by various oral microorganisms, the acid production is much less than that obtained with glucose and sucrose.[76,174,175] Coupling sugar permits very little synthesis of insoluble glucan or adherence of *S mutans* in vitro.[76] When coupling sugar is fed to rats infected with *S mutans*, the caries experience is much less than

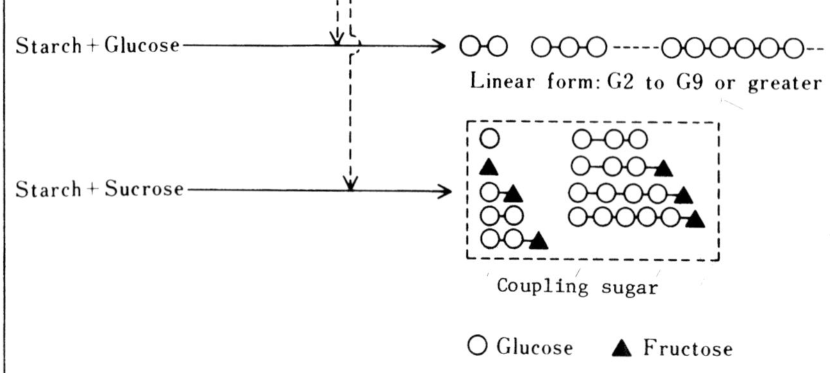

Fig 5-4 Production of coupling sugar by the action of cyclodextrin glucosyltransferase on a mixture of starch and sucrose.

that with sucrose.[77] Accordingly, coupling sugar is cariogenic, although its cariogenicity is considerably less than that of sucrose or other sugars.

Aspartame: L-aspartyl L-phenylalanine methyl ester

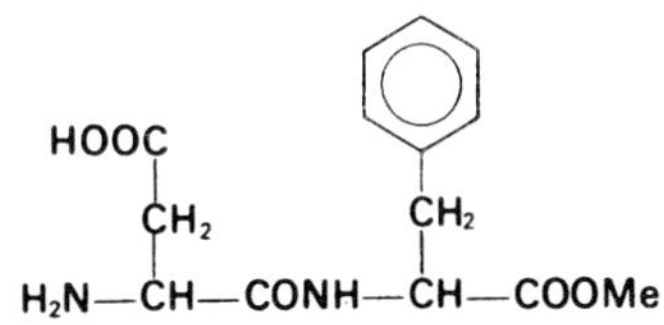

ASPARTAME

Aspartame was accidentally discovered to have a pronounced sweet taste, being about 180 times sweeter than sucrose in aqueous solution.[35,106] Subsequent research has shown that many α-amides of L-aspartic acid are sweet.[105] This dipeptide is more acceptable and relatively sweeter in low than in high concentration. It is stable in liquid form down to pH 3, but it is unstable at extreme pH ranges. This instability manifests itself as a loss of sweetness during storage. Prolonged cooking temperatures, as encountered in frying and baking, can cause significant breakdown of aspartame to diketopiperazine with a consequent loss of sweetness.[166] For this reason the Food and Drug Administration requires the product label to state that aspartame should not be used in cooking or baking.[160]

Concerns about the safety of aspartame relate to its phenylalanine and aspartate contents. Phenylketonuria (PKU), a genetic defect of phenylalanine metabolism, occurs in one in 10,000 births. For persons with PKU, if blood levels of phenylalanine are not carefully maintained below approximately 12 mg/100 ml during pregnancy and fetal development, the risk of fetal anomalies and mental retardation is exceedingly high. The manufacturers (Searle & Co; Ajinomoto Co, Inc) are required to label aspartame clearly to indicate it contains phenylalanine and that intake is restricted for such individuals. Similarly, any food products containing aspartame would have to be so labeled.[160]

The other reason for caution in approving aspartame is based on neurotoxic properties of aspartate and glutamate on the developing brain.[129] Irreversible destruction of nerve cells in the hypothalamus of newborn mice and monkeys results from a single dose of glutamate delivered by stomach tube at 0.5 and 1 g/kg, respectively. This mode of feeding has been criticized as unrealistic, and in terms of human feeding it is difficult to conceive of an individual consuming enough aspartame to cause any adverse effects.[71]

The US Food and Drug Administration (FDA) approved aspartame in 1974 but then suspended permission to market the product pending resolution of questions of safety. The reproduction and teratology studies for aspartame conducted by Searle came under question because of poor animal husbandry practices and problems in design of some of these studies. The FDA ordered an independent check, which found the company's studies valid. Final approval of aspartame for use as a tabletop sugar substitute, as a tablet, or as an additive in cereals, drink mixes, instant coffee and tea, gelatins, puddings, fillings, dairy products, and toppings was given in 1981.[160] Since the use of aspartame became widespread, various reactions have been reported. These have mostly been neurological or behavioral symptoms, particularly headaches, attributed to sensitivity to the sweetener. However, in a human double-blind crossover trial, aspartame was no more likely to produce headache than was placebo, nor were treatment-related effects detected in vital signs, blood pressure, or plasma concentrations of cortisol, insulin, glucagon, histamine, epinephrine, or norepinephrine.[140] Approval has since been extended to its use in noncarbonated fruit juices, fruit drinks, frozen stick-type confections, breath mints, and as a sweetening agent in drug products.[162,163]

Maltol (3-hydroxy-2-methyl-4-pyrone)

This organic product is derived from a number of plant materials (bark of larch trees, pine needles, chicory, and roasted malt) and is manufactured and sold in pure form.

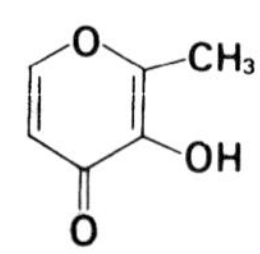

MALTOL

Maltol has a fragrant, caramel-like odor and is used as a flavoring agent and enhancer for carbohydrates generally, to impart a "freshly baked" odor and flavor to breads and cakes. In this respect, its effect has been compared to that of monosodium glutamate on proteins. One of its effects is to intensify the sweet flavor of sugar when added to certain food products in amounts varying from 30 to 3,300 ppm. Its use in the United States has been approved by the FDA.

Ammoniated glycyrrhizin

This compound is a β,β′-glucuronido-glucuronide of glycyrrhetinic acid. It is derived from licorice root (*Glycyrrhiza glabra*). Ammoniated glycyrrhizin has an intensely sweet taste, about 50 times as sweet as sucrose when used alone and 100 times as sweet when used with sucrose. Licorice root extract has been used by pharmacists for years to mask unpleasant-tasting drugs. However, because of its licorice flavor, its usefulness in the food industry is limited. In medicine it has been used as a demulcent, expectorant, and pharmaceutical vehicle.

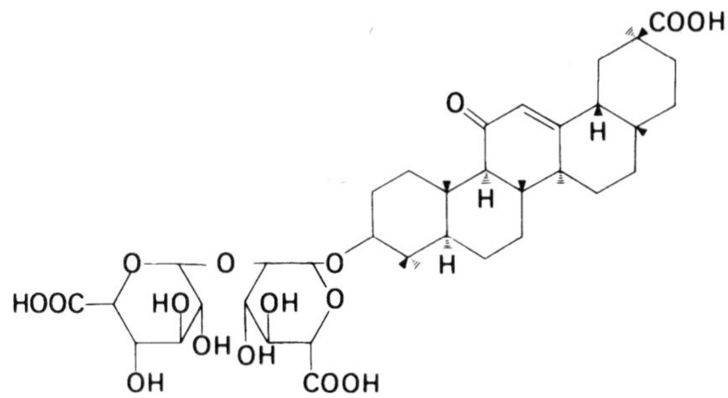

AMMONIATED GLYCYRRHIZIN

Licorice extracts and ammoniated glycyrrhizin reduce the solubility of enamel and prevent a fall in pH during incubation of saliva-glucose mixtures.[45] The latter action may be due to their inhibition of glycolysis and their direct buffering properties.

Neither maltol nor ammoniated glycyrrhizin has as yet been used in sufficient quantities to have had any material effect on the market for sugar or other sweeteners. They are of potential importance in the food industry partly because they affect sweetness.

Stevioside

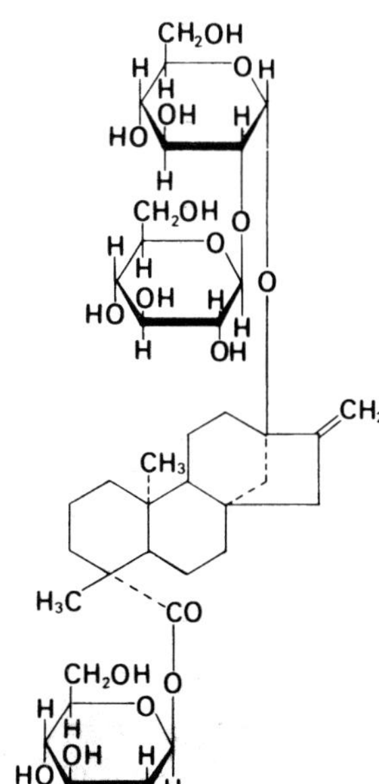

STEVIOSIDE

Stevioside is an intensely sweet, naturally occurring compound found in the leaves of a small shrub, *Stevia rebaudiana* Bertoni, also called *yerba dulce*, which grows wild in Paraguay. It is 300 times sweeter than sucrose.[14]

Stevioside is a steroid glycoside. It is a diterpenoic acid esterified to one glucose unit and combined in glycosidic linkage to two other glucose units. Work by Dorfman and Ness[43] has demonstrated some antiandrogenic activity by steviol and dihydroisosteviol, the diterpinoid acids derived from stevioside.

Dihydrochalcone sweeteners

Citrus fruits contain certain bitter substances known as flavone glycosides or dehydrochalcones. Typical examples are naringin, the chief bitter constituent of grapefruit, and neohesperidin, one of the bitter constituents of Seville oranges. Scientists at the US Department of Agriculture Research Service[155] discovered that when certain of these substances are converted into the closely related dihydrochalcones by hydrogenation in an alkaline solution, the bitterness disappears and is replaced by a sweet taste.

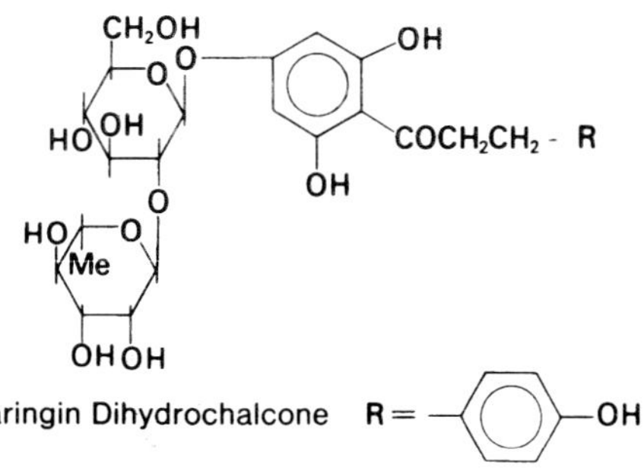

Naringin Dihydrochalcone

The sweetness of the dihydrochalcones (neohesperidin dihydrochalcone, naringin dihydrochalcone, and hesperidin dihydrochalcone) is many times greater than sucrose (see Table 5-1)[92]; however, unlike sugar, the dihydrochalcone sweetness is relatively slow in onset and is lingering. This aftertaste can be described as cooling like menthol, or licoricelike. Although the intense sweetness of neohesperidin dihydrochalcone permits the use of extremely small amounts, the lingering aftertaste presents some problems. The glycoside moiety of the dihydrochalcones is unimportant with regard to taste intensity but serves to make the molecule more soluble in water.[44]

Various combinations of neohesperidin dihydrochalcone (neo DHC) and saccharin appear to give more acceptable taste qualities. Dihydrochalcones are stable over a broad range of temperatures, in aqueous solution, and in acids at normal temperature. They are, therefore, potentially useful in fruit and carbonated beverage products.[80] Neo DHC is manufactured by California Aromatics and Flavors, Inc, and by Nutrilite Products, Inc.

Dihydrochalcones have been fed at high dosage (5% of diet) designed to reveal toxic tendencies. No ill effects have been found in multigeneration rat-feeding studies. Certain biological alterations have been detected when dogs were fed 2 g/kg/day.[67]

Dental aspects

The dehydrochalcones, but not dihydrochalcones, have been studied. In one study some of the flavones, either as the glycoside or aglycone, were fed to rats at the 1% level (sucrose 66%). Hesperidin and hesperetin methylchalcone caused significant reduction in caries.[152] However, in a subsequent study,[149] no significant inhibition of caries was found. Naringenin (0.2%), when used as a dietary supplement, significantly reduced caries in hamsters.[68]

Monellin

Dioscoreophyllum cumminsii Diels is a tropical plant indigenous to Africa. The fruit of this plant is a red berry growing in grapelike clusters and was initially called "serendipity berries" because of the unexpected finding of its intensely sweet properties.[81] The sweet sensation persists in the mouth for an unusual length of time. The sweet principle of these berries has been isolated, shown to be a soluble protein, and named "monellin."[28,111] Monellin is approximately 3,000 times sweeter than sucrose. It is the sweetest natural product known and is the first protein found to elicit a sweet taste. Its composition, structure, and properties have been studied.[112] A serious limitation to the possible industrial use of monellin is the finding that the purified protein, if left standing at room temperature, loses its sweetness within about a day. In some cases the samples became putrified.

Thaumatin

In West Africa the inhabitants have for centuries used an extract of the fruit of a shrub that grows in the rain forest, *Thaumatoccus daniellii,* to sweeten foods such as bread and palm wine.[169] Two major sweet proteins have been identified in the fruit, thaumatin I and II, with almost identical molecular weights of 22,000 and an isoelectric point of 12. They consist of 207 amino acids and have identical amino acid sequences except for five residues. These proteins are about 100,000 times sweeter than sucrose on a molar basis and 3,000 times sweeter on a weight basis. Heat denaturation or splitting of the disulfide bridges of the protein both result in complete loss of sweetness, indicating the importance of the tertiary structure of the proteins for their taste. Antibodies raised against thaumatin cross-react with monellin.

Miraculin

The active principle of miracle fruit, *Synaepalum dulcificum,* is a basic glycoprotein with a molecular weight of approximately 44,000.[22,106] This native shrub in tropical West Africa yields a small red berry that causes sour substances to taste sweet when its pulp is chewed.[81] This modifying effect lasts for some time, usually 1 to 2 hours. The purified glycoprotein itself has no inherent taste. It is believed that the protein binds to the receptors of the taste buds and modifies their function.[94] Activity of the protein is destroyed by heat, limiting its use.

Miraculin was sold as Miralin Miracle Fruit Drops (Miralin Co), to be chewed before meals or snacks. It is effective in sweetening citrus fruits, berries, yogurt, and other sour foods but does not sweeten cereals, cocoa, coffee, etc. However, because manufacturers were unable to document their claims of efficacy in weight control and reduced caloric intake, miraculin has been withdrawn from the market in the United States.

Chlorogenic acid and cynarin

The taste-modifying property of artichoke (*Cynara scolymus*) has been known for some time. Tests have shown that prior rinsing with artichoke extract makes different-tasting compounds (eg, sucrose, citric acid, quinine hydrochloride, and sodium chloride) taste sweeter. Unlike miracle fruit, the sweetening effect is not selective for acids and may affect the common solvent, water.[8] The artichoke-induced sweetness is not as long-lasting as miraculin, lasting for about 4 to 5 minutes. Two compounds, chlorogenic acid (3-caffeoylquinic acid) and cynarin (1,5-dicaffeoylquinic acid), have been isolated from artichoke and shown to be the two major active components responsible for its taste-modifying property. Chlorogenic acid is also present in green coffee beans, fruit, leaves, and

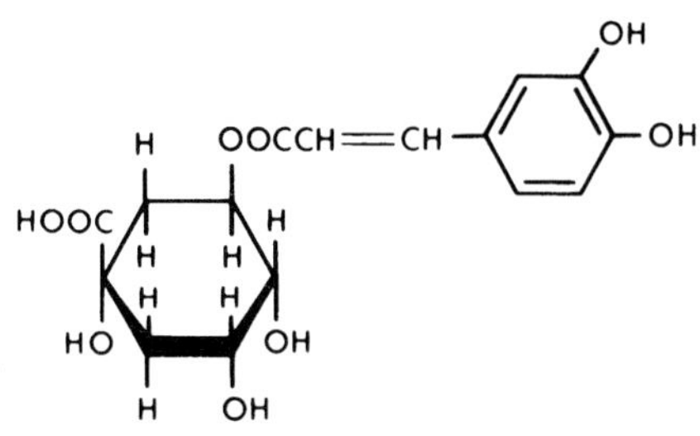

Chlorogenic Acid

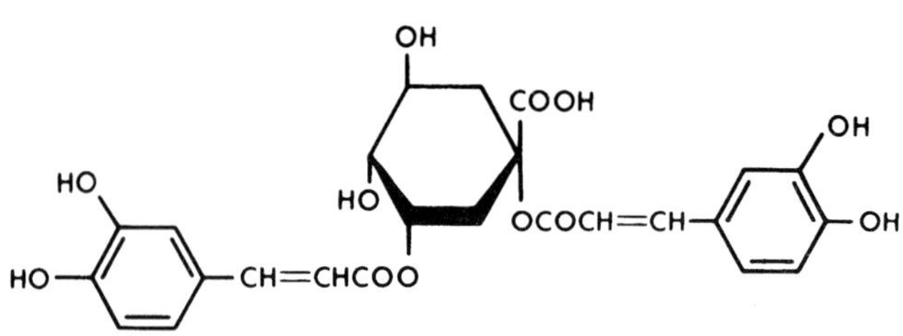

Cynarin

potatoes. Cynarin itself has a sweet taste. Because artichokes are on the GRAS (generally recognized as safe) list of the Food and Drug Administration, these compounds may find potential use as sugar substitutes.

Noncaloric sweetening agents

These are nonnutritive sweetening agents that have no caloric value and are not fermented by microorganisms of the oral cavity. Their principal use has been in the diet of those people, including diabetics, who wish to restrict their caloric intake. They are used in the food and drink industry and in medicinal preparations, dentifrices, and mouthwashes.

Noncaloric sweeteners include a wide variety of compounds. In addition to the well-known saccharin and cyclamate, there are also dulcin, suosan, 1-perillaldehyde α-antioxime, and ultrasüss. The noncaloric sweeteners are generally much sweeter than sucrose (see Table 5-1) and can, therefore, be used in smaller amounts. However, this creates problems for the food manufacturer because of their lack of bulk. Sucrose in high concentrations acts as a preservative; for example, jams contain about 75% sucrose in the liquid phase, and this prevents fungal growth. Substituting for sucrose necessitates higher standards of microbiological cleanliness by the manufacturer.

Saccharin

Discovered accidentally by Remsen and Fahlberg in 1879, saccharin was, until comparatively recently, the sweetest substance known. Saccharin has been widely used as a food additive for more than 80 years and has been preeminent as a substitute for sugar. Its sweet taste is still detectable at 1:100,000 dilution. In excess of 0.1% concentration, it tends to have a bitter taste. Saccharin is pharmacologically inert and untoward effects

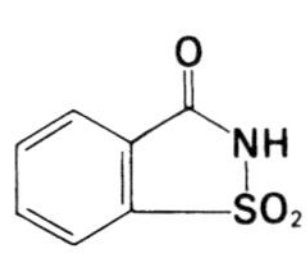

SACCHARIN

are very rare. Cases of photosensitization and allergic reactions such as urticaria have been reported.[108]

Saccharin (*o*-sulfobenzimide, $C_7H_5NO_3S$) is an aromatic organic compound used mainly in the form of its sodium salt. The consumption of saccharin has increased dramatically in many countries. About 70% of the total amount used in the United States and Canada has been used in "diet" soft drinks; 13% in dietetic foods (eg, canned fruits, gelatin desserts, jams, ice cream); 12% in products sold at retail for table use;

and the remaining 5% in miscellaneous products such as mouthwashes, cosmetics, and medicinal preparations.

Saccharin has been available commercially in a variety of forms. Most commonly it has been used as tablets containing 15, 30, or 60 mg of sodium saccharin, National Formulary. Liquid sweeteners contain either the sodium or ammonium salt. As most salts of saccharin are sweet, the taste must be due to the influence of the anion. Several powdered forms have been developed to simulate the bulk and crystalline appearance of sucrose, for example, powders containing 4% saccharin, 94% lactose, and 2% cream of tartar (Sweet 'n Low, Cumberland Packing Corp), or 3.53% calcium saccharin and 90.2% dextrin (Sugar Twin, Alberto Culver, Inc). Other competing products have been Sprinkle Sweet (Pillsbury) and Scoop (General Foods). Gum acacia or gelatin is incorporated to add bulk, the mixture is vacuum-dried, during which a porous cellular structure is induced, and finally the powder is commuted to the appropriate particle size.[136]

Saccharin is stable under most conditions of food preparation and processing, and no loss of sweetening power or development of off-flavors due to instability are encountered.

The off-taste of saccharin, detected by about 25% of the population who are sensitive to it, is intrinsic in the saccharin molecule and is not due to any trace impurities or decomposition products.

Saccharin is excreted almost quantitatively without metabolic alteration, 75% to 90% of it in the urine. Oral dose of 5 to 25 g daily may cause anorexia, nausea, and vomiting. Three studies have demonstrated that high-saccharin diets fed to rats over a long period produce bladder tumors in second-generation rats. In contrast, several studies conducted by feeding saccharin to a single generation of animals from weening until death reported negative or ambiguous results. These findings are not considered absolute proof of saccharin's safety, but they do indicate that, for a wide range of exposure in several species of animals, saccharin did not cause cancer.[125]

In 1972, the FDA set limits on the use of saccharin (1 g/day for a 155-lb person), citing the evidence that rats develop bladder tumors when fed extremely high levels of it. Saccharin was switched from the list of GRAS food additives to the interim regulated additives list. The only legal uses for saccharin were in foods for caloric control. Based on a public forum of the National Academy of Sciences in 1975, evidence was considered insufficient to determine whether saccharin is carcinogenic when administered orally.[37,122] In 1977, following a Canadian study in which experimental rats fed saccharin at 5% of the diet contracted more bladder cancer than did control rats, the FDA proposed a ban on the use of saccharin as a food additive. The possibility of a link between the use of saccharin and the risk of bladder cancer has been investigated; some studies found a weak positive association[74,75] and others found no association.[87,113,170] Two problems in all such studies are the impossibility of assessing the accuracy of the interviewee's responses and the existence of "recall bias." A causal link between use of artificial sweeteners and bladder cancer has not been established by epidemiological standards,[38] nor do the data show a consistent dose-response relationship. In eukaryotic cells, saccharin induces sister chromatid exchanges, which is a sensitive test of mutagenicity.[173] The status of saccharin as a possible over-the-counter product or prescription item is still indeterminate.

Dental aspects

Saccharin (0.5%), when used as a supplement to a cariogenic diet (56% sucrose), significantly reduced both fissure and smooth surface caries in rats, apparently by interfering with the growth of *S mutans*. The caries reductions were associated with initially reduced recovery of *S mutans* soon after saccharin supplementation began. However, the mechanism whereby saccharin inhibits growth of the organism is not understood.

Acesulfame-K

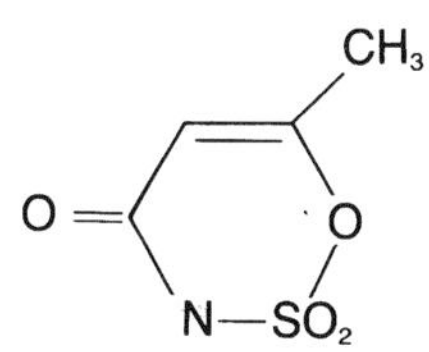

K^+

ACESULFAME-K

In 1967, in the laboratories of Hoechst AG, it was found by chance that compounds with the dihydro-oxathiazinone dioxide ring-system had a sweet taste. The quality of sweetness ranged from barely sweet and metallic to a pure sweet taste, depending on the substituents. Organoleptic properties were also altered according to which cation was in a salt-like bond with the heteronitrogen. For optimum sweetness, 3,4-dihydro-6-methyl-1,2,3 oxathiazine-4-one-2,2-dioxide potassium salt, acesulfame-K (generic name), was selected and patented.[4] In terms of sweetness, it ranks lower than saccharine, is similar to aspartame, and is about 130 times as sweet as sucrose (see Table 5-1). The sweetness is quickly perceptible and does not linger. Acesulfame-K is stable in the temperature, pH, and storage range that is likely to be encountered in foods and beverages.[96] Safety studies have found no evidence of carcinogenicity, mutagenicity, cytotoxicity, or teratogenicity. Pharmacokinetic tests indicate rapid and almost complete absorption. Excretion, preponderantly via the urine, is also complete, because the compound does not accumulate in tissues or organs.

In 1988 the FDA approved acesulfame-K for use in dry food products, including chewing gum, dry mixes for beverages, instant coffee, instant tea, gelatins, puddings, and nondairy creamers.[164] In the United States it will be marketed as Sunette® by Hoechst Celanese Corp. Its estimated cost will approximate that of equivalent sweetness of sucrose. Acesulfame-K has been approved in 20 other countries, where it is also used in soft drinks, candies, toothpastes, mouthwashes, and pharmaceutical preparations.

Cyclamate (cyclohexylsulfamate)

The sweetness of the salt, sodium cyclamate, was discovered accidentally by Michael Sveda at the University of Illinois when he became curious about the taste of a cigarette that he had laid down on some chemicals on the laboratory bench. Cyclamate is about 30 times as sweet as sucrose, has a pleasantly sweet taste, and is freely soluble in water. Commercially it was also produced and sold as the calcium salt and as a compound mixture (ten parts cyclamate, one part saccharin).

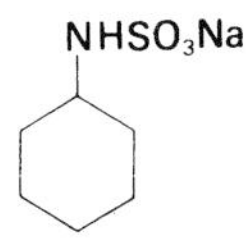

sodium cyclamate

Initially, cyclamate was quite expensive, but improved production processes, greater volume of use, and competition combined to bring the price steadily down. By 1969 it was estimated that three quarters of the population in the United States was consuming some amount of nonnutritive sweeteners. Sixty-four cents worth of cyclamates was equivalent to about $6 worth of sucrose in sweetening effect. There was, therefore, an economic incentive for industry to replace sucrose with the less expensive cyclamate in formulating food products.[154] From 1955, when cyclamate production in the United States was about 1 million pounds, until 1970 when production was in excess of 16 million pounds, the concurrent use of sucrose remained steady.[153] However, between 1947 and 1965, sucrose's share of the total sweetener consumption declined by about 6%, from 87% to 81%.[157]

In numerous acute, short-term, and chronic toxicity studies of cyclamates and of saccharin-cyclamate mixtures in several species of animals, including rats, mice, dogs, monkeys, rabbits, swine, and chickens, no adverse effects were observed *at doses or consumption levels currently taken by humans under practical circumstances.*[46]

Cyclamates at 1% dietary levels produce a minimal laxative effect. Evidence indicates that this effect is attributable to the osmotic action of unabsorbed cyclamate in the intestine. It is not felt that this effect constitutes a hazard because it may only occur occasionally, when high levels are consumed.[15]

Chronic studies in several species of animals (rats, dogs, swine, and chickens) showed that dietary levels of cyclamate in excess of 1% are necessary to suppress growth rate.

Studies in rats at doses of 2.5 g/kg/day (3% dietary levels) and in dogs at doses of up to 1.5 g/kg/day had no effect on reproductive function.

Cyclamate metabolism

When a test dose of cyclamate is given to humans or experimental animals, a large proportion is excreted unchanged. In general, less than 50% is excreted in the urine and more than 50% is excreted in the feces, though there is individual variation.

There is no evidence of accumulation of cyclamate in the body. Cyclamates have been reported to be bound to plasma proteins. There have been reports on the excretion of cyclohexylamine in the urine following oral administration of cyclamate.

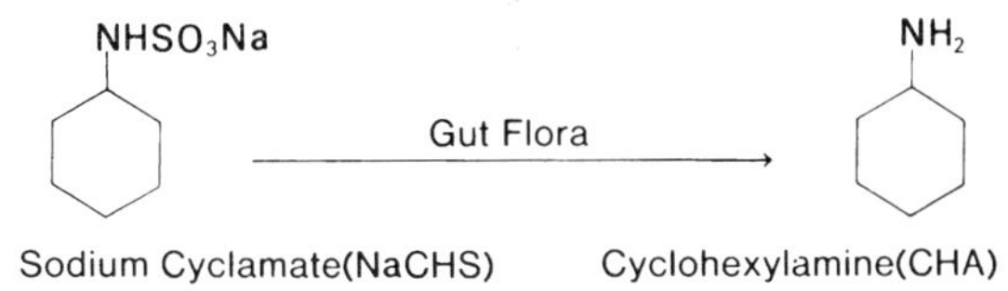

About 25% of humans can convert some of orally ingested cyclamate to cyclohexylamine. It has been established in humans, rats, and pigs that conversion is affected by microbial organisms in the lower intestinal tract.[36] The absolute amount converted increases with increasing cyclamate ingestion but in decreased proportions.

Cyclohexylamine has sympathomimetic effects, possibly mediated through the release of catecholamines. Although they are vasoconstrictors and may be hypertensive agents, it is questionable whether sufficient cyclohexylamine is produced, even by "convertors," to be pharmacologically active. However, the possibility of potentiation of other drugs or adverse effects in certain disease entities should be considered.

The greatest concern arises from the observation that when rats were injected with cyclohexylamine, there was a direct relation between dose concentration and percentage of spermatogonial and bone marrow cells showing chromosomal breaks.[95] Single chromatid breaks predominated with infrequent exchange figures. This type of chromosomal abnormality may have potential mutagenic, teratogenic, and carcinogenic significance. The effects have yet to be determined.

Cyclamate can induce chromosome breaks in both leukocytes and monolayer cultures of human skin and cancer cells in vitro.[148] Saccharin tested in the same system did not increase chromosomal breaks. The demonstration of cytogenetic damage to germinal and somatic cells is presumptive evidence of a genetic hazard.[50]

Carcinogenesis—removal of cyclamates from the market

In October 1969, the Secretary of Health, Education and Welfare (HEW) banned the use of cyclamates in drinks and foods, effective from January 1970.[153] Cyclamates were taken off the GRAS list but remained available to people with such conditions as obesity and diabetes. Cyclamates were no longer classified as "food additives" but as new drugs that require proof of efficacy (eg, that they will cause weight reduction).[131] On August 14, 1970, the sale of all cyclamates was forbidden in the United States. The initial action was taken under the relevant United States legislation—the Food and Drug Amendments of 1958, the so-called Delaney Clause of the Food, Drug and Cosmetics Act. This act requires that any food additive shown to cause cancer in man or any animal at any usage level cannot be marketed for general use.

The ultimate decision to ban cyclamates was based on the finding that cyclamate (and cyclamate-saccharin compound) when embedded with cholesterol in a pellet in mouse bladders, or fed to rats at a dosage 50 times the daily maximum recommended for humans by the World Health Organization, induced bladder cancer. Experiments detected bladder cancer in 7 of 20 male rats thus treated. The animals received daily amounts equivalent to the total cyclamate contained in at least 500 eight-ounce bottles of a typical diet soft drink. The justification for such high dosage was to improve the chances of cancer detection. Solids (eg, sodium stearate) can induce bladder cancer. Furthermore, a common rat bladder parasite also induces cancer.

Although cyclamates and saccharin have been implicated in animal carcinogenesis, there is little evidence linking these agents with human disease. In a patient-control (retrospective) study of transitional cell carcinoma of the urinary bladder and use of these sweeteners, no positive relationship could be established; if anything, cancer patients were less likely than controls to give a history of ingesting diet desserts, diet soft drinks, and noncaloric sweeteners.[110] Cyclamates had been widely used prior to 1970 without any influence on bladder carcinoma rates in the United States.[25] Recently a panel of scientists assembled by the National Cancer Institute reviewed more than 20 new animal-feeding studies and concluded that there was no firm evidence that cyclamate causes cancer, birth defects, or genetic damage. Cyclamate and saccharin may be tumor promoters rather than true carcinogens. In the absence of a carcinogen, animals fed these sweeteners have a low incidence of bladder tumors. However, in animals receiving a single dose of carcinogen and eating diets containing either of these sweeteners, the incidence of bladder tumors was very high.[104] Because of unresolved safety questions as to the risk of cancer in humans, the FDA has maintained the 1969 ban on cyclamates. In 1980, after extensive appeals, Abbott Laboratories (the principal manufacturer) finally dropped efforts to return cyclamate sweeteners to the American market. Cyclamates continue to be sold in Canada and several European and Latin American nations.

The history of the ban on cyclamates is an interesting example of a combination of economic and political pressures and inept government actions.[10] When the sale of noncaloric sweet beverages made significant inroads into the consumption of sucrose-containing drinks, the sugar industry started supporting research into the effects of noncaloric sweeteners. With the findings of carcinogenesis, the Secretary of HEW had no choice in banning the sale of cyclamates as a food additive; nevertheless he delayed implementation of the ban to allow sale of existing stocks of artificially sweetened goods. Obviously, the counter-pressure from the drug industry must have been influential.

The question that must be raised is, why has the sale of tobacco and cigarettes not been banned by the government? Their role in carcinogenesis at human levels of consumption is much better established.[165]

Dulcin (sucrol; valzin; *p*-phenetolcarbamide 4-ethoxyphenylurea)

Dulcin was first synthesized in 1883. It consists of lustrous needles with a very sweet taste, about 250 times as sweet as sucrose. Its solubility is 1 to 800. At one time dulcin was employed as a noncaloric sweetening

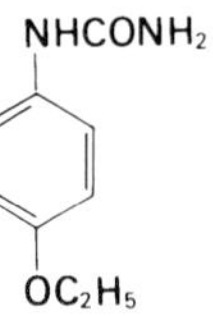

DULCIN

agent. Unfortunately, dulcin was toxic to experimental animals after prolonged consumption, possibly because of amino-phenol produced in vivo. Dulcin is prohibited in the United States and in the United Kingdom. Lethal dose (LD) in dogs, orally: 1.0 g/kg.

Aldoximes

Perillartine (perilla sugar) is about 200 times as sweet as sucrose. Originally studied as a perfume, it was found to have a very sweet taste and has been used as a sweetening agent in Japan. In spite of its insecticidal power, it is harmless to higher animals, especially humans. When ingested, it is conjugated with glucuronic acid and excreted. Perillartine has limited applicability because of its low solubility in water, although it is soluble in alcohol and ether. It is synthesized chemically from the neutral essential oil of pine root oil. LD_{50} orally in rats: 2.5 g/kg.

A systematic search of oximes analogous to the little-used sweetener, perillartine, has revealed a potentially useful new sweetener.[1] This compound, aldoxime V SRI, 4-(methoxymethyl)-1,4-cyclohexadiene-1-carboxaldehyde, *syn*-oxime, has 450 times the sweetening power of sucrose and has good water solubility. Preliminary toxicity and human safety studies have proven favorable, and in vitro tests have shown no evidence of mutagenicity. LD_{50} orally in rats: 1 g/kg.

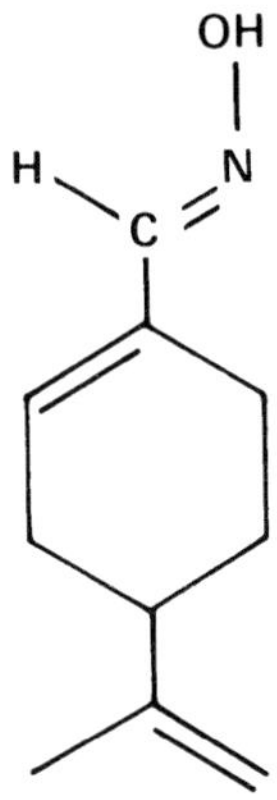

Perillartine

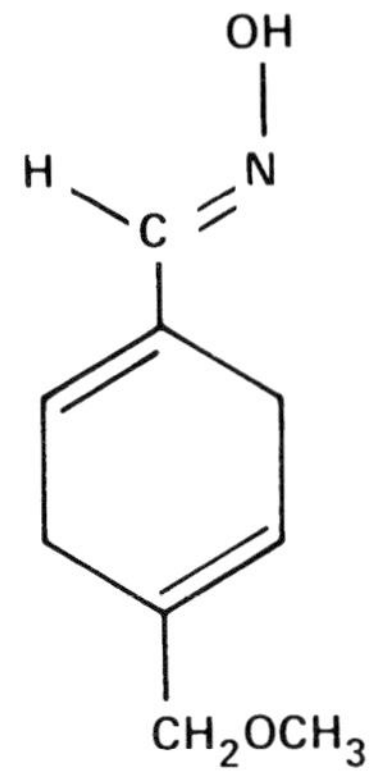

"SRI Oxime V"

5-Nitro-2-propoxyaniline (2-amino-4-nitrophenyl *n*-propyl ether; 1-propoxy-2-amino-4-nitrobenzene; P-4000; ultrasüss)

Ultrasüss is slightly soluble (136 mg/l); it is stable in boiling water and in dilute acid. It is the sweetest substance known, being 4,000 times as sweet as sucrose and leaving no bitter aftertaste. The sweetness depends on the ether substituent (propyl>ethyl>methyl). Acute toxicity data are not available. This compound is used as a sweetener in some European countries but is banned in the United States because of possible carcinogenic effects.

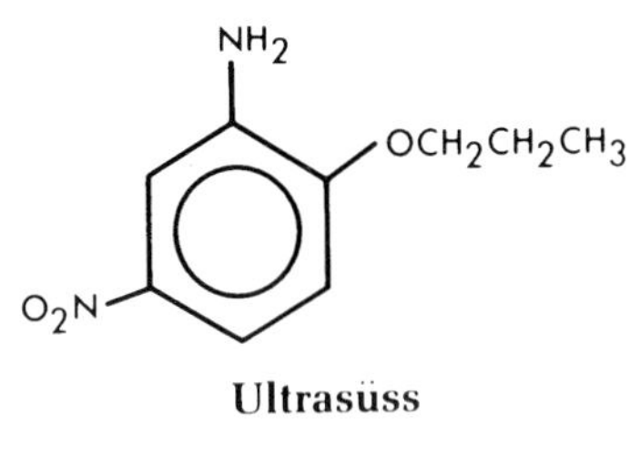

Ultrasüss

Miscellaneous sweet compounds

Compounds such as 6-substituted-tryptophans,[91] 4β, 10α-dimethyl-1,2,3,4,5,10 hexahydrofluorene-4α, 6-dicarboxylic acid,[150] and suosan are very sweet. No industrial applications of these compounds have been established.

Discussion

Consumer acceptance of sugar substitutes and nonnutritive sweeteners depends on the fact that the product will be consumed for its own sake and not as a therapeutic agent or for other special dietary values. Consumers of products containing nonnutritive sweeteners are those who *want* to use them, not those who *must*.[136]

It is virtually impossible to duplicate the flavor, texture, and other characteristics of a sugar-sweetened product with a nonnutritive sweetener. Manufacturers can hope for equal acceptability rather than exact duplication. In baked goods, problems arise of texture development with good flavor. Cookies baked with nonnutritive sweeteners, even with the addition of bulking agents, tend to be hard and tough. In cakes it is extremely difficult to get any reasonable development of moistness, crumb structure, and overall volume. In products such as jams, fruit syrups, and condensed milk, sucrose provides an osmotic preservative protection. If sucrose is replaced, the risk of microbiological spoilage is increased, unless other corrective measures are adopted.[21] Even more stringent microbiological control is required during the manufacturing process in the absence of sucrose.

Some of the problems of texture and bulk may be overcome in the near future by combining the use of sugar substitutes with bulking agents. Polydextrose (Pfizer) is a water-soluble, low-calorie bulking agent that contributes to the bulk and texture normally obtained with sugars in many food products, particularly desserts, confections, and baked goods. Chemically, polydextrose is a randomly bonded polymer of glucose containing minor amounts of sorbitol end groups and bound citric acid; its average molecular weight is 1,500.[12] Polydextrose has been approved by the FDA for use in accordance with good manufacturing practices as a bulking agent, formulation aid, and texturizer in baked goods, baking mixes, chewing gum, confections and frostings, salad dressings, frozen desserts, and hard and soft candy.[161]

In order to be an acceptable sweetener of commercial utility, a substance must:

1. Have sufficient sweetening power
2. Be nontoxic
3. Be reasonably inexpensive
4. Be thermostable (ie, resist cooking temperatures)

Although a fascinating variety of sweet chemicals exist (see Table 5-1), most have no practical use because they do not satisfy all of the above criteria. The demise of cyclamates from the commercial market and the limitation on the amount of saccharin that may be consumed accentuate the problem of what suitable sucrose substitutes a dentist can safely recommend to a highly caries-prone patient. Aspartame is the first sweetener to be approved by the FDA in almost 25 years. A vigorous and continual search for harmless, nonfermentable, acceptable sweeteners is imperative. The latest candidates, the dihydrochalcones, monellin, miraculin, xylitol, aldoxime, and coupling sugar, bear watching. Some dentists do not consider that sugar substitutes are of great importance in a preventive dentistry program. Many may advise their patients who have rampant caries to restrict the frequency of sucrose intake without suggesting any alternatives. This does not solve the problem for people who simply cannot control cravings for candies and sweet foods and continue to overindulge. A safe, noncariogenic sweetener is still very much needed for these patients.

Chapter review

- List the four basic taste modalities.
- State how the sweetness of a substance is measured.
- Rank the common mono- and disaccharides in increasing order of sweetness.
- Give some examples of noncaloric sweetening agents and indicate which is the sweetest.
- Indicate how sorbitol is fermented by *Streptococcus mutans.*
- Indicate which happens faster, acid formation by dental plaque using *(1)* sorbitol or *(2)* other mono- and disaccharides as substrate.
- List the hazards of ingesting excessive amounts of sorbitol.
- Contrast the Lycasin (Roslagen) and xylitol (Turku) sugar studies.
- State the chemical and biological properties of xylitol. Explain its potential role in caries prevention.
- Rank the commercially available sweeteners in increasing order of cost, based on comparable sweetening power.
- Indicate why cyclamates were removed from the GRAS list of food additives.
- State the current annual disappearance of sucrose per capita in the United States, and percentage of total caloric intake this represents.
- State why disappearance of sucrose per capita and consumption of sucrose per capita differ.
- Give the composition, sweetness, uses, and cariogenicity of high-fructose corn syrup and coupling sugar.
- State the composition, sweetness, uses, and other relevant properties of aspartame.
- State, roughly, the proportion of manufactured sucrose used by industry.
- Give some examples of consumable items containing "hidden sugars."

Selected readings

Beck, K.M. 1980. Nonnutritive sweeteners: saccharin and cyclamate. In *CRC Handbook of Food Additives,* 2nd ed, vol. II, T.E. Furia (ed), Cleveland, Ohio: Chemical Rubber Co, pp. 125–185.

Birch, G.G., Green, L.F., and Coulson, C.B. (eds) 1971. *Sweetness and Sweeteners.* London: Applied Science Publications, Ltd.

Crosby, G.A., DuBois, G.E., and Wingard, R.E. 1979. The design of synthetic sweeteners. *Drug Design* 8:215–310.

Crosby, G.A., and Furia, T.E. 1980. New sweeteners. In *CRC Handbook of Food Additives,* 2nd ed, vol. II, T.E. Furia (ed), Cleveland, Ohio: Chemical Rubber Co, pp. 187–227.

Guggenheim, B. (ed) 1979. *Health and Sugar Substitutes.* Basel: S. Karger.

Hough, C.A.M., Parker, K.J., and Vlitos, A.J. (eds) 1979. *Developments in Sweeteners-1.* London: Applied Science Publications, Ltd.

Jukes, T.H. 1986. Sugar and health. *Wld Rev Nutr Diet* 48:137–194.

Morris, J.A. 1976. Sweetening agents from natural sources. *Lloydia* 39:25–38.

Nabors, L. O'B., and Gelardi, R.C. (eds) 1986. *Alternative Sweeteners.* New York: Marcel Dekker.

National Academy of Sciences. 1975. *Sweeteners: Issues and Uncertainties.* Academy Forum. Fourth of a Series. Washington, D.C.

Salant, A. 1972. Nonnutritive sweeteners. In *CRC Handbook on Food Additives,* 2nd ed, T.E. Furia (ed), Cleveland, Ohio: Chemical Rubber Co, pp. 523–585.

Shaw, J.H., and Roussos, G.G. (eds) 1978. *Sweeteners and Dental Caries.* Sp. Suppl., Feeding, Weight and Obesity Abstracts. Washington, D.C.: Information Retrieval, Inc.

Sipple, H.L., and McNutt, K.W. (eds) 1974. *Sugars in Nutrition.* New York: Academic Press.

Stegink, L.D., and Filer, L.J. (eds) 1984. *Aspartame Physiology and Biochemistry.* New York: Marcel Dekker.

Weiffenbach, J.M. (ed) 1977. *Taste and Development. The Genesis of Sweet Preference.* Bethesda, Md.: Department of Health, Education, and Welfare publication No. NIH 77–1068.

References

1. Acton, E.M., and Stone, H. 1976. Potential new artificial sweetener from study of structure-taste relationships. *Science* 193:584–586.
2. American Pharmaceutical Association. 1982. "Sugar-free" preparations by therapeutic category. In *Handbook of Non Prescription Drugs,* 7th ed, Washington, D.C.: American Pharmacological Association, pp. 289–292.
3. Anonymous. 1979. Sugar-free liquid preparations. *American Druggist* July:62–65.
4. Arpe, H.J. 1979. Acesulfame-K, a new noncaloric sweetener. In *Health and Sugar Substitutes,* B. Guggenheim (ed), Basel: S. Karger, pp. 178–183.
5. Aykroyd, W.R. 1967. *Sweet malefactor. Sugar, Slavery and Human Society.* London: Heinemann.
6. Bär, A. 1988. Caries prevention with xylitol. *World Rev Nutr Diet* 55:1–27.
7. Bär, A., and Ritzel, G. (eds) 1985. Xylitol and oxalate. Metabolic studies in animals and man. *Int J Vit Nutrit Res* 55 (Suppl. 28): 1–152.
8. Bartoshuk, L.M., Lee, C.H., and Scarpellino, R. 1972. Sweet taste of water induced by artichoke *(Cynara scolymus). Science* 178:988–989.
9. Batzinger, R.P., Ou, S.Y.L., and Bueding, E. 1977. Saccharin and other sweeteners. Mutagenic properties. *Science* 198:944–946.
10. Bazell, R.J. 1970. Cyclamates. House report charges administrative alchemy at HEW. *Science* 170:419–420.
11. Beck, K.M. 1969. Sweeteners, non-nutritive. In *Encyclopedia of Chemical Technology,* 2nd ed, H. Mark, J. McKetta, and D. Othmer (eds), New York: John Wiley & Sons, pp. 593–607.
12. Beereboom, J.J. 1982. Polydextrose. A low calorie sugar replacement. In *Foods, Nutrition and Dental Health,* vol. 2, J.J. Hefferren and H.M. Koehler (eds), Park Forest South, Ill.: Pathotox Publishers, Inc, pp. 97–106.
13. Beidler, L.M. 1971. The physical basis of the sweet response. In *Sweetness and Sweeteners,* G.G. Birch, L.F. Green, and C.B. Coulson (eds), London: Applied Science Publications, Ltd, pp. 81–94.
14. Bell, F. 1954. Stevioside. A unique sweetening agent. *Chemy Ind* pp. 897–898.

15. Berryman, G.H., Hazel, G.R., Taylor, J.D., Sanders, P.F., and Weinberg, M.S. 1968. A case for safety of cyclamate and cyclamate-saccharin combinations. *Am J Clin Nutr* 21:688–692.
16. Birkhed, D., Edwardsson, S., Alden, M.L., and Frostell, G. 1979. Effects of three months frequent consumption of hydrogenated starch hydrolysate (Lycasin), maltitol sorbitol and xylitol on human dental plaque. *Acta Odontol Scand* 37:103–115.
17. Birkhed, D., Edwardsson, S., Svensson, B., Moskovitz, F., and Frostell, G. 1978. Acid production from sorbitol in human dental plaque. *Arch Oral Biol* 23:971–975.
18. Bosso, J.A., and Pearson, R.E. 1973. Sugar content of selected liquid medicinals. *Diabetes* 22:776–784.
19. Bowen, W.H., Eastoe, J.E., and Cock, D.J. 1966. Effect of sugar solutions on pH of plaque in caries active monkeys. *Arch Oral Biol* 11:833–837.
20. Brody, S., and Wolitzk, D. 1983. Lack of mood changes following sucrose loading. *Psychosomatics* 24:155–162.
21. Brooks, M. 1970. Sugar substitutes and their significance for dental health. *Dent Health* 30:46–52.
22. Brouwer, J.N., van der Wel, H., Francke, A., and Henning, G.J. 1968. Miraculin, the sweetness-inducing protein from miracle fruit. *Nature* 220:373–374.
23. Brown, A.T., and Bowles, R.D. 1977. Polyol metabolism by a caries-conducive *Streptococcus*. Purification and properties of a nicotinamide adenine dinucleotide-dependent mannitol-1-phosphate dehydrogenase. *Infect Immun* 16:163–173.
24. Brown, A.T., and Wittenberger, C.L. 1973. Mannitol and sorbitol catabolism in *Streptococcus mutans*. *Arch Oral Biol* 18:117–126.
25. Burbank, F., and Fraumeni, J.F. 1970. Synthetic sweetener consumption and bladder cancer trends in the United States. *Nature* 227:296–297.
26. Cabanac, M. 1971. Physiological role of pleasure. *Science* 173:1103–1107.
27. Cabanac, M., and Duclaux, R. 1970. Obesity. Absence of satiety aversion to sucrose. *Science* 168:496–497.
28. Cagan, R.H. 1973. Chemostimulatory protein. A new type of taste stimulus. *Science* 181:32–35.
29. Cagan, R.H. 1974. The biochemistry of sweet sensation. In *Sugars in Nutrition*, H.L. Sipple and K.W. McNutt (eds), New York: Academic Press, pp. 19–36.
30. Cameron, A.T. 1947. The taste sense and relative sweetness of sugars and other sweet substances. Science Report Series No. 9. New York: Sugar Research Foundation.
31. Carlsson, J. 1968. A numerical taxonomic study of human oral streptococci. *Odontol Revy* 19:137–160.
32. Cantor, S.M. 1978. Patterns of use of sweeteners. In *Sweeteners and Dental Caries*, J.H. Shaw and G.G. Roussos (eds), Feeding, Weight and Obesity Abstracts (Suppl.), Washington, D.C.: Information Retrieval, Inc, pp. 111–129.
33. Charlton, G., Fitzgerald, R.J., and Keyes, P.H. 1971. Hydrogen ion activity in dental plaque of hamsters during metabolism of sucrose, glucose and fructose. *Arch Oral Biol* 16:655–662.
34. Clark, R., Hay, D.I., Schram, C.J., and Wagg, B.J. 1961. Removal of carbohydrate debris from teeth by salivary stimulation. *Br Dent J* 111:244–48.
35. Cloninger, M.R., and Baldwin, R.E. 1970. Aspartylphenylalanine methyl ester. A low-calorie sweetener. *Science* 170:81–82.
36. Collings, A.J. 1971. The metabolism of sodium cyclamate. In *Sweetness and Sweeteners*, G.G. Birch, L.F. Green, and C.B. Coulson (eds), London: Applied Science Publications, Ltd, pp. 51–68.
37. Coon, J.M. 1975. Saccharin toxicology. In *Sweeteners: Issues and Uncertainties*, Academy Forum. Fourth of a Series. Washington, D.C.: National Academy of Science, pp. 133–140.
38. Cordle, F., and Miller, S.A. 1984. Using epidemiology to regulate food additives: saccharin case-control studies. *Pub Hlth Rep* 99:365–369.
39. Cornick, D.E.R., and Bowen, W.H. 1972. The effect of sorbitol on the microbiology of dental plaque in monkeys *(M. irus)*. *Arch Oral Biol* 17:1637–1648.
40. Dalderup, L.M., and Visser, W. 1969. Influence of extra sucrose in daily food on the life span of Wistra albino rats. *Nature* 222:1050–1052.
41. Dastoli, F.R., and Price, S. 1966. Sweet-sensitive protein from bovine taste buds. Isolation and assay. *Science* 154:905–907.
42. Deutsch, E.W., and Hansch, C. 1966. Dependence of relative sweetness of hydrophobic bonding. *Nature* 211:75.
43. Dorfman, R.I., and Ness, W.R. 1960. Anti-androgenic activity of dihydroisosteviol. *Endocrinology* 67:282–285.

44. DuBois, G.E., Crosby, G.A., and Saffron, P. 1977. Nonnutritive sweeteners. Taste-structure relationships for some new simple dihydrochalcones. *Science* 195:397–399.
45. Edgar, W.M. 1978. Reduction in enamel dissolution by licorice and glycyrrhizinic acid. *J Dent Res* 57:59–64.
46. Editorial. 1969. More on cyclamates. *Am J Clin Nutr* 22:228–231.
47. Edwardsson, S. 1968. Characteristics of caries-inducing human streptococci resembling *Streptococcus mutans*. *Arch Oral Biol* 13:637–646.
48. Elwood, P.C., Waters, W.E., Moore, S., and Sweetnam, P. 1970. Sucrose consumption and ischaemic heart disease in the community. *Lancet* 1:1014–1016.
49. Emslie, R.D., and Sinclair, L. 1961. Effect on dental caries of sorbitol in the diet of sialadenectomized rats. *J Dent Res* 40:1283.
50. Epstein, S.S., Hollaender, A., Lederberg, J., Legator, M., Richardson, H., and Wolff, A.H. 1969. Wisdom of cyclamate ban. *Science* 166:1575.
51. Estoe, J.E., and Bowen, W.H. 1967. Some factors affecting pH measurements on tooth surfaces in monkeys. *Caries Res* 1:59–68.
52. Feigal, R.J., Jensen, M.E., and Mensing, C.A. 1981. Dental caries potential of liquid medications. *Pediatrics* 68:416–419.
53. Feigal, R.J., Gleeson, M.C., Beckman, T.M., and Greenwood, M.E. 1984. Dental caries related to liquid medication intake in young cardiac patients. *J Dent Child* 51:360–362.
54. Fewkes, D.W., Parker, K.J., and Vlitos, A.J. 1971. Sucrose. *Sci Prog* 59:25–39.
55. Frostell, G. 1964. Quantitative determination of the acid production from different carbohydrates in suspension of dental plaque material. *Acta Odontol Scand* 22: 457–475.
56. Frostell, G. 1965. Substitution of fermentable sugars in sweets. In *Nutrition and Caries Prevention*, G. Blix (ed), *Symposia of Swedish Nutrition Foundation III*, pp. 60–66.
57. Frostell, G. 1971. The caries-inducing properties of Lycasin in comparison to sucrose. *Dtsch Zahnaertzl Z* 26:1181–1187.
58. Frostell, G., Blomlöf, L., Blomqvist, T., Dahl, G.M., Edward, S., Fjellstöm, A., Henrikson, C.O., Larje, O., Nord, C.E., and Nordenvall, K.J. 1974. Substitution of sucrose by Lycasin® in candy. "The Roslagen Study." *Acta Odontol Scand* 32:235–254.
59. Frostell, G., Keyes, P.H., and Larson, R.H. 1967. Effect of various sugars and sugar substitutes on dental caries in hamsters and rats. *J Nutr* 93:65–76.
60. Glinsmann, W.H., Irausquin, H., and Park, Y.K. 1986. Evaluation of the health aspects of sugars contained in carbohydrate sweeteners. Report of sugars task force. *J Nutrit* 116(Suppl. 11): S1–S216.
61. Grande, F. 1975. Sugar and cardiovascular disease. *World Rev Nutr Diet* 22:248–269.
62. Grunberg, E., Beskid, G., and Brin, M. 1973. Xylitol and dental caries. Efficacy of xylitol in reducing dental caries in rats. *Int J Vitam Nutr Res* 43:227–232.
63. Gryboski, J.D. 1966. Diarrhea from dietetic candy. *N Engl J Med* 275:718.
64. Guggenheim, B. 1968. Streptococci of dental plaque. *Caries Res* 2:147–163.
65. Gülzow, H.J. 1968. *Comparative Biochemical Studies on the Degradation of Sorbitol by Oral Microorganisms*. Thesis. Munich: Carl Hanser Verlag.
66. Gülzow, H.J. 1971. Sorbitabbau in Speichel und in den Zahnbelagen des Menschen. *Dtsch Zahnaerztl Z* 26:1121–1128.
67. Gumbman, M.R., and Gould, D.H. 1977. Two-year study of neohesperidin dihydrochalcone in dogs. Report, West. Reg. Res. Center, U.S. Department of Agriculture.
68. Gustafsson, B.E., and Krasse, B. 1958. The caries reducing effect of naringenin and protamine in hamsters. *Acta Odontol Scand* 16:355–361.
69. Gutschmidt, J., and Ordynsky, G. 1961. Bestimmung des Süssungsgrades von Xylit. *Dtsch Lebansm Rundschau* 12:321.
70. Haaren, M.R.T. van, and Lukassen, J. 1973. Cariogenicity of sugar substitutes. Limitation of frequency controlled feeding in rats. *J Dent Res* 52:602–603.
71. Harper, A.E. 1975. Aspartame. In *Sweeteners: Issues and Uncertainties*, Academy Forum. Fourth of a Series. Washington, D.C.: National Academy of Science, pp. 182–188, 193–195.
72. Hockett, R.C. 1950. "Natural" and refined sugars. *J Calif State Dent Assoc, Nevada State Dent Assoc* 26:72–84.
73. Hollingsworth, D.F., and Greaves, J.P. 1967. Consumption of carbohydrates in the United Kingdom. *Am J Clin Nutr* 20:65–72.
74. Hoover, R.N., and Strasser, P.H. 1980. Artificial sweeteners and human bladder cancer. *Lancet* 1:837–840.
75. Howe, G.R., Burch, J.D., Miller, A.B., Morrison, B., Gordon, P., Weldon, L., Chambers, L.W., Fodor, G., and Winsor, G.M. 1977. Artificial sweeteners and human

bladder cancer. *Lancet* 2:578–581.
76. Ikeda, T. 1982. Sugar substitutes. Reasons and indications for their use. *Int Dent J* 32:33–43.
77. Ikeda, T., Shiota, T., McGhee, J.R., Otake, S., Michalek, S.M., Ochiai, K., Hirasawa, S., and Sugimoto, K. 1978. Virulence of *Streptococcus mutans*. Comparison of the effects of a coupling sugar and sucrose on certain metabolic activities and cariogenicity. *Infect Immun* 19:477–480.
78. Imfeld, T. 1977. Evaluation of the cariogenicity of confectionery by intra-oral wire telemetry. *Helv Odontol Acta* 21:437–464.
79. Imfeld, T., and Mühlemann, H.R. 1977. Evaluation of sugar substitutes in preventive cariology. *J Prev Dent* 4:8–14.
80. Inglett, G.E., Krbechek, L., Dowling, B., and Wagner, R. 1969. Dihydrochalcone sweeteners—sensory and stability evaluation. *J Food Sci* 34:101–103.
81. Inglett, G.E., and May, J.F. 1968. Tropical plants with unusual taste properties. *Econ Bot* 22:326–331.
82. Isokangas, P. 1987. Xylitol chewing gum in caries prevention. A longitudinal study on Finnish school children. *Proc Finn Dent Soc* 83(Suppl. 1):1–117.
83. Jenkins, G.N. 1966. The refinement of food and caries. *Adv Oral Biol* 2:67–100.
84. Kandelman, D., Bär, A., and Hefti, A. 1988. Collaborative WHO xylitol field study in French Polynesia. I. Baseline prevalence and 32-month caries increment. *Caries Res* 22:55–62.
85. Kandelman, D., and Gagnon, G. 1987. Clinical results after 12 months from a study of the incidence and progression of dental caries in relation to consumption of chewing-gum containing xylitol in school preventive programs. *J Dent Res* 66:1407–1411.
86. Karle, E., and Büttner, W. 1971. Kariesbefall im Tieversuch nach Verabreichung von Sorbit, Xylit, Lycasin und Calciumsaccharosephosphat. *Dtsch Zahnaerztl Z* 26:1097–1108.
87. Kessler, I.I., and Clark, J.P. 1978. Saccharin, cyclamate and human bladder cancer. *J Am Med Assoc* 240:349–355.
88. Keyes, P.H. 1969. Present and future measures for dental caries control. *J Am Dent Assoc* 79:1395–1404.
89. Kieckenbuch, W., Gziem, W., and Lang, K. 1961. Die Verwertbarkeit von Xylit als Nahrungskohlenhydrat und seine Verträglichkeit. *Klin Wochenschr* 39:447–448.
90. Kitahata, S., and Okada, S. 1975. Transfer action of cyclodextrin glycosyltransferase on starch. *Agr Biol Chem* 39:2185–2191.
91. Kornfeld, E.C., Suarez, T., Edie, R., Brannon, D.R., Fukada, D., Sheneman, J., Todd, G.C., and Secondino, M. 1974. 6-Substituted-tryptophans, a new class of potent synthetic sweetening agents. 167th Meeting. American Chemical Society, Los Angeles, Calif., Abstr. 41.
92. Krbechek, L., Inglett, G., Holik, M., Dowling, B., Wagner, R., and Riter, R. 1968. Dihydrochalcones. Synthesis of potentially sweetening agents. *J Agr Food Chem* 16:108–112.
93. Kurihara, K., and Beidler, L.M. 1968. Taste modifying protein from miracle fruit. *Science* 161:1241–43.
94. Kurihara, K., and Beidler, L.M. 1969. Mechanisms of action of taste modifying protein. *Nature* 222:1176–1179.
95. Legator, M.S., Palmer, K.A., Green, S., and Petersen, K.W. 1969. Cytogenic studies in rats in cyclohexylamine, a metabolite of cyclamate. *Science* 165:1139–1140.
96. Lipinski, G.W. 1986. Acesulfame-K. In *Alternative Sweeteners*, L. O'Brien Nabors and R.C. Gelardi (eds), New York: Dekker, pp. 89–102.
97. Loesche, W.J., Earnest, R., Grossman, N.S., and Corpron, R. 1984. The effect of chewing xylitol gum on the plaque and saliva levels of *Streptococcus mutans*. *J Am Dent Assoc* 108:587–592.
98. Mahdihassan, S. 1981. A comparative study of the word sugar and its equivalence in Hindustani and as traceable to Chinese. *Am J Chinese Med* 9:187–192.
99. Mäkinen, K.K. 1972. Enzyme dynamics of a cariogenic streptococcus. The effect of xylitol and sorbitol. *J Dent Res* 51:403–408.
100. Mäkinen, K.K. 1972. The role of sucrose and other sugars in the development of dental caries. A review. *Int Dent J* 22:363–386.
101. Mäkinen, K.K. 1985. New biochemical aspects of sweeteners. *Int Dent J* 35:23–35.
102. Mäkinen, K.K., and Scheinin, A. 1975. Turku sugar studies. The administration of the trial and the control of the dietary regimen. *Acta Odontol Scand* 33 (Suppl. 70): 105–127.

103. Martinsson, T. 1973. Socio-odontologic investigation of school children with high and low caries frequency. *Odontol Revy* 24 (Suppl. 24): 1–23.
104. Marx, J.L. 1978. Tumor promoters. Carcinogenesis gets more complicated. *Science* 201:515–518.
105. Mazur, R.H., Goldkamp, A.H., James, P.A., and Schlatter, J.M. 1970. Structure-taste relationships of aspartic acid amides. *J Med Chem* 130:1217–1221.
106. Mazur, R.H., Schlatter, J.M., and Goldkamp, A.H. 1969. Structure-taste relationships of some dipeptides. *J Am Chem Soc* 91:2684–2691.
107. Mellinghoff, C.H. 1961. Über die Verwendbarkeit des Xylit als Ersatzzucker bei Diabetikern. *Klin Wochenschr* 39:447.
108. Miller, R., White, L.W., and Schwartz, H.J. 1974. A case of episodic urticaria due to saccharin ingestion. *J Allergy Clin Immunol* 53:240–242.
109. Moncrieff, R.W. 1967. *The Chemical Senses.* Cleveland, Ohio: CRC Press, pp. 486–543.
110. Morgan, R.W., and Jain, M.G. 1974. Bladder cancer, beverages and artificial sweeteners. *Can Med Assoc J* 11:1067–1070.
111. Morris, J.A., and Cagan, R.H. 1972. Purification of monellin, the sweet principle of *Dioscoreophyllum cumminsii. Biochim Biophys Acta* 261:114–122.
112. Morris, J.A., Martenson, R., Deibler, G., and Cagan, R.H. 1973. Characterization of monellin, a protein that tastes sweet. *J Biol Chem* 248:534–539.
113. Morrison, A.S., and Buring, J.E. 1980. Artificial sweeteners and cancer of the lower urinary tract. *N Engl J Med* 302:537–541.
114. Moskowitz, H.R., Kluter, R.A., Westerling, J., and Jacobs, H.L. 1974. Sugar sweetness and pleasantness. Evidence for different psychological laws. *Science* 184:583–585.
115. Moskowitz, H.R. 1978. Psychological correlates of sugar consumption. In *Health and Sugar Substitutes,* B. Guggenheim (ed), Basel: S. Karger, pp. 10–16.
116. Mouton, C., Scheinin, A., and Mäkinen, K.K. 1975. Effect on plaque of a xylitol-containing chewing-gum. *Acta Odontol Scand* 33:27–31.
117. Mühlemann, H.R. 1969. Sucrose-free, tooth protective and noncariogenic bonbons and sweets. *Schweiz Monatschr Zahnheilkd* 79:117–45.
118. Mühlemann, H.R., and De Boever, J. 1970. Radiotelemetry of the pH of interdental areas exposed to various carbohydrates. In *Dental Plaque,* W.M. McHugh (ed), Edinburgh: Livingstone Press, pp. 179–186.
119. Mühlemann, H.R., Regolati, B., and Marthaler, T.M. 1970. The effect on rat fissure caries of xylitol and sorbitol. *Helv Odontol Acta* 14:48–50.
120. Mühlemann, H.R., Schmid, R., Noguchi, T., Imfeld, T., and Hirsch, R.S. 1977. Some dental effects of xylitol under laboratory and in vivo conditions. *Caries Res* 11: 263–276.
121. Muller, E.G. 1972. The sugar industry. In *Quality Control in the Food Industry,* vol. 3, S.M. Herschdoerfer (ed), New York: Academic Press, pp. 227–258.
122. Munro, I.C., Stavrie, B., and Lacombe, R. 1974. The current status of saccharin. In *Toxicology Annual,* C.L. Winek and S.P. Shanor (eds), New York: Marcel Dekker, pp. 71–91.
123. Newbrun, E. 1967. Sucrose, the arch criminal of dental caries. *Odontol Revy* 18: 373–386.
124. Newbrun, E., Hoover, C., Mettraux, G., and Graf, H. 1980. Comparison of dietary habits and dental health of subjects with hereditary fructose intolerance and control subjects. *J Am Dent Assoc* 101:619–626.
125. Newel, G.R. 1981. Artificial sweeteners and cancer. In *Nutrition and Cancer: Etiology and Treatment,* G.R. Newel and N.M. Ellison (eds), New York: Raven Press, pp. 273–278.
126. Nilsson, B., Holm, A.-K., and Sjöström, R. 1982. Taste thresholds, preferences for sweet taste and dental caries in 15-year-old children. *Swed Dent J* 6:21–27.
127. Nizel, A.E. 1981. *Nutrition in Preventive Dentistry: Science and Practice.* 2nd ed. Philadelphia: W.B. Saunders, pp. 453–475.
128. Nordsieck, F.W. 1972. The sweet tooth. *Am Sci* 60:41–45.
129. Olney, J.W. 1975. Another view of aspartame. In *Sweeteners: Issues and Uncertainties,* Academy Forum. Fourth of a Series. Washington, D.C.: National Academy of Science, pp. 189–195.
130. Paul, O., MacMillan, A., McCean, H., and Park, H. 1968. Sucrose intake and coronary heart disease. *Lancet* 2:1049–51.
131. Pines, W.L. 1975. The cyclamate story. *FDA Consumer* 8:19–27.
132. Rateitschak-Pluss, E.M., and Guggenheim, B. 1982. Effect of a carbohydrate-free diet and sugar substitutes on dental plaque accumulation. *J Clin Periodontol* 9:

239–251.

133. Roberts, I.F., and Roberts, G.J. 1979. Relationship between medicine sweetened with sucrose and dental disease. *Br Med J* 2:14–16.
134. Roe, F.J.C. 1984. Perspectives in carbohydrate toxicology with special reference to carcinogenicity. *Swed Dent J* 8:99–111.
135. Rosenmann, E., Teitelbaum, A., and Cohen, A.M. 1971. Nephropathy in sucrose-fed rats. *Diabetes* 20:803–810.
136. Salant, A. 1972. Non-nutritive sweeteners. In *CRC Handbook on Food Additives*, 2nd ed, T.E. Furia (ed), Cleveland, Ohio: Chemical Rubber Co, pp. 523–585.
137. Scheinin, A., and Banoczy, J. 1985. Xylitol and caries: the collaborative WHO oral disease preventive programme in Hungary. *Int Dent J* 35:50–57.
138. Scheinin, A., and Mäkinen, K.K. 1972. Effect of sugars and sugar mixtures on dental plaque. *Acta Odontol Scand* 30:235–257.
139. Scheinin, A., and Mäkinen, K.K. 1975. Turku sugar studies. I-XXI. *Acta Odontol Scand* 33:Suppl. 70.
140. Schiffman, S.S., Buckley, C.E., Sampson, H.A., Massey, E.W., Baraniuk, J.N., Follett, J.V., and Warwick, Z.S. 1987. Aspartame and susceptibility to headache. *N Engl J Med* 317:1181–1185.
141. Selby, K., and Taggart, J. 1971. The industrial potential of cereal-based sweeteners. In *Sweetness and Sweeteners*, G.G. Birch, L.F. Green, and C.B. Coulson (eds), London: Applied Science Publications, Ltd, pp. 130–138.
142. Shallenberger, R.S. 1971. Molecular structure and taste. In *Gustation and Olfaction*, G. Ohloff and A.F. Thomas (eds), New York: Academic Press, pp. 126–232.
143. Shallenberger, R.S., and Acree, T.E. 1967. Molecular theory of sweet taste. *Nature* 216:480–482.
144. Shannon, I.L., and Edmonds, E.J. 1977. The physician's role in reducing patients' exposure to sucrose. *Tex Med* 73:52–58.
145. Shaw, J.H., and Griffiths, D. 1960. Partial substitution of hexitols for sucrose and dextrin in caries-producing diets. *J Dent Res* 39:377–384.
146. Souney, P.F., Cyr, D.A., Chang, J.T., and Kaul, A.F. 1983. Sugar content of selected pharmaceuticals. *Diabetes Care* 6:231–240.
147. Sreebny, L.M. 1982. Sugar availability, sugar consumption and dental caries. *Community Dent Oral Epidemiol* 10:1–7.
148. Stone, R., Lamson, E., Chang, Y.S., and Pickering, K.W. 1969. Cytogenetic effects of cyclamates on human cells in vitro. *Science* 164:568–569.
149. Strålfors, A. 1967. Inhibition of hamster caries by phenolic compounds. *Arch Oral Biol* 12:1375–1378.
150. Tahara, A., Nakata, T., and Ohtsuka, Y. 1971. New type of compound with strong sweetness. *Nature* 233:619–620.
151. Tanzer, J.M., and Slee, A.M. 1983. Saccharin inhibits tooth decay in laboratory models. *J Am Dent Assoc* 106:331–333.
152. Thomson, D.T., Vogel, J.J., and Phillips, P.H. 1965. Certain organic substances and their effect upon the incidence of dental caries in the cotton rat. *J Dent Res* 44: 596–599.
153. U.S. Congress, House Committee on Government Operations. 1970. *Cyclamate Sweeteners, Hearing Before a Subcommittee on Government Operations*. June 10, 1970. 91st Cong., 2nd Session, Washington, D.C.: U.S. Government Printing Office.
154. U.S. Congress, House Committee on Government Operations. 1970. *Regulation of Cyclamate Sweeteners*. Oct. 8, 1970. House Report 91–1585. 91st Cong., 2nd Session, Washington, D.C.: U.S. Government Printing Office, p. 3.
155. U.S. Department of Agriculture, Agricultural Research Service. 1968. *Dihydrochalcone Sweeteners*. CA 74-18. June. Washington, D.C.: U.S. Government Printing Office.
156. U.S. Department of Agriculture, Economic Research Service. 1965. *The Sweetener Market—Trends and Prospects*. NFS 114. November. Washington, D.C.: U.S. Government Printing Office.
157. U.S. Department of Agriculture, Economic Research Service. 1967. *Noncaloric Sweeteners: Their Position in the Sweetener Industry*. AER 113. May. Washington, D.C.: U.S. Government Printing Office.
158. U.S. Department of Agriculture, Economic Research Service.1968. *Food Consumption. Prices, Expenditures*. Washington, D.C.: U.S. Government Printing Office.
159. U.S. Department of Agriculture, Economics and Statistics Service. 1981. *Sugar and Sweetener Report* 6:1–49.
160. U.S. Department of Health and Human Services, Food and Drug Administration. 1981. Aspartame. Commissioner's final decision. *Federal Register* 46:38285–38308.

161. U.S. Department of Health and Human Services, Food and Drug Administration. 1981. Polydextrose. Food additives permitted for direct addition to food for human consumption. *Federal Register* 46:30080–30081.
162. U.S. Department of Health and Human Services, Food and Drug Administration. 1986. Food additives permitted for direct addition to food for human consumption: aspartame. *Federal Register* 51:42999–43002.
163. U.S. Department of Health and Human Services, Food and Drug Administration. 1987. Aspartame as an inactive ingredient in human drug products: labeling requirements. *Federal Register* 52:2108–2111.
164. U.S. Department of Health and Human Services, Food and Drug Administration. 1988. Food additives permitted for direct addition to food for human consumption: acesulfame potassium. *Federal Register* 53:28379–28383.
165. U.S. Department of Health, Education, and Welfare. 1971. *The Health Consequences of Smoking.* A report to the Surgeon General. Washington, D.C.: U.S. Government Printing Office.
166. U.S. Department of Health, Education, and Welfare, Food and Drug Administration. 1974. Aspartame. *Federal Register* 39:27317–27320.
167. U.S. Senate. 1973. *Sugar in Diet, Diabetes and Heart Diseases.* Hearings before the Select Committee on Nutrition and Human Needs. April 30, May 1–2, 1973. Washington, D.C.: U.S. Government Printing Office, p. 146.
168. U.S. Senate. 1977. *Dietary Goals for the United States.* Select Committee on Nutrition and Human Needs. Washington, D.C.: U.S. Government Printing Office.
169. van der Wel, H. 1971. Thaumatin, the sweet-tasting protein from *Thaumatococcus daniellii* Benth. Olfaction and Taste. IV. D. Schneider (ed). Proceedings 4th International Symposium, pp. 226–233.
170. Walker, A.M., Dryer, N.A., Friedlander, E., Loughlin, J., Rothman, K.J. and Kohn, H.I. 1982. An independent analysis on non-nutritive sweeteners and bladder cancer. *Am J Public Health* 72:376–381.
171. Washüttl, J., Riederer, P., and Bancher, E. 1973. A qualitative and quantitative study of sugar-alcohols in several foods. *J Food Sci* 38:1262–1263.
172. Winter, G.B. 1968. Sucrose and cariogenesis. *Br Dent J* 124:407–411.
173. Wolff, S., and Rodin, B. 1978. Saccharin-induced sister chromatid exchanges in Chinese hamster and human cells. *Science* 200:543–545.
174. Yamada, T., Igarashi, K., and Mitsutomi, M. 1980. Evaluation of cariogenicity of glycosylsucrose by a new method to measure pH and under human dental plaque in situ. *J Dent Res* 59:2157–2162.
175. Yamada, T., Kimura, S., and Igarashi, K. 1980. Metabolism of glucosylsucrose and maltosylsucrose by *Streptococcus mutans. Caries Res* 14:239–247.
176. Yudkin, J. 1968. Dietary intake of carbohydrate in relation to diabetes and atherosclerosis. In *Carbohydrate Metabolism and Its Disorders*, F. Dickens, P.J. Randle, and W.J. Whelan (eds), New York: Academic Press, pp. 169–184.
177. Yudkin, J. 1969. Dental decay is preventable. Why not prevented? *Br Dent J* 127: 425–429.
178. Yudkin, J. 1972. *Sweet and Dangerous.* New York: P.H. Wyden, Inc.
179. Yudkin, J., and Morland, S. 1967. Sugar intake and myocardial infarction. *Am J Clin Nutr* 20:503–506.
180. Zengo, A.N., and Mandel, I.D. 1972. Sucrose tasting and dental caries in man. *Arch Oral Biol* 17:605–607.
181. Zöllner, N., and Wolfram, G. 1973. Sucrose in human nutrition. In *The Role of Sugar in Modern Nutrition,* Naringsforskning 17 (Suppl. 9):22–25.

Chapter 6

Dental Deposits

Then Job answered and said . . .
and I am escaped with the skin of my teeth.

Job 19:20

On eruption, teeth are covered by organic structures of embryonic origin. These structures usually are soon worn away, although remnants may be retained. Shortly after eruption, organic deposits form on the surfaces of teeth. These acquired deposits contain substances such as organic acids, bacterial antigens, cytotoxic agents, and hydrolytic enzymes, which are capable of causing dental caries or periodontal disease.[244] It is now known that significant differences exist, particularly in the microflora, between odontopathic and periodontopathic deposits.[87,240] Bibby[10] emphasized the considerable variations in the nature of the organic layerings on tooth surfaces:

> What is truly remarkable is the continuing tendency of so many . . . to attribute to plaque a uniformity of structure and function which surely does not exist.

In the fourth century BC, Aristotle related soft, adherent food deposits to tooth decay, but it was not until the advent of the microscope in the seventeenth century that "animalcules" (microorganisms) were seen in these dental deposits. Antony van Leeuwenhoek, a draper and sheriff's chamberlain in Delft, recognized the limitations of mechanical oral hygiene in removing these deposits.[41]

> Yet notwithstanding, my teeth are not so cleaned thereby (rubbing with rag and salt) but what there sticketh or groweth between my front ones and my grinders a *little white matter* which is as thick as if 'twere wetted flour. [Italics added.]

Van Leeuwenhoek saw large numbers of living (motile) cells in scrapings from teeth[41]:

> I judge for myself (howbeit I clean my mouth like I've already said) that all the people living in our United Netherlands are not as many as the living animalcules that I carry in my own mouth this very day.

Subsequent descriptions of these microbial deposits on teeth refer to "a slime coating of *denticolae*" (Ficinus, 1847) and "coatings of leptothrix" (Leber and Rottenstein, 1867). In 1897, Williams demonstrated microscopically the presence of a thick, feltlike mass of microorganisms covering the surface where decay had started.[258] The following year G. V. Black introduced the term *gelatinous microbial plaque* to describe microbial colonies on the surface of teeth.[18]

In recent years dental plaque has been investigated morphologically, microbiologically, immunologically, and chemically. It has been the theme of numerous workshops and symposia* as well as the subject of frequent reviews.† The attention devoted to dental plaque is a reflection of important new developments and insights concerning its role in dental diseases. Supragingival and fissure plaques play an integral role in the caries process, and subgingival plaques are necessary for the development of periodontal disease.

Terminology

Many names have been given to the organic materials or structures on the surface of teeth, including several broad terms such as "tooth accumulated materials,"[206] "dental surface coatings,"[115] and "dental deposits."[206] Before consideration of the specific structures, some related terms frequently used in the past are defined (*Random House Dictionary*, 1966):

Accretion:	an increase by natural growth or by gradual external addition; accumulation.
Coating:	a layer of any substance spread over a surface.
Cuticle:	a superficial integument or membrane.
Deposit:	something precipitated, delivered, and left, or thrown down, as by a natural process; a natural accumulation.
Integument:	a natural covering (as skin, shell, or rind); any covering, coating, enclosure.
Pellicle:	a thin skin or membrane; film, scum.
Plaque:	a thin flat plate (from French plaquier: to plate).

The early nomenclature was quite confusing because older descriptions were based on inconsistent interpretation of observations by light microscopy. This confusion has been partly resolved by a classification that distinguishes structures of embryonic origin from those acquired after eruption and proposes a limited number of names (Table 6-1).[39]

Primary enamel cuticle

Ameloblasts were thought to secrete a film after completion of amelo-

*References 151, 164, 189, 195, 234.
†References 23, 25, 38, 63, 97, 137, 184, 202, 259.

Table 6-1 Terminology of integuments of enamel*

Description	Previous names	Recommended name
Structures of embryonic origin		
Acellular layer	Inner structureless layer of Nasmyth's membrane Primary enamel cuticle Enamel capsule Enamel cuticle Nasmyth's membrane	Primary enamel cuticle†
Cellular layer	Outer cellular layer of Nasmyth's membrane Cuticula dentis United enamel epithelium Reduced enamel epithelium Inner zone epithelium Epithelial attachment cells Dental cuticle Reduced dental epithelium	Reduced enamel epithelium
Structures acquired after eruption		
Cuticle acquired after eruption	Mucin plaque Acquired cuticle Plaque and film Dental cuticle Enamel cuticle Brown pellicle Acquired enamel cuticle Post-eruption cuticle	Acquired pellicle
Food debris	Materia alba Sordes Food debris	Food debris
Dense bacterial layer	Plaque Materia alba Muco-bacterial film	Dental plaque
Calcified material	Calculus Tartar	Calculus

*Adapted from Dawes et al.[38]
†Existence questioned (see text).

genesis. However, electron microscopic observations of developing teeth have failed to substantiate the existence of this structure.[115]

Reduced enamel epithelium

This endogenous coating on the surface of newly erupted enamel consists of postsecretory ameloblasts attached to the enamel surface by hemidesmosomes and a basal lamina.

Acquired pellicle

The acquired pellicle is an acellular, homogeneous organic film that forms on enamel and other hard surfaces by selective adsorption of salivary proteins. Its formation, composition, and function will be discussed in more detail later.

Food debris

As the name implies, this material consists of food remnants adhering to the teeth and is usually present only transiently after meals. Obsolete terms such as *sordes* (literally, dirt) or *materia alba* (literally, white matter) are confusing since they have also been used to describe plaque. Distinguishing *materia alba* from plaque by its supposed susceptibility to being washed away by a water spray and the resistance of plaque to such treatment is an oversimplification. For example, some food debris, such as meat fibers that become wedged interdentally, cannot be sprayed away. Conversely, mild washing procedures can displace the loosely structured organisms on the surface of plaque.[118] The important difference is that food debris is made up mostly of food, whereas plaque is essentially a bacterial mass.

Dental plaque

Different definitions of dental plaque have been offered,* but none is more figurative than that of Mandel[139]: "A bacterial aspic with millions of organisms standing shoulder to shoulder." A more formal definition has been formulated by Löe[112]:

> Plaque is the soft, nonmineralized, bacterial deposit which forms on teeth (and dental prostheses) that are not adequately cleaned.

These definitions justifiably stress the bacterial component of plaque. Counts of 2×10^{11} microorganisms/g have been reported in direct smears of plaque. Strålfors centrifuged streptococci to pack them and counted 3×10^{11} organisms/g.[236] In other words, two thirds of plaque must consist of bacteria. Similar conclusions have been reached based on morphometric analyses of the condensed microbial layer of plaque, which indicate 70% of the area is composed of microorganisms and 30% of intercellular material.[204]

*References 69, 149, 166, 206, 235, 259.

The mouth contains a number of ecological niches. To discuss the microbial composition of plaque, it is first necessary to define its source. Supragingival plaque is that growing on surfaces of teeth at or above the free gingival margin. Subgingival plaque refers to the microbial flora apical to the free gingival margin. Earlier studies made no attempt to separate these two: the plaque was simply called gingival sulcus or dentinogingival plaque.[244] There is no reason to expect supragingival plaque to be identical to plaque in the gingival sulcus. Similarly, plaque in occlusal fissures differs from supragingival plaque found on smooth surfaces. While there are some similarities between these plaques, differences do exist in their microflorae. Dental plaque is a microbial community formed by interaction between microorganisms and their environment. Together with the environment, plaque constitutes a structural and functional unit, a microbial ecosystem.[30]

Dental calculus

Dental calculus is plaque in which mineralization has involved both the plaque matrix and the microorganisms. However, the free surface of calculus usually harbors living bacteria.

Acquired pellicle

Formation

The acquired pellicle is a biofilm formed posteruptively by adsorption of salivary proteins or glycoproteins to tooth surfaces.[146,228,247] Adsorption of proteins to hydroxyapatite is a well-known physicochemical phenomenon that biochemists have used for many years to purify proteins. Pellicle formation is not restricted to teeth. Pellicle can form on polyethylene strips ligated to the teeth,[140] on glass beads exposed to saliva,[227] on various restorative materials,[230] and on dentures. Manly[143] described a brown, structureless film accumulating on teeth of persons using nonabrasive dentifrices. It is now known that, regardless of the type of dentifrice used, acquired pellicle forms rapidly on solid surfaces exposed to the oral environment.

The adsorption of proteins to a surface has several significant consequences that change many of the physical and chemical properties of the adsorbant as well as the adsorbate. The changes include alteration in the secondary and tertiary structure and solubility of the adsorbed proteins. The chemical reactivity of, and the diffusion through, enamel are also changed as a consequence.

Morphologically the formation of acquired pellicle can be followed in vivo by taking repeated replicas of the same tooth surface with silicone rubber impressions and examining the replicas by scanning electron

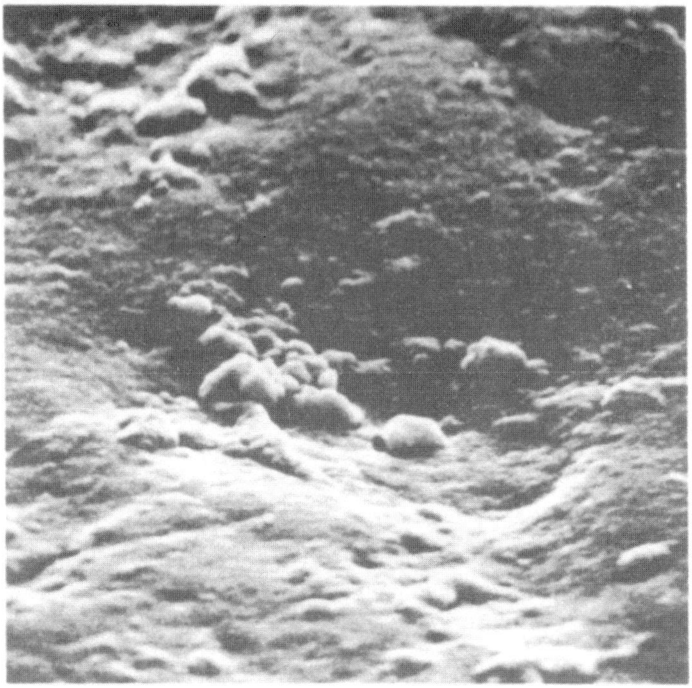

Fig 6-1 Defects on the enamel surface, revealing organic material not removed by polishing (SEM, original magnification × 3,020). (Courtesy of C.A. Saxton.)

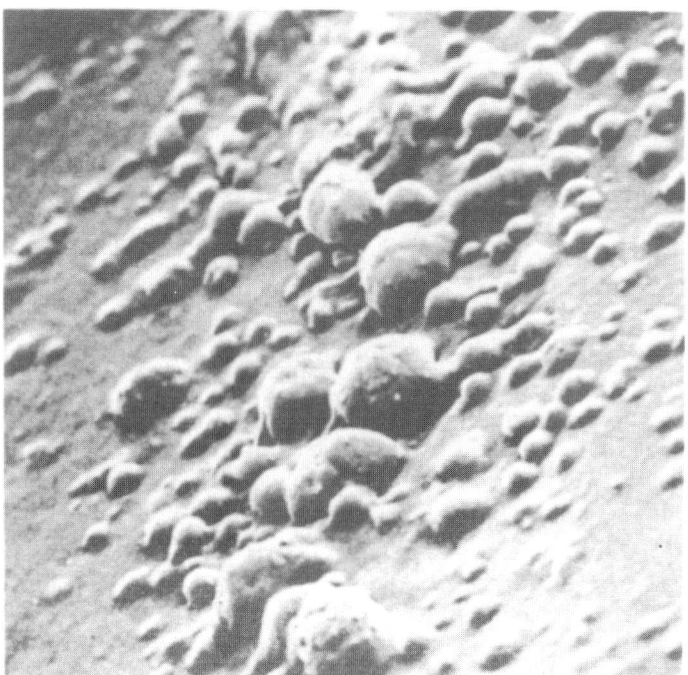

Fig 6-2 Crevicular region 20 minutes after polishing. Globular deposits have settled on the enamel surface (SEM, original magnification × 1,105). (Courtesy of C.A. Saxton.)

microscopy.[199,200] Immediately after cleaning and polishing, scratches and some material remaining in enamel defects are evident (Fig 6-1). Dome-shaped masses of amorphous material, ranging in size from 5 to 20 μm, form on this surface within 20 minutes (Figs 6-2 and 6-3). These early deposits already contain bacteria[224]; the microflora will be described subsequently under "Formation and development of dental plaques," (see page 211). After 1 hour, globular deposits are present in greater numbers, and some have coalesced. After 24 hours, they have coalesced completely, the whole tooth surface becoming covered with amorphous material (Fig 6-4). After 48 hours, filamentous and coccal microorganisms can be recognized (Fig 6-5).[45]

Stereomicroscopy has also been used to examine the pellicle. A film of acquired pellicle and some bacteria, having weak affinity for fuchsin stain, is visible 24 hours after teeth have been cleaned.[17] Gradually, material (plaque) that stains more intensely forms first in enamel cracks, then extends over the tooth surface. After 1 to 4 days, small, discrete, hemispherical accumulations (30 to 60 μm) occur scattered on the tooth surface, especially in cracks and along the gingival margin. These accumulations are bacterial plaque colonies.

In vivo there is no finite conversion of acquired pellicle to plaque. There is a transition from teeth covered with acquired pellicle to teeth covered with pellicle and plaque, the two developing contemporaneously.

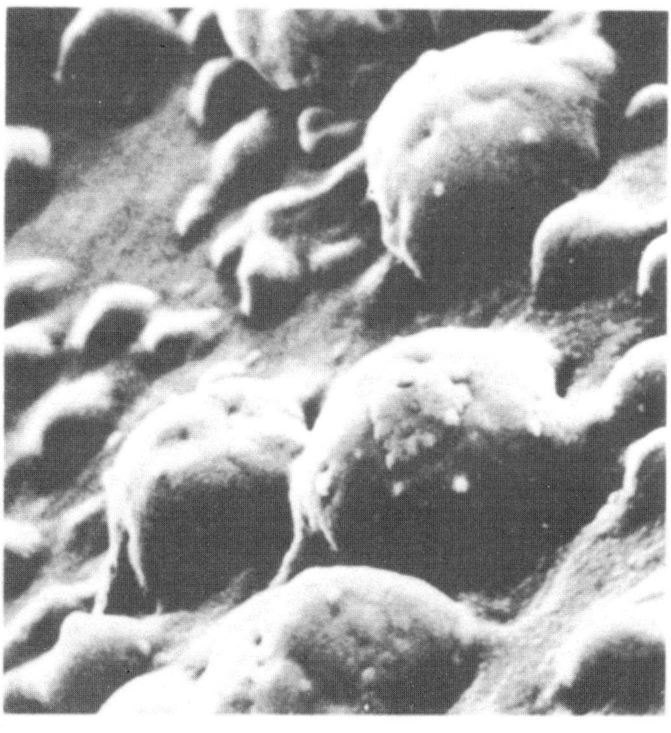

Fig 6-3 High magnification of globular deposit (shown in Fig 6-2) formed during 20-minute exposure in the mouth. A number of small spherical protuberances seen on the large globules are possible oral microorganisms (SEM, original magnification ×2,665). (Courtesy of C.A. Saxton.)

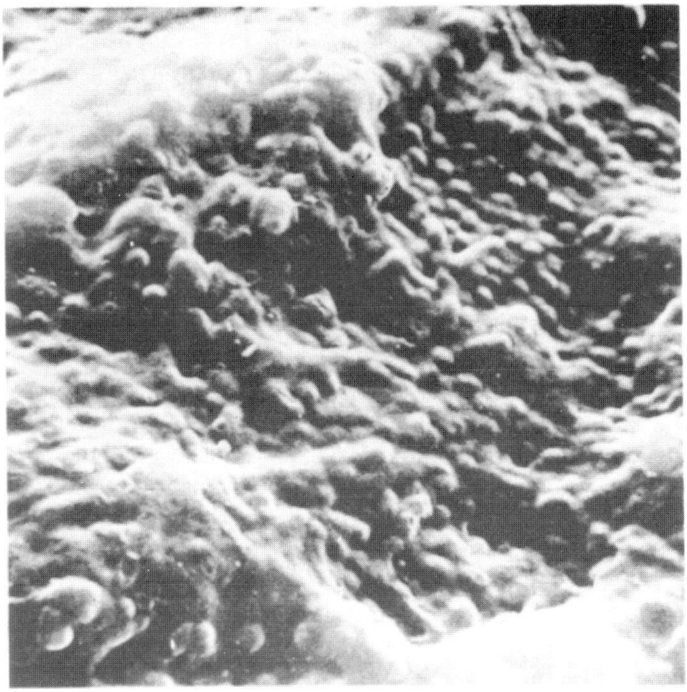

Fig 6-4 After 24 hours the globules appear to have coalesced, forming an uneven continuous surface (SEM, original magnification ×2,220). (Courtesy of C.A. Saxton.)

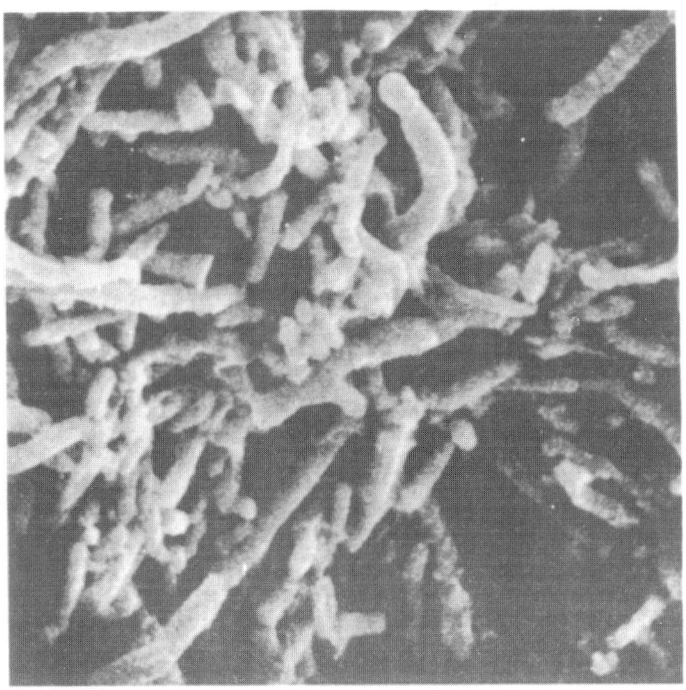

Fig 6-5 After 48 hours filamentous and coccal organisms are recognizable. Generally, the bacteria are covered by matrix (saliva) and the interface is featureless. Replica was obtained following twice rinsing with water (SEM, original magnification ×2,665). (Courtesy of C.A. Saxton.)

Nevertheless, acquired pellicle does have an independent existence.[204] Unlike plaque, bacteria are not required for pellicle formation.[145,152] In vitro, acquired pellicle will form on enamel immersed in saliva containing antibiotics to inhibit bacterial growth, or in saliva from which bacteria have been removed by filtration. The most convincing proof that bacteria are not necessary for pellicle formation is that pellicle is found on teeth of germ-free animals.[117]

Histological appearance

The acid-insoluble portion of the acquired pellicle, when removed from the tooth, appears as a translucent, diaphanous structure. Histochemically, it stains positively for carbohydrates, proteins, and lipids.[140,149] These staining properties have been interpreted as evidence that the acquired pellicle is composed of salivary glycoproteins. The staining reactions alone are not adequate proof of the composition of the pellicle, but they serve to confirm the conclusion of chemical analyses (see "Composition" of pellicle, page 186).

Pellicle appears acellular and faintly granular when seen under established plaque in transmission electron micrographs (Fig 6-6). It may have a scalloped surface (Fig 6-7).[2,203] These scalloped spaces frequently contain bacterial ghosts and debris. Newly formed (2-hour) pellicle is fairly uniform in thickness, 100 to 700 nm, and is without recesses or notches in the outer border.[226] It increases in thickness during the first 24 hours of formation, mostly at night.[111] Pellicles of unknown age may vary in thickness from 50 to 1,000 nm. Three different morphological types—globular, fibrillar, and granular—form on hydroxyapatite splints. The surface properties of these splints, however, are not the same as those of enamel. The nature of the surface of solids has an important influence on the type of proteins they adsorb[227] and may account for these different morphological types.

A subsurface pellicle, consisting of dendritic processes that spread into the intercrystalline spaces and extend 1 to 3 μm into the enamel, may be found beneath the surface pellicle.[3,109,152] Some consider this as representing the earliest appearance of caries[34] or an arrested lesion.

Composition

A brief acid treatment can remove acquired pellicle from cleaned extracted teeth. The acid-insoluble portion of the pellicle becomes detached from the tooth and can be teased away so that it floats off as a membrane, very much as originally described by Alexander Nasmyth in 1839. Some of the pellicle dissolves in the acid; this is not visible but can be detected chemically.

Total pellicle can be obtained in vivo by scaling the enamel surface of teeth that have been pumiced 1 or 2 hours previously. The scrapings

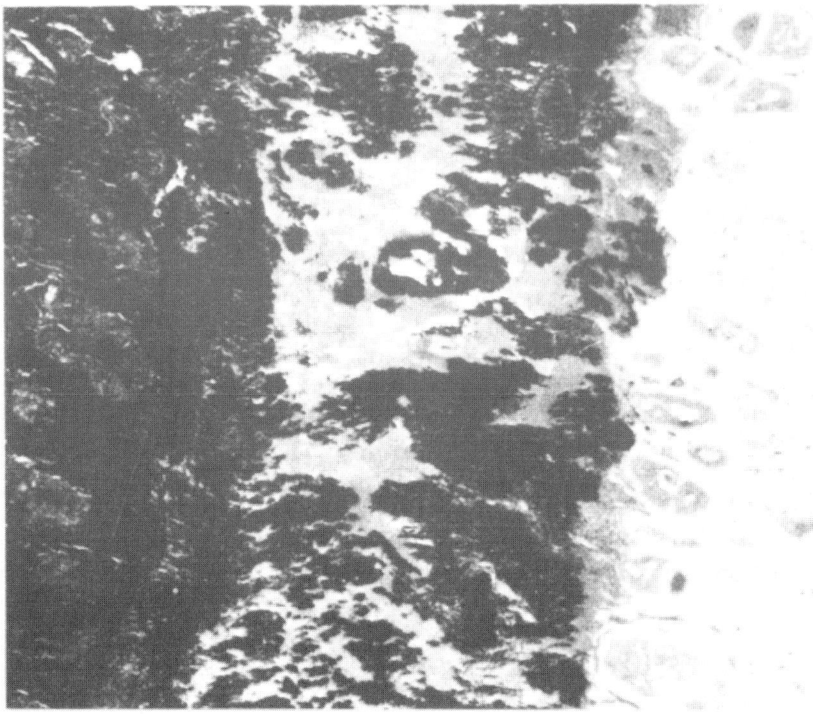

Fig 6-6 Acquired pellicle located between supragingival calculus and plaque. The pellicle is partly mineralized (TEM, original magnification × 17,500). (Courtesy of H. Schroeder.)

are carefully trapped on glass wool with a pipette connected to a suction device.[228]

According to chemical analyses, amino acids account for 45% to 50%

$$\text{clean erupted teeth} \xrightarrow[\text{5 min}]{\text{0.6 N.HCl}} \begin{cases} \nearrow \text{insoluble pellicle} \\ \searrow \text{soluble pellicle} \end{cases} \text{total pellicle}$$

of the insoluble pellicle.[1-3,108] Anthrone-reacting carbohydrates amount to 10% to 15% of the dry weight; this includes hexoses, pentoses, and hexuronic acids but not amino sugars. There is a high proportion of acidic amino acids (about 20% of the total amino acids), a high alanine content, and a low content of sulfur amino acids. Often there are traces of rhamnose, muramic, and diaminopimelic acids. These acids are characteristic of bacterial cell walls. Accordingly, Armstrong[2] concluded that the insoluble pellicle is comparable to a mixture of salivary glycoproteins and bacterial cell walls.

Total pellicle (acid-soluble and acid-insoluble) characteristically has a

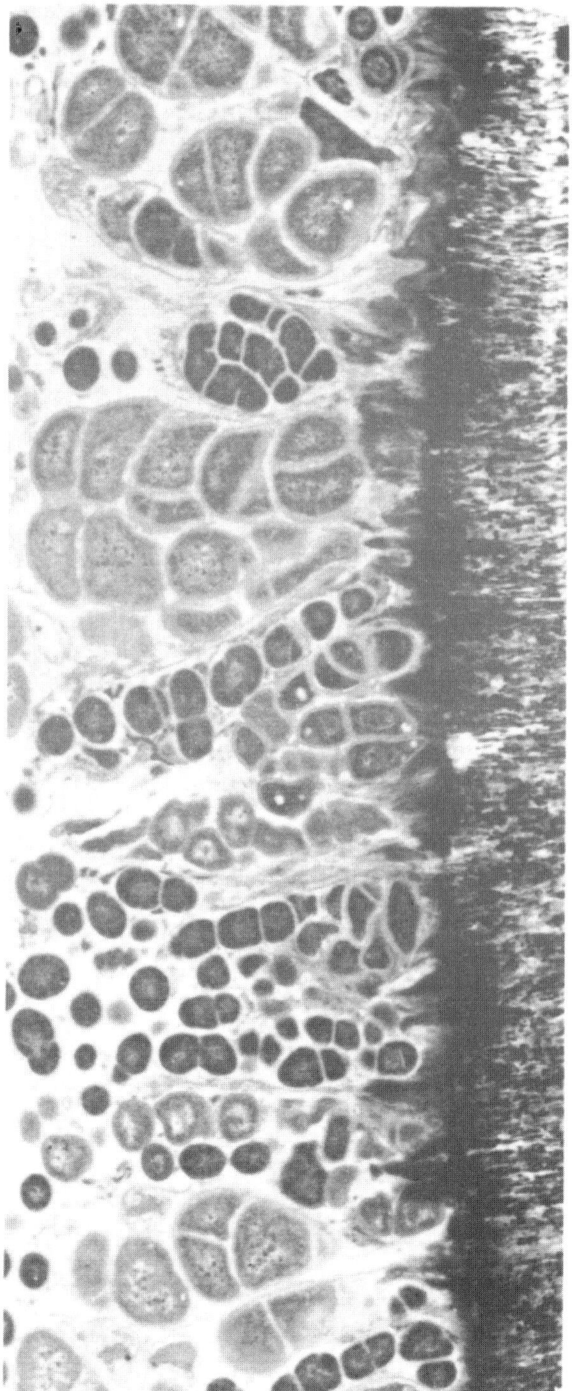

Fig 6-7 Tooth plaque interface showing an electron-dense scalloped pellicle. Note the fibrillar material between the cells (original magnification ×9,000). (Courtesy of H. Schroeder.)

high content of glycine, serine, and glutamic acid (42% of total amino acids), followed by aspartic acid, proline, alanine, and leucine (each more than 6% of total amino acids). The total pellicle has a low sulfur and aromatic amino acid content.[145-147] Muramic and diaminopimelic acids are not chemically detectable in freshly formed (2-hour) pellicle,[228] indicating the absence of a measurable amount of bacterial cell wall components.

The carbohydrate composition of total pellicle includes glucose, galactose, glucosamine, galactosamine, mannose, and fucose.[145,146,148,226] Acquired pellicle contains 23% lipids, mainly glycolipids (13%); neutral lipids and phospholipids together make up an additional 5%.[215]

The foregoing chemical analyses indicate that there are some similarities between the chemical composition of acquired pellicle and mixed saliva or salivary glycoprotein, although important differences exist. The relative abundance of acidic amino acids demonstrates a selective adsorption of proteins to the tooth surface from saliva.

A more specific approach to the identification of proteins in pellicle is based on their antigenic determinants, which can be recognized by immunofluorescent staining techniques.[103,104,181] Up to ten different proteins have been identified in pellicles. The proportion of each protein is highly dependent upon the subject, each of whom presents a characteristic profile of pellicle proteins. The typical salivary proteins, such as amylase, lysozyme, and IgA, are consistently detected in both pellicle and plaque. Albumin, IgG, and IgM are frequently encountered in pellicle. Enzymatic activity of lysozyme and amylase has also been demonstrated in acquired pellicle grown for 2 hours in vitro.[182] Similar pellicles formed in vivo lack this activity, presumably because these enzymes are rapidly denatured. Blood group and virus hemagglutination inhibition activities are present in acquired pellicle.

Function

Various biological functions have been attributed to acquired pellicle, including:

1. Healing, repairing, or protecting the enamel surface
2. Imparting selective permeability to the enamel
3. Influencing the adherence of specific oral microorganisms to the tooth surface
4. Serving as a substrate or nutrient for the plaque organisms that have colonized on the tooth surface

Most of these suggestions are speculative, but some are supported by direct experimental data. The protective function, mostly hypothetical, is based on the observation of organic material replacing lost inorganic crystallites.[247] Enamel coated with saliva is less permeable and less susceptible to acid attack in vitro,[152,159] causing formation of subsurface rather than surface lesions. The presence of a pellicle influences the adherence of organisms to enamel or restorative materials. Adherence will increase in some cases and decrease in others, depending on both the type of organisms and the type of surface (enamel, resin, cement, zinc phosphate cement, etc).[103,179,183] Pellicle is generally considered an initial step in the formation of microbial plaque. Histologically the acquired pellicle may appear scalloped and thin underneath established dental plaque. This has led some people to postulate that pellicle or adsorbed glycoproteins on the tooth surface can be utilized for bacterial metabolism.[3,102,171]

Summary

Acquired pellicle is an organic deposit that forms naturally by selective adsorption of proteins from saliva. If removed by cleaning and polishing, it rapidly re-forms on the tooth surface. Bacteria are not required for this process, but settle on the pellicle almost as soon as it forms. The pellicle thereby influences the bacterial colonization on the tooth surface and the formation of dental plaque.

Morphology of dental plaque

General features

Far from being "an invisible film," plaque can be seen on exposed surfaces of teeth as a white or off-white accumulation of variable thickness, depending on its location and the extent and frequency of oral hygiene. Plaque is thin in the gingival sulcus (subgingival plaque) because of anatomical constraints. Above the gingiva, if it is not controlled it can become very thick, resembling microbial colonies growing on agar plates (Fig 6-8). Pioneer plaque colonies usually start growing at enamel cracks and surface irregularities. They coalesce and become continuous along the gingival margin (Fig 6-9), the rate of spread varying from individual to individual. When permitted, plaque will form up to the height of contour of the tooth and fill the interproximal spaces, tapering to nothing at the contact areas.[84] Pits and fissures of erupted teeth and the gingival sulcus are never completely free of plaque. Growth on occlusal surfaces and above the height of contour is somewhat limited by mastication. Chewing coarse food has no effect on plaque in interproximal or gingival areas, and eating fibrous vegetables between meals does not prevent plaque formation.[229] The type of diet—its content and consistency—

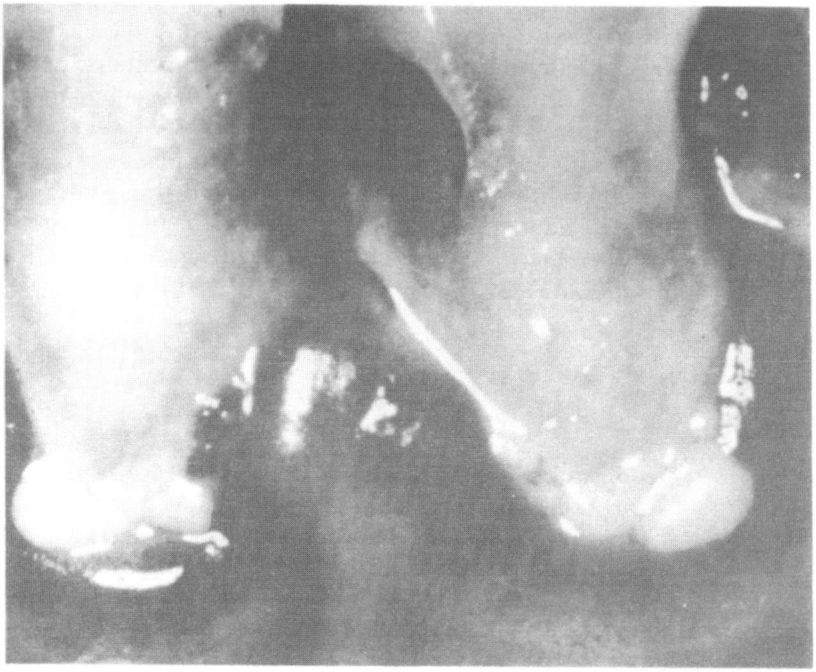

Fig 6-8 Supragingival plaque resembling microbial colonies growing on agar plates. This plaque is unstained and of unknown age. Note the interproximal recurrent caries on the lower incisors and the inflamed edematous gingivae. (Courtesy of J. Egelberg.)

does influence the rate of accumulation and thickness of early plaque. For example, frequent ingestion of sucrose in the absence of oral hygiene promotes a voluminous plaque.[30]

Most early attempts to examine the histology of plaque were limited by the use of thick sections and the poor resolution of the light microscope. Early descriptions emphasized the presence of leptotrichiae and filamentous organisms rather than cocci. *Leptotrichia buccalis* has dimensions of 2 μm × 20 μm, compared with a typical *Streptococcus,* which is 1 μm × 0.6 μm.[24] The structure of plaque depends on the arrangement of the microorganisms, some of which have a diameter about 1 μm; therefore, only sections thinner than this can reveal the relationship between cells.

With the advent of electron microscopy a clearer picture of plaque structure emerged, particularly of the spatial arrangement of the organisms. However, there are also limitations to this technique. The ultrastructural classification of bacteria in plaque is only approximate, accounting for three main types: coccoid, rod-shaped, and filamentous. Distinctly shaped organisms, such as spirochetes, can be identified, and gram-positive and gram-negative cell walls can sometimes be distin-

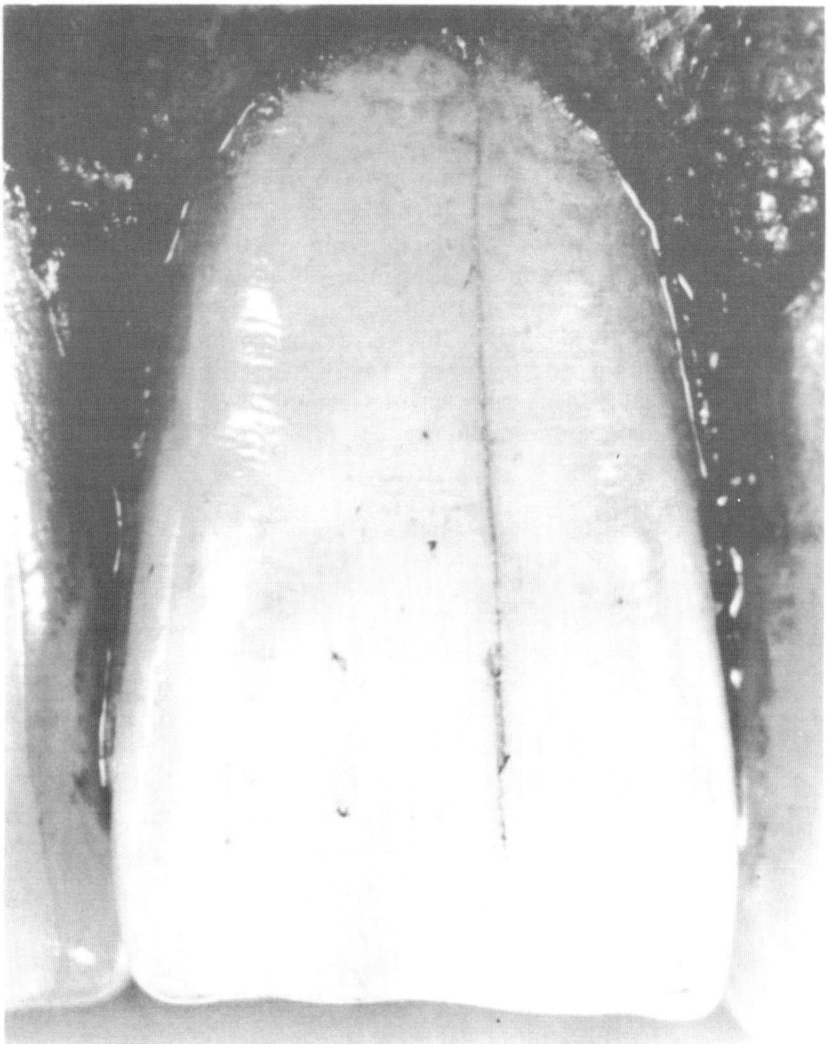

Fig 6-9 Plaque growth 24 hours after cleaning, on a central maxillary incisor of a patient who is an "abundant" plaque former. Note the spread along the gingival margin, the crack, and other surface defects (original magnification ×20). (Courtesy of A.D. Eastcott.)

guished.[114,119] Nevertheless, most organisms cannot be taxonomically identified by ultrastructural criteria.

Supragingival smooth surface plaque

For descriptive purposes, supragingival plaque can be conveniently subdivided into four areas: *(1)* plaque/tooth interface, *(2)* condensed microbial layer, *(3)* body of the plaque, and *(4)* plaque surface.

Plaque/tooth interface

The most common arrangement is that bacteria settle on acquired pellicle. The pellicle may be fairly thick and continuous (see Fig 6-6), it may be scalloped with bacterial cells occupying the scalloped areas (see Fig 6-7), or it may appear as a thin, electron-dense, discontinuous layer (Fig 6-10). In some locations no pellicle can be discerned, so that the microorganisms are in direct contact with the hydroxyapatite crystals of enamel (Fig 6-11). When this occurs the enamel surface may have a scalloped outline, suggestive of an active bacterial invasion.[54] Occasionally, plaque may form near the gingival margin on the remnants of the reduced enamel epithelium.

Condensed microbial layer

This term, introduced by Schroeder and collaborators,[204,205] refers to a layer of very densely packed coccoid organisms, from 3 to 20 cells thick (see Figs 6-7 and 6-10; Fig 6-12). Actively dividing cells can be seen, although some cells have unusually thick walls, suggesting a low multiplication rate.[254]

The condensed microbial layer varies in thickness. It may arise from the original microorganisms that settle on the pellicle and grow at different rates but eventually fuse. The columnar appearance of some microcolonies (see Fig 6-7) may be due to restricted lateral growth and/or requirement of nutrients, so that only vertical growth is possible. Plaque growth at this stage is analogous to the proliferation of skyscrapers in crowded cities.[119]

Body of the plaque

This occupies by far the largest portion of the plaque (Figs 6-12 to 6-15). It consists of different species of microorganisms, normally in clusters and rather haphazardly arranged except for the filamentous organisms, which tend to line up at right angles to the tooth surface in a palisade (Fig 6-16).

Plaque surface

The surface layer is more loosely packed than the rest of the plaque, with wide intercellular spaces (Figs 6-12 and 6-19). A great variety of organisms may be seen on the free surface of plaque (Figs 6-17 to 6-19). They may be coccoid, rodlike, or "corncob" formations.[84,85] These latter measure 3 to 4 μm across and consist of a filament coated by a single, closely packed layer of cocci (Fig 6-20). Similar formulations were described in early literature as the reproductive phase of the filamentous

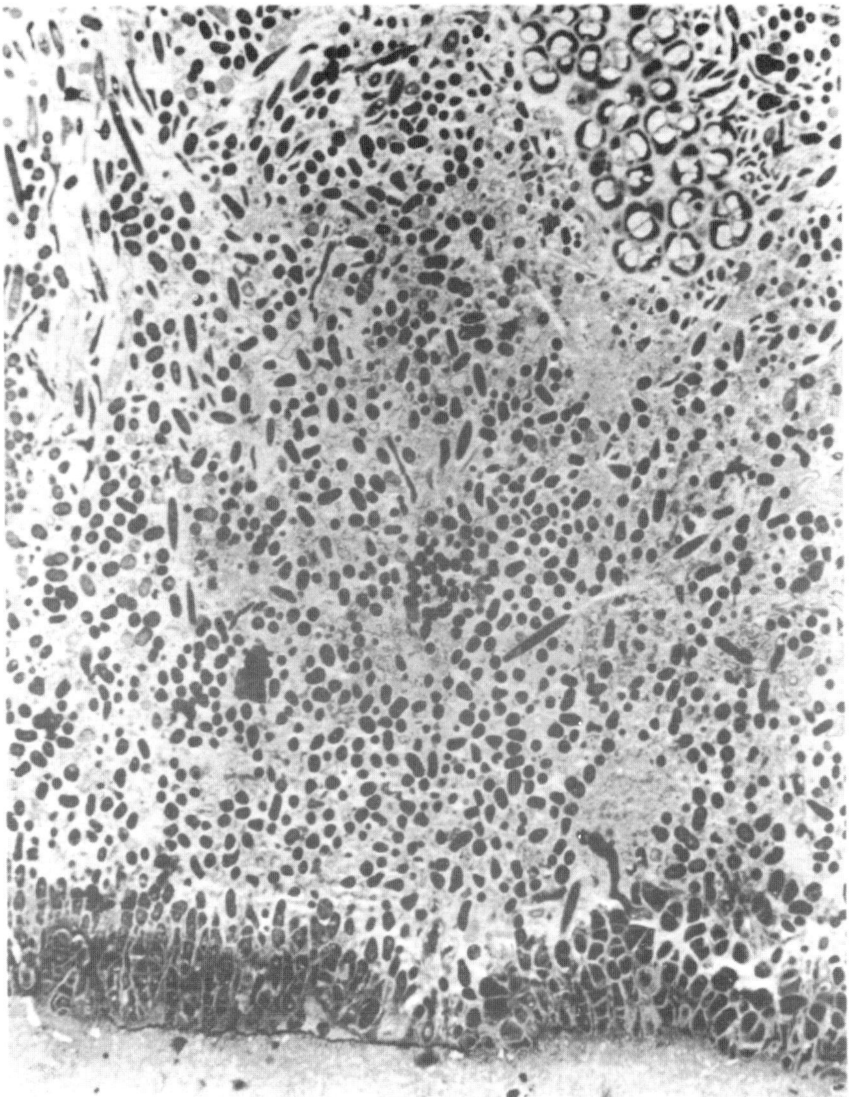

Fig 6-10 Part of a 7-day-old interdental plaque grown on enamel. The enamel matrix *(bottom)*, appearing as a fine meshwork, is covered by a thin electron-dense and discontinuous pellicle. Immediately above this is the condensed microbial layer which is covered by a layer of coccoid and filamentous micro-organisms and probably *Neisseria*. The intermicrobial space is electron-lucent and reveals cell remnants (original magnification ×6,500). (Courtesy of H. Schroeder.)

bacterium *Leptothrix racemosa*. Based on their ultrastructure, the cocci and filaments belong to different genera. The "cob" and the "kernels" have distinctly different cytoplasmic and cell wall features.[118,119] The

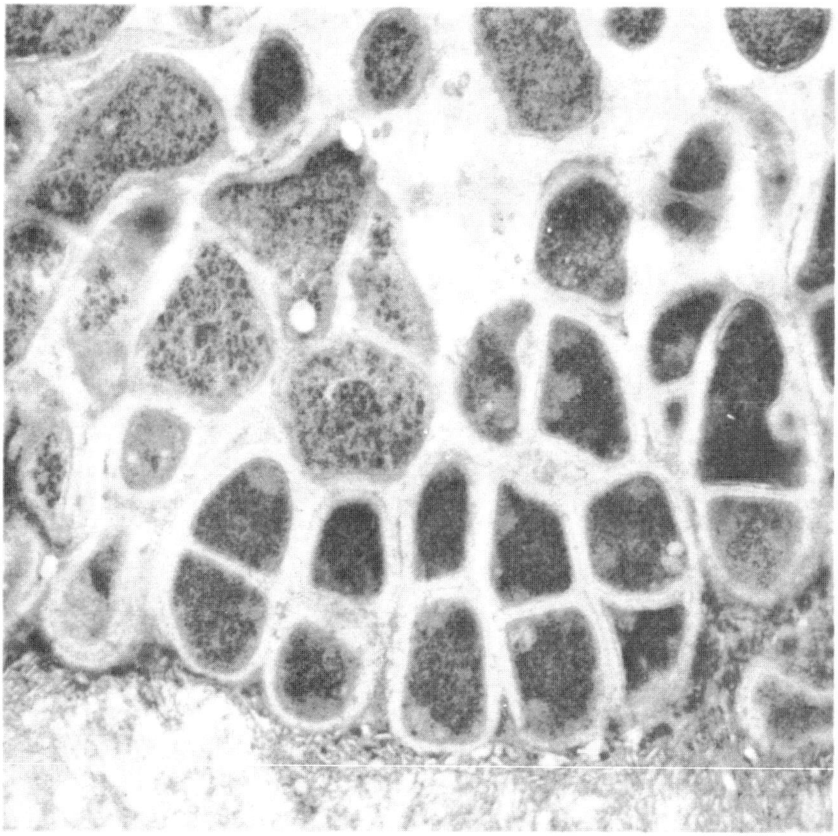

Fig 6-11 Higher magnification of plaque-enamel border. Microorganisms that divide in horizontal planes are in direct contact with enamel (original magnification ×30,000). (Courtesy of H. Schroeder.)

filamentous portion in this epiphytic arrangement has been identified as *Bacterionema matruchotii*[160] or *Fusobacterium nucleatum*,[107] and the cocci as *Streptococcus sanguis*[162,163,239] and *Streptococcus mitior*.[163] The "corncob" configuration is a readily identifiable example of an in vivo bacterial adhesive interaction.[172] The "corncob" streptococci adhere to *B matruchotii* by means of a polar tuft.[161]

In addition to the cellular components of plaque there exists an intercellular matrix material that may be granular, globular, or fibrillar. It consists of proteins and extracellular polysaccharides, some of which are important in interbacterial adherence. At the plaque/tooth interface, the plaque matrix material may seem continuous with the acquired pellicle.[55]

Subgingival plaque

In young children, subgingival plaque around premolars extracted

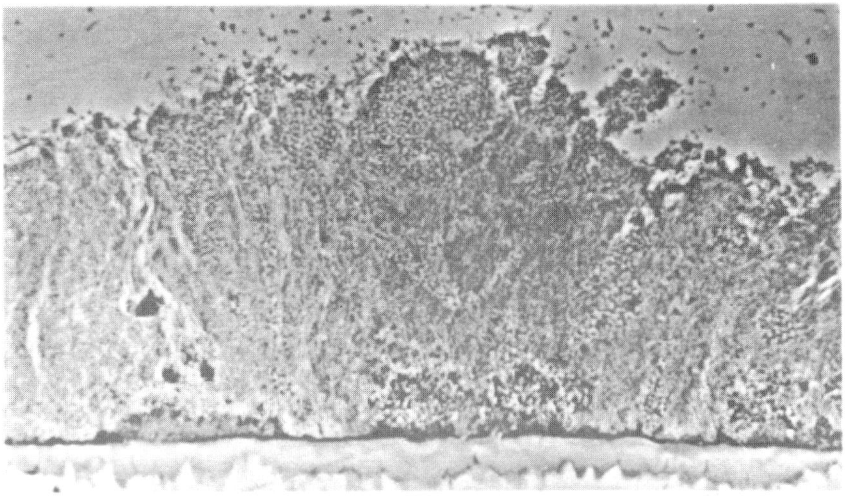

Fig 6-12 Thick section of plaque on enamel surface. A pellicle separates the plaque from the enamel. (Phase contrast micrograph, original magnification ×560). (Courtesy of H. Schroeder.)

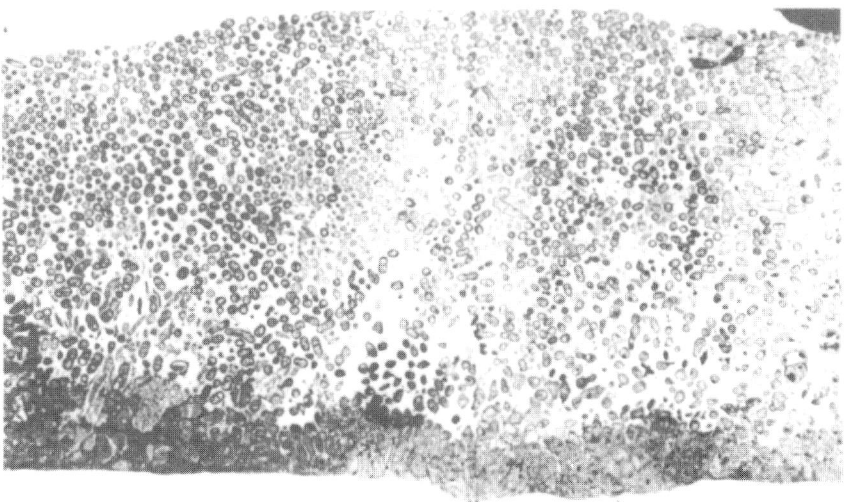

Fig 6-13 Thin section of plaque made of different bacterial species—predominantly coccoidal. Condensed microbial layer at tooth/plaque interface (original magnification ×3,000). (Courtesy of H. Schroeder.)

within 3 years after eruption may appear as *(1)* a loose arrangement of mostly cocci, *(2)* a condensed arrangement of cocci and rods, or *(3)* a dense arrangement of cocci covered by a layer of filamentous organisms. The intercellular matrix may be either fibrillar or granular. Viable or dead neutrophilic granulocytes may cover the free surface.[204]

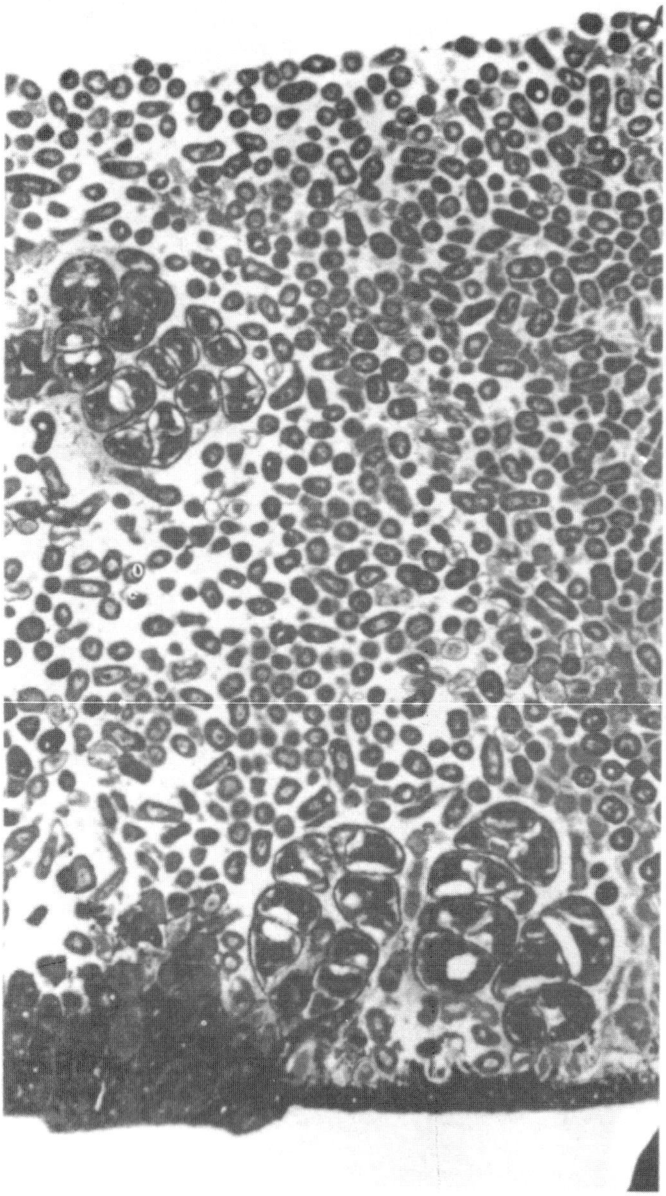

Fig 6-14 Dense aggregation of microorganisms at the enamel surface *(lower left)*. Coccoid organisms within the bulk of the plaque are more loosely packed (original magnification ×6,500). (Courtesy of H. Schroeder.)

The subgingival plaque presents a more varied picture in adults, presumably because they have pockets of different depths. The matrix is sparse, although organisms often may be associated with fine fibrils. Filamentous organisms, bacilli, and cocci are numerous. In addition, spirochetes of different dimensions are found in plaque of periodontally involved teeth.[172] The periodontal status depends on the morphological

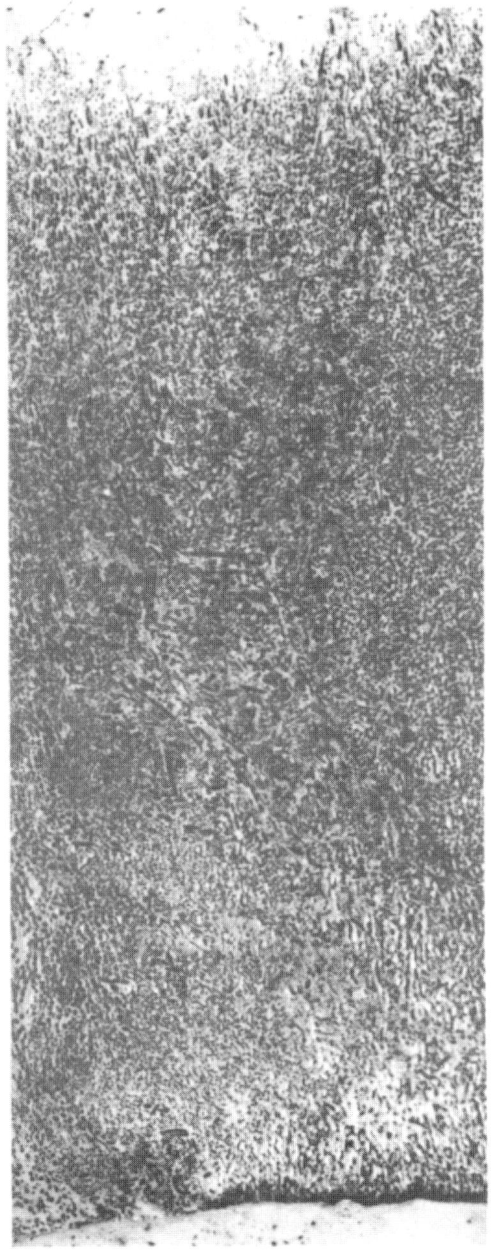

Fig 6-15 Seven-day-old plaque grown in vivo on a mesial enamel surface. Filamentous and coccoid organisms appear in colonies. Section approximately 6 to 8 μm thick. Specimen stained with uranyl and lead salts (original magnification ×580). (Courtesy of H. Schroeder.)

types colonizing the apical region. Adherent plaque does not extend to the base of the pocket, but unattached organisms appear to float in a "soup" of gingival exudate.

Listgarten[114] has noted morphological differences in the flora associated with varying degrees of periodontal disease. Healthy gingival sites have a flora composed of predominantly gram-positive cocci. Isolated

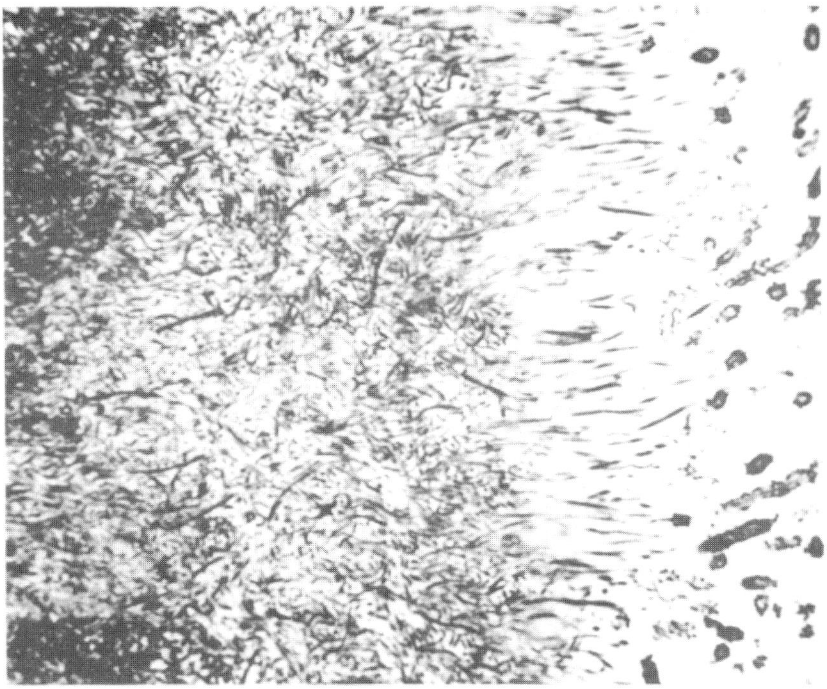

Fig 6-16 Supragingival plaque on a periodontally involved tooth. Dense predominantly filamentous bacterial mass in the body of the plaque. Filaments arranged perpendicularly to the tooth in a palisade toward the plaque surface. "Corncob" formations extend from the surface (original magnification ×850). (Courtesy of M. Listgarten.)

filamentous or branching forms and some gram-negative bacteria can be seen, whereas spirochetes and flagellated cells are rarely found. In the absence of pockets, the plaque is confined to the enamel surface.

Gingivitis samples reveal flagellated cells with spirochetes within a predominantly gram-negative flora at the bottom of the sulcus. In contrast, in periodontitis relatively few cells adhere to the root surface, and there is an increase in gram-negative and flagellated cells and in medium-sized spirochetes. A distinctive "bristle-brush" or "test-tube brush" formation may be found near the plaque surface. These structures consist of a large filamentous cell forming a central axis, with multiple "bristles" of gram-negative rods or short filaments perpendicular to the central axis. In juvenile periodontitis (periodontosis), pockets contain a relatively sparse, predominantly gram-negative flora.

A clear example of the dependence of plaque flora on environment has been observed in beagle dogs. Biopsies of teeth and gingivae from beagle dogs with gingivitis show a defined structure of the in situ plaque proceeding from the orifice to the base of the gingival sulcus. At the orifice the flora comprises a dense mixed population. Within the pocket,

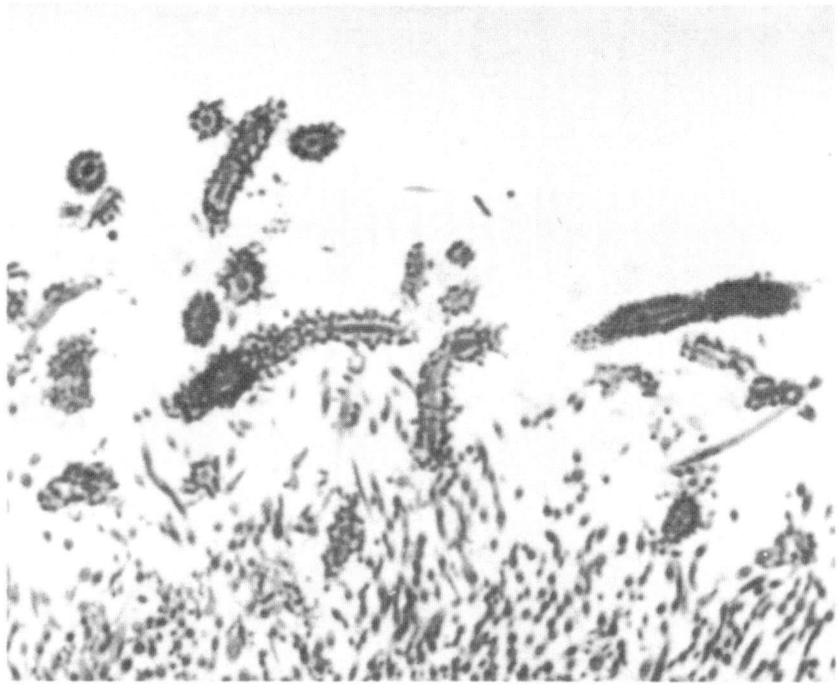

Fig 6-17 Magnified view of "corncob." The corncobs consist of a central filamentous microorganism surrounded by adherent coccoid cells. Some are seen in cross-section and others are cut longitudinally. Methylene blue and toluidine blue (original magnification × 1,500). (Courtesy of M. Listgarten.)

spirochetes and other gram-negative organisms are present. The spirochetes are closely arranged in a parallel fashion perpendicular to the root. Toward the base of the pocket, spirochetes are loosely arranged and randomly oriented.[220]

Fissure plaque

Plaque within fissures is distinctly different from that described on smooth surfaces.[204] Fissures contain microorganisms and food particles. A more limited number of morphological types occur in fissure than in smooth surface plaque. Gram-positive cocci and short rods predominate in a homogeneous matrix, with occasional yeast cells. Palisading and branching filaments are absent within the fissures, although filaments may colonize at the orifice. Empty, ghostlike cell wall structures intermingle with viable cells in some areas (Fig 6-21), while other sites are loosely packed with viable cells. Mineralization may occur within and around the bacteria.[54,245]

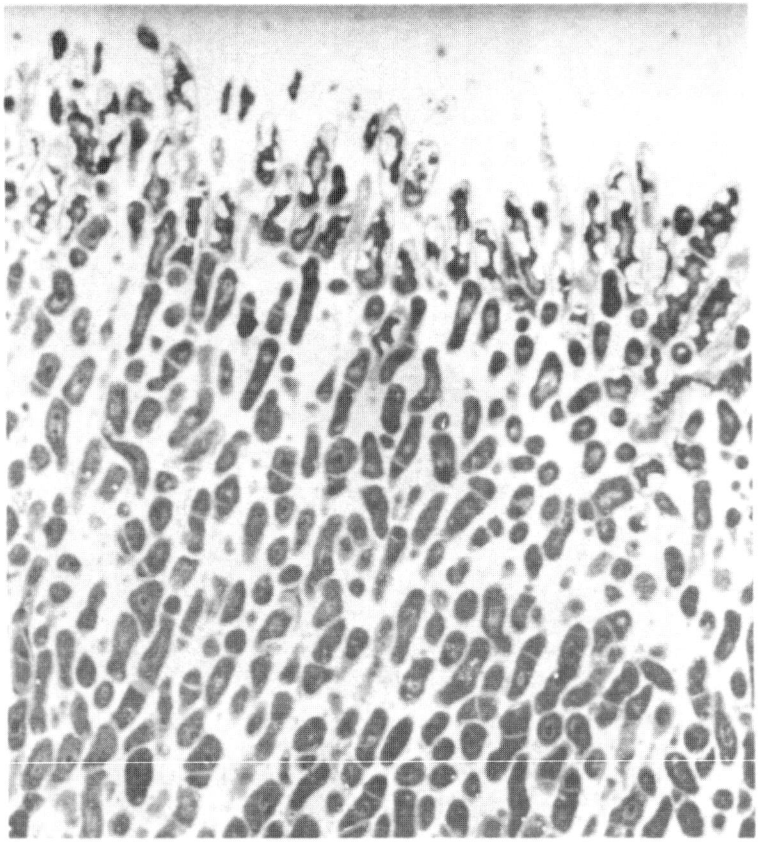

Fig 6-18 Free surface of plaque composed of unidentified organisms. The wide intercellular space appears structureless (original magnification ×6,000). (Courtesy of H. Schroeder.)

Microbiology of dental plaque

Methods of study

There are major technical difficulties in obtaining representative plaque samples and in dispersing, cultivating, identifying, and quantifying the microbial components.[29,70,141] Socransky[221] has facetiously enunciated the "First Law of Oral Biology": A plaque sample will not satisfy anybody—it is either pooled or too small, unrepresentative, too young or too old.

There is no single "correct" method of examining the complex and variable microflora of dental plaque. All approaches require some compromise. The traditional viable cell-counting techniques have been employed extensively. More recently, specific organisms have been identified and quantitated in plaque smears using indirect immunofluores-

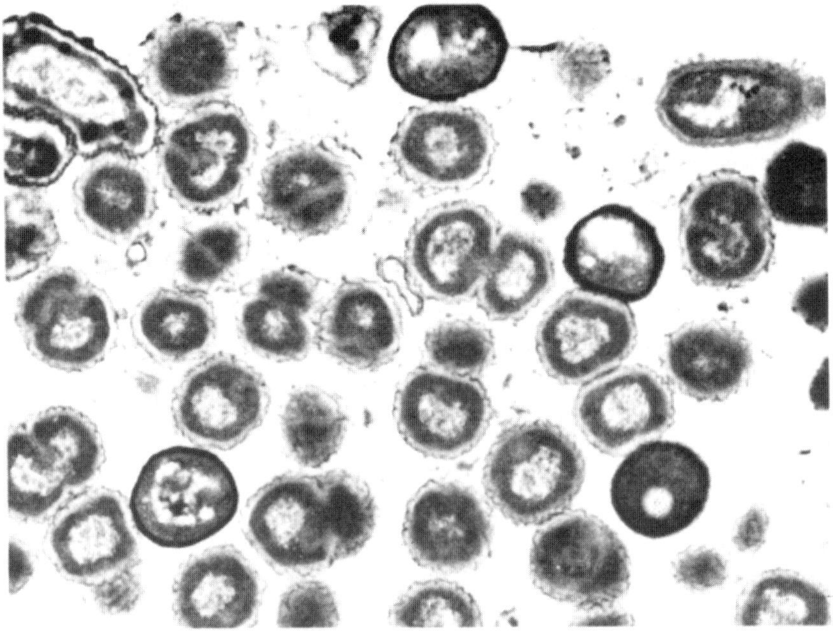

Fig 6-19 Free surface of plaque composed of coccoid gram-positive *(heavily stained cell walls)* and unidentified gram-negative microorganisms. Specimen treated with thiosemicarbazide-osmium and stained with uranyl and lead salts (original magnification ×20,000). (Courtesy of H. Schroeder.)

cence microscopy.[32] With the increasing availability of monoclonal antibodies, these methods will become useful for clinical identification of specific cariogenic and periodontopathic organisms. Using viable counting techniques assumes that each cell in the sample gives rise to one colony, that the media will sustain all types of bacteria in the sample, and that one colony does not inhibit the growth of others. DNA hybridization tests have also recently become available for studying the flora in periodontal pockets. The pocket is sampled with paper points to which the bacteria adhere. These cells are then lysed to release their DNA, which is "melted" (heated) to unwind the two strands of double helix. A labeled DNA probe that hybridizes only with the complementary DNA of a specific pathogen is then used to quantify the levels of pathogen, if present.

Sampling procedure

Because the oral cavity consists of a number of ecological niches, the flora on the tongue, mucosa, tonsils, occlusal fissures, smooth surfaces of teeth, and subgingival sulcus are each unique. Even a single tooth constitutes several distinct microenvironments.[58,68,253] In the past, pooled

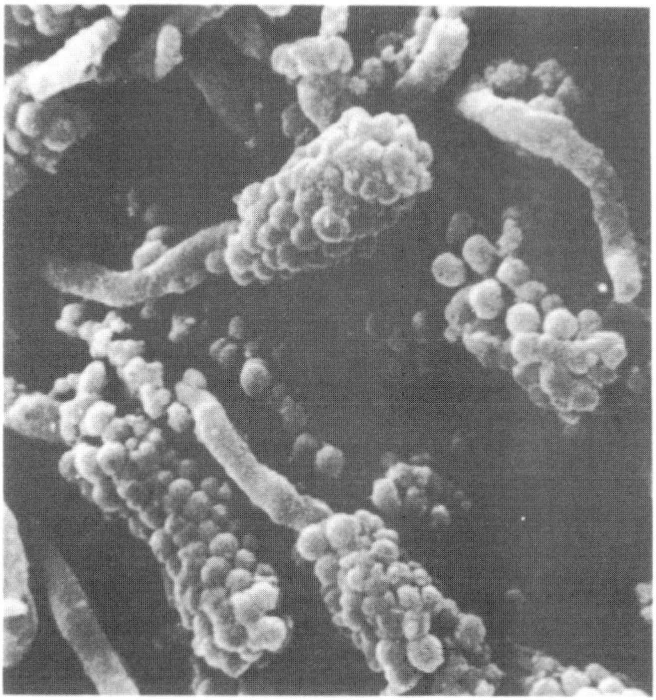

Fig 6-20 Filamentous microorganisms coated with cocci, illustrating adherence of different species to each other (SEM, original magnification ×5,250). (Courtesy of C.A. Saxton.)

plaque (combined samples from several teeth) has been used. Such samples obscure important site variations.

Specimens have generally been obtained from accessible smooth or interproximal surfaces of teeth with dental explorers, scalers, abrasive strips, floss, or plastic "spoons" fashioned from disposable micropipette tips. Fissure plaque has been collected with explorers, fine probes or wires, or disposable injection needles. Subgingival plaque has been obtained using adsorbent paper joints or by an anaerobic sampling device consisting of a needle flushed with nitrogen and bearing a fine barbed broach surrounded by calcium alginate fibers that adsorb the bacteria.[175] It is now possible by such methods to sample specific sites on the tooth or in the gingival sulcus.

Once collected, the plaque sample must be transported from the clinic to the laboratory for processing. Several transport media have been devised, including viability-preserving microbistatic medium,[158] reduced transport fluid (RTF),[134] and a simple broth containing glucose, serum, and cysteine.[21] Anaerobic storage in plastic bags, which can be sealed and contain an anaerobic generator, enhances survival of plaque flora between collection and culture.[76] However, irrespective of what transport fluid is used and what environmental conditions prevail (temperature, oxygen tension), recovery of viable bacteria decreases the longer plaque is stored before processing.

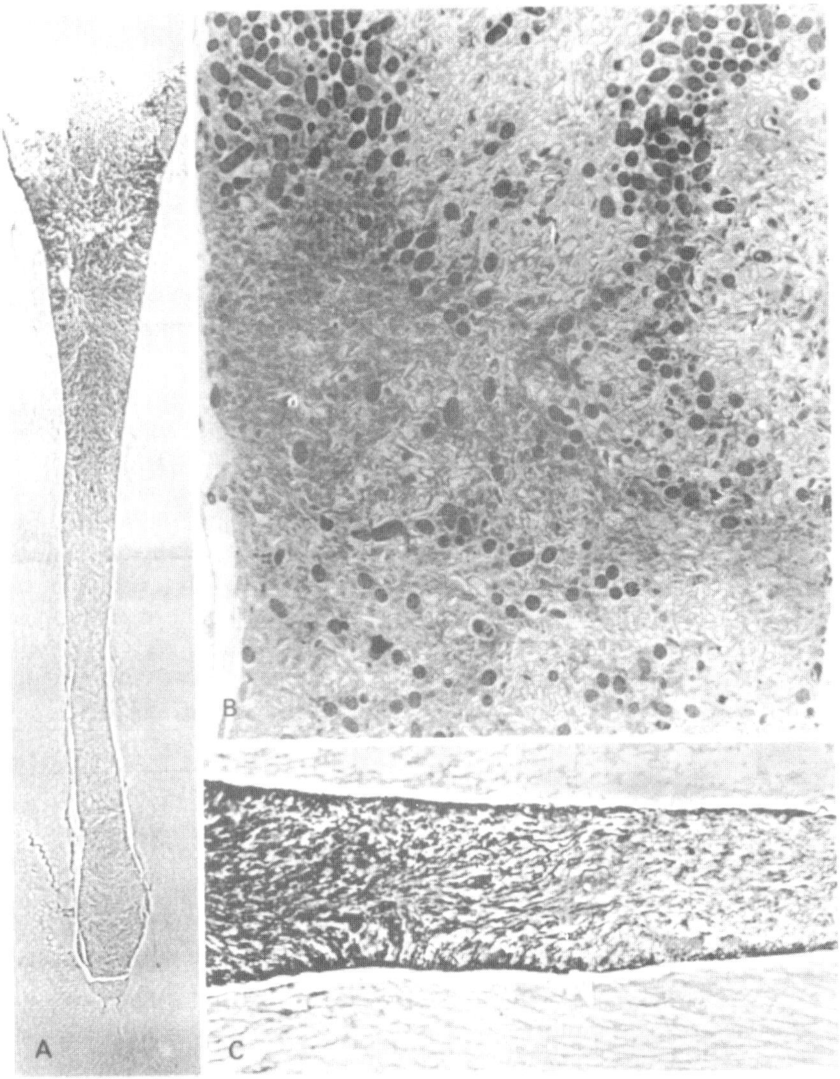

Fig 6-21 *(A)* Survey of dental plaque situated within a deep, narrow fissure of a premolar (×200). *(B)* The upper half of the fissure is filled with dark material, the lower half is less dense (×640). *(C)* Higher magnification reveals a plaque consisting of mostly ghostlike membrane and cell wall structures (TEM, original magnification ×4,700). (Courtesy of H. Schroeder.)

Dispersion

As was seen in the section on "Morphology of dental plaque," the organisms are somewhat haphazardly arranged in aggregates surrounded by an interbacterial matrix. In order to separate and quantitate the cells, they should be uniformly suspended, thus allowing representative dilutions and platings. Chemical agents such as ethylenediaminetetraacetic acid, employed in RTF, chelate calcium and facilitate separation of some bacterial aggregates. Most frequently, physical methods have been employed to disperse the zoogleal plaque clusters. These methods include sonic oscillation, vortex mixing, grinding or homogenizing, shaking with glass beads, and repeated forceful expulsion from hypodermic syringes.

Different types of plaques require different treatments. For example, subgingival plaque has a looser structure and presumably can be dispersed with mild force. More vigorous efforts are necessary to separate the tightly packed supragingival plaque, where many of the cells are stuck together by insoluble extracellular polysaccharides. Ultimately the conditions used are a compromise aimed at maximizing dispersion while minimizing loss of viability.

Studies on the effect of ultrasonic energy on the survival of pure cultures of microorganisms demonstrate this point (Fig 6-22, *A*).[190] Spirochetes and gram-negative filaments are much more sensitive, whereas gram-positive rods (actinomycetes) and cocci (streptococci) are more resistant to the lethal effects of sonic treatment. When organisms are released from plaque aggregate, they will be killed exponentially at a specific rate that is characteristic of the toughness of the cell wall of that group (Fig 6-22, *B*). Periodontopathic plaque, containing large numbers of the more fragile gram-negative motile rods,[175] requires extremely gentle dispersal methods. Cariogenic plaque, containing adherent *Streptococcus mutans* and *S sanguis*, needs more prolonged sonic treatment to separate these streptococci.

Isolation and culture conditions

Anaerobic procedures can more than double the survival and recovery of the total plaque flora.[62,141,216,257] An anaerobic environment is particularly important during sample dispersion, dilution, and cultivation, and preferably should also be maintained during plating. More fastidious anaerobes also require prereduced culture media to ensure a low oxidation-reduction potential. Anaerobiosis has been achieved by continuously flushing tubes with oxygen-free gas during isolation procedures or by performing these procedures within an anaerobic chamber. The vast majority of plaque organisms are facultative; some are strict anaerobes (the proportion depending on the site, that is, more subgingivally than supragingivally); very few, if any, are obligate aerobes.[141,224] Clearly no single environment can support the optimal growth of all organisms residing in plaque.

The percent viable recovery is expressed as the ratio of the total viable cell count to the number of cells that can be counted in a direct smear of the sample, multiplied by 100. For example, if the viable cell count is 1.23×10^{11} cells/g wet weight and the direct cell count is 2.47×10^{11} cells/g wet weight, the viable recovery is 50%.[186] Use of aerobic procedures exclusively yielded only 10% recovery of viable cells from subgingival plaque. This increased to 20% when the cultures were incubated

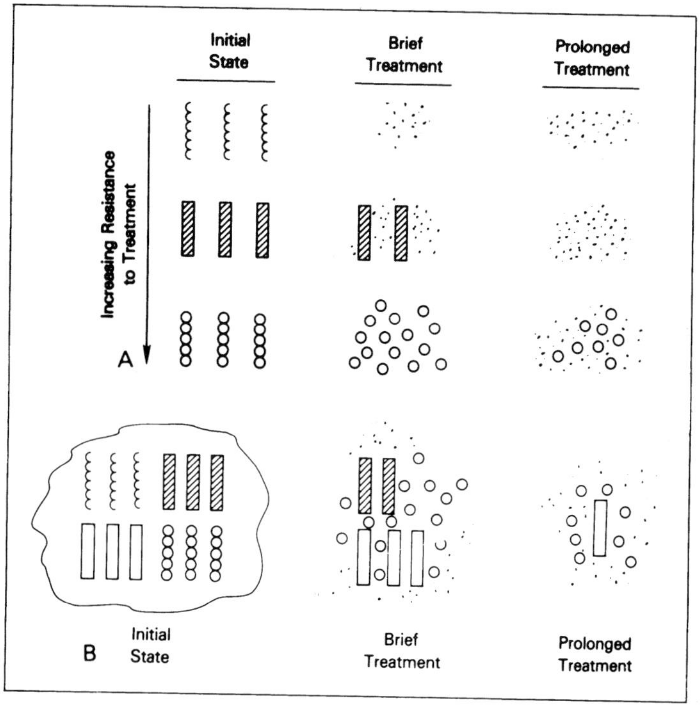

Fig 6-22 *(A)* Events in the sonic treatment of pure cultures of microorganisms. Even brief exposure to ultrasonic energy can rupture the cell walls of some spirochetes (⌇) and gram-negative rods (▨). Streptococci (8) are much more resistant. *(B)* Model of events in the sonic treatment of plaque. Following brief treatment, some of the susceptible organisms will be killed whereas others will not be adequately dispersed. Prolonged treatment may destroy some of the more resistant cells as well. (Courtesy of S. Robrish.)

anaerobically in a Brewer jar, all other steps being performed on the open bench. Maximum recovery, 70%, was achieved by ensuring that dispersal, dilution, and plating were all done anaerobically (Fig 6-23, *A*).[62] Somewhat similar results of 60% viable recovery were obtained from supragingival plaque by anaerobic dispersion and cultivation. Using several enriched culture media could raise this to 75% (Fig 6-23, *B*).[141] Some 25% to 30% of cells seen in direct microscopic counts are lost on culture, in part because dispersion was incomplete and in part because some cells stick to glassware (pipettes, rods) used during dilution and plating. The remainder just may not grow on the available media or may already have been dead.

A combination of nonselective and selective media are commonly used. The selective media are useful for quantitating certain species and for isolating those present only in small numbers. Details of some of these methods are covered in chapters 3 and 8.

Identification and quantitation

Several genera of plaque microorganisms, such as *Streptococcus*[29] and *Actinomyces,* are well defined. Unfortunately, taxonomic classification is difficult within several broad groups such as gram-positive rods, anaerobic gram-negative rods, and aerobic gram-negative cocci.[70] Many plaque isolates cannot readily be identified by current criteria. Nevertheless,

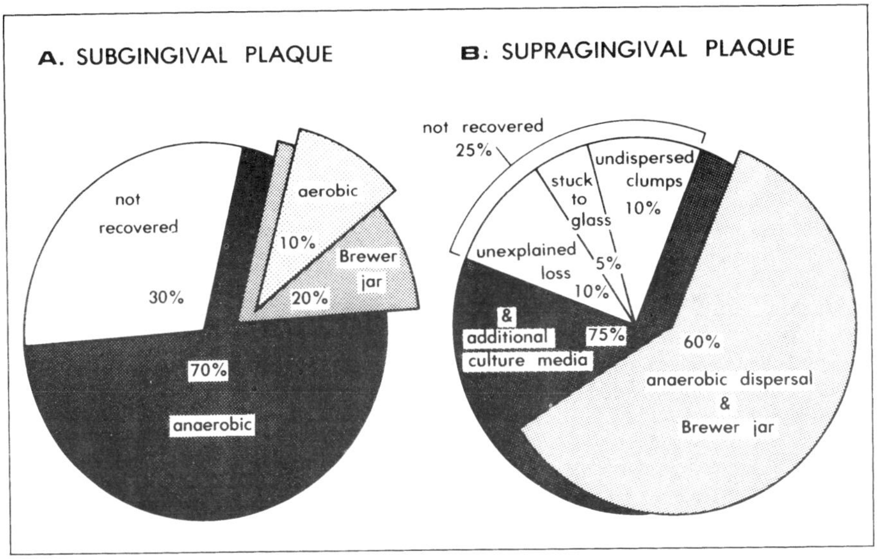

Fig 6-23 Percent viable recovery of microorganisms. *(A)* Percent viable recovery of subgingival plaque. Aerobic samples were processed and cultured aerobically. Brewer jar samples were processed aerobically and cultured anaerobically. Anaerobic samples were processed and cultured entirely anaerobically. (Data from Gordon et al.[62]) *(B)* Percent recovery of supragingival plaque. All samples were sonicated anaerobically, diluted and plated in the open, then incubated anaerobically. (Data from Manganiello et al.[111])

most isolates can be identified to the genus level and many to the species level. The latter may require not only morphological, physiological, and biochemical tests but also end product analyses and even serology and analyses of cell wall components.

Microbiological data can be collected qualitatively, simply by determining absence or presence of an organism in plaque or frequency of isolation per population. Collecting quantitative data is much more difficult. Sometimes the quantity of organisms has been expressed as numbers per weight or volume, or more commonly as a percentage of the total viable count. Additionally, cell counts can be in proportion to the deoxyribonucleic acid or protein content of the original plaque suspension.

Microbial composition of plaque

Plaque consists of a mélange of organisms that varies depending not only on the site and the customary diet but also on how much time the plaque has had to "mature." Bacteria that have been isolated from the oral cavity are shown in Table 6-2. Occasionally other organisms have been found, but it is likely that these are transient inhabitants and not

Table 6-2 Some microbial genera and species in the human oral cavity*

Gram positive bacteria		Gram negative bacteria	
Aerobes and facultative anaerobes	Anaerobes	Aerobes and facultative anaerobes	Anaerobes
		COCCI	
Streptococcus *S gordonii* *S milleri* *S mitis* *S mutans* *S oralis* *S salivarius* *S sanguis* *S sobrinus* *S vestibularis* ***Staphylococcus*** *S epidermidis* ***Stomatococcus*** *S mucilaginosus* ***Micrococcus*** ***Aerococcus***	***Peptostreptococcus*** *P anaerobius* *P asaccharolyticus* *P magnus* *P micros* *P prevotii*	***Moraxella*** *M catarrhalis* ***Neisseria*** *N flavescens* *N mucosa* *N sicca* *N subflava*	***Veillonella*** *V alcalescens* *V parvula* ***Acidaminococcus*** *A fermentans*
		RODS	
Actinomyces *A naeslundii* *A viscosus* ***Corynebacterium*** *C matruchotii* ***Rothia*** *R dentocariosa* ***Lactobacillus*** *L acidophilus* *L brevis* *L buchneri* *L casei* *L cellobiosus* *L delbrueckii* *L fermentum* *L plantarum* *L salivarius*	***Actinomyces*** *A israelii* *A meyeri* *A odontolyticus* ***Eubacterium*** *E alactolyticum* *E brachy* *E lentum* *E nodatum* *E saburreum* *E timidum* ***Lactobacillus*** *L catenaforme* *L crispatus* *L minutus* ***Bifidobacterium*** *B dentium* *B eriksonii* ***Propionibacterium*** *P acnes* *P freudenreichii* *P jensenii* *P propionicus* ***Clostridium***	***Haemophilus*** *H aphrophilus* *H influenzae* *H parainfluenzae* *H paraphrophilus* *H segnis* ***Actinobacillus*** *A actinomycetemcomitans* ***Capnocytophaga*** *C gingivalis* *C ochracea* *C sputigena* ***Eikenella*** *E corrodens* ***Campylobacter*** *C sputorum*	***Bacteroides*** *B buccae* *B buccalis* *B denticola* *B endodontalis*† *B forsythus* *B gingivalis*† *B gracilis* *B heparinolyticus* *B loescheii* *B intermedius* *B melaninogenicus* *B oris* *B oralis* *B veroralis* *B zoogleoformans* ***Fusobacterium*** *F nucleatum* *F periodonticum* ***Leptotrichia*** *L buccalis* ***Campylobacter*** *C concisus* ***Selenomonas*** *S sputigena* ***Wolinella*** *W recta* *W curva*

Other organisms

Mycoplasma	***Treponema***	***Candida***	***Entamoeba***	***Trichomonas***
M orale *M salivarium* *M hominis* *M pneumoniae*	*T denticola* *T macrodentium* *T oralis* *T vincentii*	*C albicans*	*E gingivalis*	*T tenax*

*Adapted from J. Carlsson and Approved Lists of Bacterial Names, *Internat J System Bact* 35:387–407, 1985.
†Proposed reclassification as a new genus, *Porphyromonas* (Shah, H.N. and Collins, M.D. *Internat J System Bact* 38:128–131, 1988).

part of the commensal flora.[69] Although there is tremendous heterogeneity and variation in plaque flora, certain trends are discernible.

Supragingival microbiota

Supragingival plaque contains mostly gram-positive facultative anaerobes. *S sanguis* is the most commonly found streptococcus and constitutes about 10% of the cells.[246] *Actinomyces viscosus, Actinomyces naeslundii,* and *Actinomyces israelii* are found in almost all plaque samples.[246] Other gram-positive species that are regularly detected include *Streptococcus mitis, S mutans* (very much localized), *Rothia dentocariosa, Peptostreptococcus* species, and *Staphylococcus epidermidis.* Gram-negative species found include *Veillonella alcalescens, Veillonella parvula, Fusobacteria,* and *Bacteroides oralis.*

Subgingival microbiota

Mature plaque from a healthy gingival sulcus comprises about 50% to 85% gram-positive cocci and rods, 15% to 30% gram-negative cocci and small rods, 8% each of fusobacteria and filaments, and about 2% spirochetes.[92,218] *Actinomyces* and *Streptococcus* species are the major components of the cultivable flora.[128,218,238,257] *Bacteroides melaninogenicus* is more frequently isolated from the gingival sulcus than elsewhere in the mouth, consisting of about 5% of the isolates.[57,136,257] Spirochetes of the genera *Treponema* and *Borrelia* are indigenous to the gingival sulcus area.[129] Although they are seen frequently in electron micrographs of subgingival plaque, they have only rarely been cultivated. These organisms are highly sensitive to oxygen and will only grow under conditions of low oxidation-reduction potential (Eh). Some require the presence of other organisms to supply essential growth factors and cannot be isolated. They merit further study. Spirochetes are rarely found in children with healthy gingivae, but they increase in numbers with age.[220]

Young patients with juvenile periodontitis (periodontosis) or adults with a rapidly progressing form of periodontitis have a significantly different subgingival flora.[175,176,217,219,240] Gram-negative anaerobic and microaerophilic rods increase dramatically, comprising 40% to 78% of the total cultivable microbiota. The microbiota of juvenile periodontitis lesions is characterized by saccharolytic gram-negative microorganisms of six distinct groups: *(1)* anaerobic vibrios, *(2) Capnocytophaga (Bacteroides ochraceus), (3)* tiny anaerobic rods, *(4) Bacteroides*-like organisms, *(5)* surface translocating organisms, and *(6) Actinobacillus actinomycetemcomitans.* Advanced periodontitis microbiota is characterized by the presence of large numbers of asaccharolytic microorganisms including *F nucleatum, B melaninogenicus, Eikenella corrodens, Bacteroides corrodens, Bacteroides buccae,* and anaerobic vibrios.

Despite significant advances in cultural techniques, particularly for strict anaerobes, the culture and identification of bacterial species in subgingival plaque are fraught with great difficulty. Spirochetes, which

CELL TYPE	NORMAL pocket depth 2mm	DISEASED pocket depth 7mm
COCCI	74	22
RODS	16	18
FILAMENTS	2	2
FUSIFORMS	5	6
MOTILE	0.3	13
SPIROCHETES	2	38
MOTILE/NON-MOTILE	1/49	1/1

Fig 6-24 Percentage distribution of plaque flora in health and periodontal disease using darkfield microscopy. (Courtesy of Listgarten and Helldén.[116])

are considered important periodontal pathogens, have generally not been cultured successfully. Accordingly, investigators have increasingly used darkfield microscopy, a noncultural approach, to quantitate the proportions of microorganisms in the subgingival crevice, based on their morphological appearance and on whether the organisms are motile or nonmotile.[112,116] A clear-cut difference in the microbial composition of healthy and periodontally diseased areas has been demonstrated. The proportion of motile rods and spirochetes is significantly higher at diseased sites than at healthy sites (Fig 6-24).

Based both on data from cultural studies of subgingival microflora and on darkfield microscopic examination from selected sites, certain species of microorganisms can be correlated with various forms of periodontal diseases, as summarized in Table 6-3.

Formation and development of dental plaques

The rate of growth and amount of plaque formed are influenced by physical factors such as uneven tooth surfaces, carious lesions, ill-fitting margins of restorations, and irregularities in the positioning of the teeth. However, even in the absence of such conditions plaque will grow on the teeth of individuals who cease using oral hygiene methods.

Based on both morphological[119,140] and microbiological[79,125,188,224,238] sequential analyses, a better understanding has been gained of the events

Table 6-3 Organisms of probable etiological significance in various types of periodontal disease

Disease	Location	Organisms
Gingivitis	Supragingival plaque	*Actinomyces viscosus* *Actinomyces israelii* *Capnocytophaga gingivalis*
	Subgingival plaque	*Fusbacterium nucleatum* *Veillonella parvula* *Campylobacter sputorum* Spirochetes (small)
Acute necrotizing ulcerative gingivitis	Subgingival plaque	*Fusobacterium* sp. *Bacteroides intermedius* *Selenomonas* sp. Spirochetes (intermediate size)
	Gingival tissues	Spirochetes (intermediate size)
Chronic periodontitis	Subgingival plaque	*Bacteroides intermedius* *Eikenella corrodens* Fusiform bacteroides *Eubacterium* sp. Spirochetes
Rapidly destructive periodontitis	Subgingival plaque	*Bacteroides gingivalis* *Wolinella recta* Fusiform bacteroides *Fusobacterium nucleatum* *Selenomonas sputigena* *Bacteroides gracilis* *Bacteroides buccae* *Actinobacillus actinomycetemcomitans* *Eikenella corrodens* Spirochetes (intermediate size)
Juvenile periodontitis	Subgingival plaque	*Actinobacillus actinomycetemcomitans* *Capnocytophaga ochraceus* *Bacteroides intermedius* *Eubacterium saburreum* Anaerobic *Vibrio* sp. Spirochetes

involved in plaque formation, especially on clean supragingival enamel surfaces. For convenience of description these events can be considered as three phases: *(1)* initial colonization, *(2)* rapid bacterial growth, and *(3)* remodeling. In actuality, though, these are progressive phases gradually changing and not sharply defined.

Initial colonization occurs during the first 8 hours after a tooth surface has been cleaned, and it involves the deposition of bacteria derived from the saliva or the buccal and lingual mucous surfaces adjacent to the tooth. This process is both rapid and selective, different bacterial species adsorbing to the acquired pellicle with different efficiencies.[58,59] In part this selective adsorption is determined by the surface components of the bacteria that are complementary to the pellicle. Salivary constituents, particularly high molecular weight glycoproteins, are also important; most of the isolates of early dental plaque are strongly agglutinated in the presence of saliva. Hydrophobic interactions between cell surface and pellicle are involved in the adherence of *S sanguis*.[167]

Because of its importance in the caries process, much attention has been devoted to the initial colonization by *S mutans*. Although sucrose greatly favors the colonization by *S mutans*, it is now recognized that the organism can adhere independently of sucrose, and it has been postulated that this is mediated either by the interaction of components on the surface of the organism with blood group-reactive salivary glycoproteins in the acquired pellicle, or by an electrostatic interaction between teichoic acids on the bacterial cell surface, calcium ions, and acid salivary glycoproteins.[191] However, experiments using saliva-coated hydroxyapatite at various concentrations of calcium ions do not support this latter role for teichoic acid/calcium bridging in the initial adherence step. Convincing evidence from a number of different sources indicates that proteins on the surface of *S mutans* are critical in this initial sucrose-independent adherence, because organisms that have been pretreated by proteases have greatly reduced adherence.[157,231] The nature of both the bacterial surface protein and the salivary receptive protein involved in adherence in the acquired pellicle is unknown. The adherence of *S mutans* is perceived as a two-reaction process in which initial weak attachment occurs between bacterial cell proteins and salivary glycoproteins of the acquired pellicle and is followed by cellular accumulation mediated by sucrose-dependent glucans and cell surface receptor ligands (adhesins)[231] (Fig 6-25). In other words, the adherence of selected oral streptococci initially involves nonspecific, low-affinity, very rapid binding reactions followed by specific, high-affinity, slower, but stronger attachment to the acquired pellicle.[232] According to one hypothesis, the bacterial enzyme glucosyltransferase plays a crucial role in sucrose-induced plaque formation. This enzyme can adsorb to acquired pellicle and also exists on the cell surface of *S mutans*. Newly synthesized glucan chains, produced by glucosyltransferase both on the bacteria and on the tooth surface, interact (pack) and form a strong binding mechanism.[193]

Rapid bacterial growth occurs between 8 hours and 2 days after a prophylaxis. Those organisms that have become firmly attached to the pellicle multiply as local accumulations of several layers of bacteria held together by interbacterial adherence. Extracellular glucans have been shown to facilitate homologous intercellular adherence of *S mutans* and aggregation of *A viscosus*, as discussed in chapters 3 and 4. However, these polysaccharides are not a universal glue and do not seem to be important in the accumulation of all plaque bacteria.

The remodeling phase of plaque starts after about 2 days and contin-

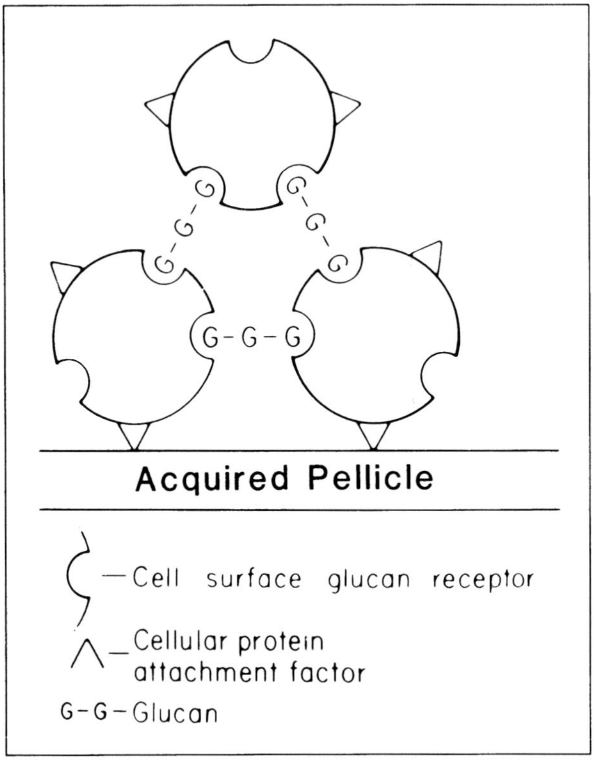

Fig 6-25 Schematic diagram of proposed model of *S mutans* adherence that illustrates *(1)* the interaction between bacterial surface proteins and acquired pellicle (sucrose-independent, weak), and *(2)* the glucan-mediated cell-to-cell accumulation (sucrose-dependent, strong). (Courtesy of Staat et al.[231])

ues indefinitely, because the bacterial mass is not a static entity. At this stage, the total number of organisms remains relatively constant, but the microbial composition becomes more complex. The general pattern is one of early dominance by streptococci, followed by a shift toward a more anaerobic and filamentous flora, particularly by the *Actinomyces* species. In the gingival sulcus region, curved and spiral-shaped organisms as well as spirochetes occur 1 to 2 weeks after plaque develops.[83] Some of these shifts are illustrated in Fig 6-26, based on pooled plaque from the labial surface of incisors sampled 1, 3, 5, 7, and 9 days after they had been polished.[188] *Streptococcus, Neisseria,* and *Actinomycetales* (probably *R dentocariosa*) constitute most of the viable early plaque colonies. By 9 days streptococci are still predominant, closely followed by *Actinomyces.* A pronounced increase occurs in *Veillonella* and *Fusobacterium,* both anaerobes. The sequential shift from streptococci to *Actinomyces* and subsequent inclusion of various gram-negative bacteria such as *Bacteroides, Fusobacterium,* and *Treponema* may be due to highly specific and ordered coaggregation bridges of partner cell-types.[99]

These alterations in the developing plaque flora are examples of *autogenic succession,* which refers to the ability of the resident microbial population to change the environment to such a degree that it is replaced by other species more suited to the modified environment. As plaque forms on a cleaned tooth surface the Eh falls (Fig 6-27). Extremely low

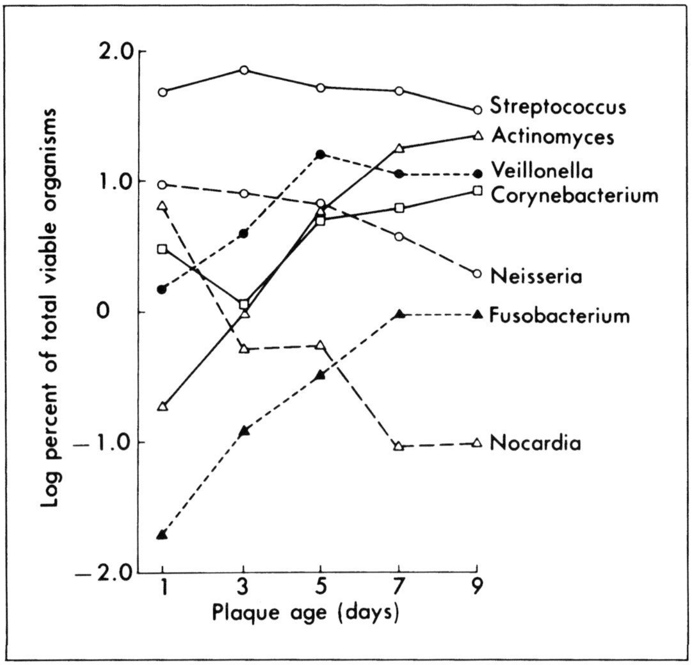

Fig 6-26 Relative proportions of selected organisms in developing supragingival plaque on the labial surface of incisors. Plaque samples were obtained 1, 3, 5, 7, and 9 days after thorough prophylaxis. (Courtesy of Ritz.[188])

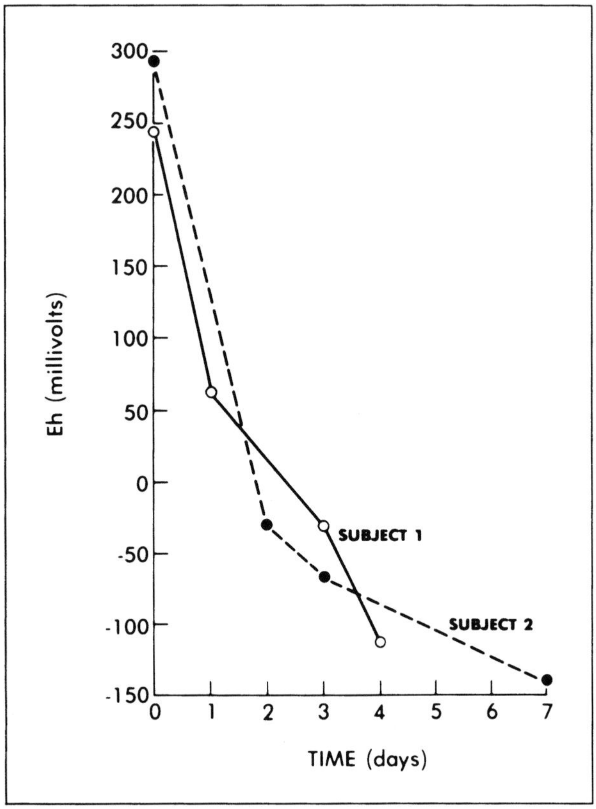

Fig 6-27 Fall in oxidation-reduction potential, Eh, in developing dental plaque of two subjects. Plaque was allowed to form over measuring electrodes attached to veneers of enamel mounted on a fixed bridge pontic. (Adapted from Kenney and Ash.[93])

Eh's have been located in established dental plaque by oxidation-reduction indicators such as benzyl viologen, methylene blue, and triphenyl tetrazolium chloride[88,223] and by direct potentiometric measurements.[93,197] Different plaque organisms have varying ability to reduce the Eh. Bacterial evolution of hydrogen sulfide[248] and hydrogenase-containing organisms may be responsible. Lowering of the Eh contributes to successional alterations in the flora of the gingival sulcus associated with the appearance of clinical signs of gingivitis.

Direct measurements of the oxygen tension (pO_2) in periodontal pockets show a narrow range (5 to 27 mm Hg), with deeper pockets tending to contain less oxygen than shallow sites. No pockets were completely anaerobic.[153]

Chemical composition of plaque

There have been numerous studies on the chemical composition of dental plaque, some emphasizing the carbohydrate components, others the proteins, and still others the inorganic constituents, especially calcium, phosphorus, and fluoride. Plaque contains about 80% water and 20% solids.[78,106] Proteins are the major component, 40% to 50% of the dry weight of plaque; carbohydrates account for 13% to 18% and lipids for 10% to 14%. This composition of plaque approximates that of washed streptococcal cells, although plaque is higher in protein and lipid components (Table 6-4).[208] About four times as much protein can be extracted from dental plaque as from an equal weight of a mixture of the predominant microorganisms cultured from plaque.[53] Presumably the additional protein is due to salivary proteins in the plaque matrix. The higher lipid content is consistent with an accumulation of gram-negative microaerophilic and anaerobic organisms in plaque as it matures. Veil-

Table 6-4 Comparison of chemical composition of supragingival dental plaque and *Streptococcus sanguis*

Component	Plaque	*S sanguis*
	% wet wt	
Water	80	84
Ash	10	7
Organic		9
	% dry wt	
Protein	40-50	21
Carbohydrate	13-18	19
Lipid	10-14	5
RNA		4
DNA		1

lonellae and fusobacteria contain lipopolysaccharides and are about 20% to 30% lipid.[98] The carbohydrate and protein content of plaque are subject to wide variations, depending on dietary considerations.[31,36]

Fractionation of plaque

Attempts to separate dental plaque into cellular and acellular fractions have been only partially successful.[106,213] One approach has been mechanical dispersion of an aqueous suspension of plaque followed by filtration. The amount of carbohydrate in the acellular (plaque matrix) phase is more than twice that in the cellular fraction. A real dilemma exists in trying to extract polysaccharides from the plaque matrix without including intracellular and cell wall carbohydrates. Aqueous extraction procedures leave behind the insoluble glucans. Very dilute alkali may dissolve all the insoluble glucans, whereas concentrated alkali removes not only extracellular material but also cellular components.

Carbohydrates of plaque

Glucose is the main carbohydrate found in hydrolyzed extracts of plaque.[78] Appreciable amounts of arabinose, ribose, galactose, and fucose can be detected. Much of the carbohydrate exists in the form of extracellular polymers, either as glucans (homopolymers of glucose), fructans (homopolymers of fructose), or heteropolysaccharides, all of which are synthesized by different plaque microorganisms (Table 6-5). The glucans occur either as dextrans, predominantly α-(1→6) linked, or as "mutans," which are mostly α-(1→3) linked. The latter may serve a skeletal function in plaque, much like that of cellulose in plants. In addition, an amylose-type glucan, mostly α-(1→4) linkage, is made by *Neisseria* species.[15,194]

Table 6-5 Plaque microorganisms forming extracellular polysaccharides

Glucans	Fructans	Heteropolysaccharides
Streptococcus sanguis	*Actinomyces viscosus*	*Actinomyces viscosus*
Streptococcus mutans	*Streptococcus mutans*	*Lactobacillus buchneri*
Streptococcus salivarius	*Streptococcus salivarius*	*Lactobacillus cellobiosus*
Streptococcus mitior		*Lactobacillus casei*
Lactobacillus casei		
Lactobacillus acidophilus		
Neisseria sp.		

The fructans made by *Streptococcus salivarius* and *A viscosus* are of the levan type with (2→6)-linked β-fructofuranoside residues, whereas *S mutans* produces an inulin-type fructan with (1→2)-linked β-fructofuranoside residues.[16] Glucans and fructans serve as a reservoir of fermentable carbohydrate for plaque metabolism. The function of glucan in adherence and coherence of selective organisms has already been discussed. *A viscosus* forms extracellular heteropolysaccharide composed mainly of *N*-acetylglucosamine (62%) together with galactose (7%), glucose (4%), and uronic acid (3%).[73,194]

In addition to extracellular polymers, carbohydrates exist in plaque as peptidoglycans of bacterial cell walls and as intracellular glycogen. Production and storage of intracellular iodophilic polysaccharides of the glycogen-amylopectin type are properties common to many bacteria.[100,251,252] For some strains of *S mutans* the synthesis of intracellular polysaccharides appears to be an important trait determining their virulence.[242] In the absence of exogenous fermentable carbohydrates, organisms with intracellular polysaccharides can continue acid production by degrading their intracellular carbohydrate reserves (see Fig 4-9). The amount of intracellular polysaccharide in plaque will, therefore, be related to how long it was before the last exogenous fermentable carbohydrate was ingested.

Proteins of plaque

The proteins found in plaque originate from bacteria, saliva, or gingival fluid. Several salivary proteins, such as amylase, lysozyme, IgA, IgG, and albumin have been identified in plaque.[75,103,243] They may be intact or degraded, and considerable variation in these proteins is found among individuals.[74] The topography and distribution of the immunoglobulins (IgG, IgA, IgM), particularly at the apical plaque border, suggest that they mainly derive from the gingival fluid.[173]

Bacterial proteins of plaque have been recognized by the fluorescent antibody technique or by their enzymatic activities. The latter include glucosyltransferase, glucanhydrolase, hyaluronidase, phosphatase, and protease.[177,225] The significance of these enzymes in plaque is not clear. The antibodies may serve an immune function, and the proteins contribute to buffering in plaque.

Inorganic components of plaque

The inorganic content of plaque depends on its location and age.[38] Plaque contains calcium, phosphate, and fluoride in higher concentrations than those of saliva. Aqueous extraction can remove all the inorganic phosphate in early plaque but only 5% of the calcium. The fluoride concentration in plaque (14 to 20 ppm) is higher than in saliva (0.01 to

0.05 ppm) or in drinking water (usually 0 to 1 ppm).[214] Most of the fluoride is bound either to inorganic component[14,214] or to bacteria.[82] As the pH of plaque falls during fermentation, more free fluoride ions are released.[12] Potentially this would favor cariostasis by resisting a further decrease in plaque pH and/or by inducing the formation of fluoridated apatite.

Pathogenic potential of plaque

The plaque microflora can cause pathological changes in either the teeth (crown or roots) or the supporting structures (periodontium) (Table 6-6). Dental caries, the destruction of the hard tissues of the tooth, is primarily due to the formation of various organic acids that are capable of dissolving the mineral components of the teeth. The metabolic pathways whereby these acids are formed and their presence in plaque have been discussed in chapter 1. Other plaque products potentially injurious to the host include low molecular weight metabolites, such as ammonia, hydrogen sulfide, methylmercaptan, toxic amines, indole, and skatole. Some of the plaque enzymes, which may be of either bacterial or host cell-lysosomal origin, are capable of degrading the periodontal connective tissues. In addition, high molecular weight cytotoxic products, such as lipopolysaccharides and peptidoglycans of the bacterial cell walls and

Table 6-6 Pathogenic constituents of dental plaque

Substances inducing direct tissue damage	
Organic acids	Protease
Indole	Collagenase
Ammonia	Hyaluronidase
Hydrogen sulfide	β-Glucuronidase
Methyl mercaptan	Neuraminidase
Toxic amines	Chondroitin sulfatase
Phospholipase A and C	
Inflammation-inducing substances	
Chemotactic substances (polypeptides)	
Activators of complement cascade	
Histamine	
Mitogens	
Substances inducing indirect tissue damage by host immunological response	
Endotoxin	
Peptidoglycan	
Polysaccharide	
Bacterial antigens	

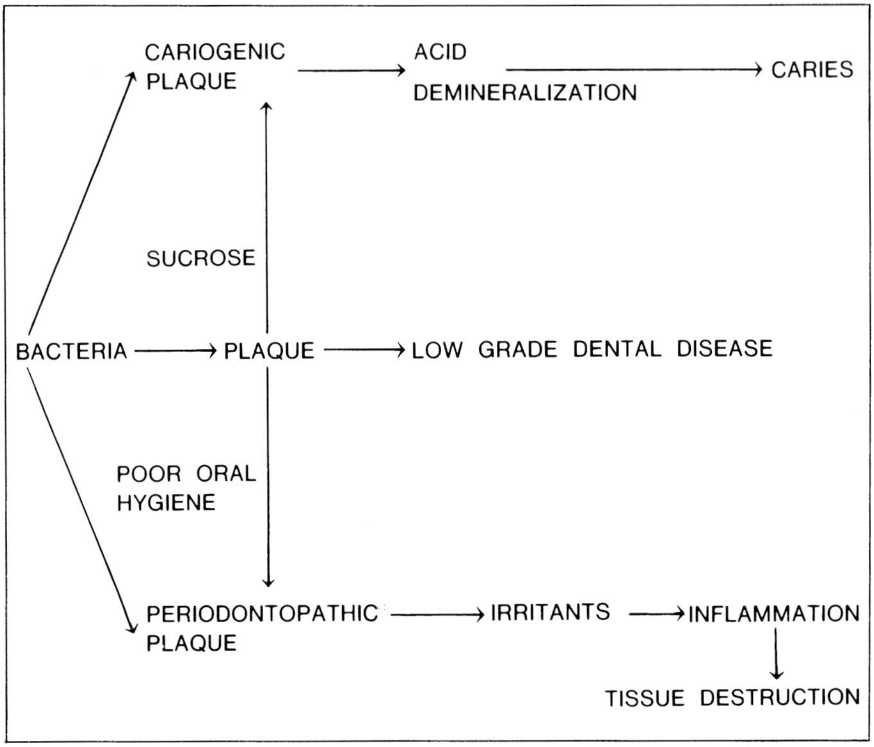

Fig 6-28 Simplified diagram showing the different pathogenic potential of dental plaques.

membranes, may penetrate the junctional epithelium and sensitize the host tissues, thereby initiating and maintaining an inflammatory response. A more detailed discussion of the pathogenic and immune mechanisms involved in periodontal disease is available elsewhere[202] and is not appropriate in a text on cariology.

Having considered some of the individual components of plaque, one must also examine the pathogenic potential of plaque as a whole. Are the harmful effects simply due to an increase in numbers of bacteria and the plaque mass, or are they due to an increased virulence of the flora? The answer will influence the strategy for prevention or control of the diseases caused by dental plaques. A simplistic model is that bacteria form plaque (Fig 6-28). A high-sucrose diet favors establishment of a cariogenic flora, acid formation, demineralization, and caries. With poor oral hygiene a periodontopathic plaque forms, and bacterial irritants cause inflammation and tissue loss. In addition, some plaques have no, or very low-grade, pathogenic potential.

Loesche[129] has drawn attention to the two prevailing philosophies concerning prophylaxis or therapy of plaque-related dental diseases. These are called the *nonspecific plaque hypothesis* (NSPH) and the *specific plaque hypothesis* (SPH). The nonspecific plaque hypothesis states that caries and periodontal disease result from the elaboration of noxious products by the entire plaque flora. It is easy to see how the NSPH came about; after all, many organisms are acidogenic, releasing lactic or other organic acids within the plaque. Similarly, ammonia, hydrogen sulfide, hydrolytic enzymes, antigens, and other cytotoxic products are formed by a wide spectrum of the plaque flora. The NSPH assumes there is a host threshold for these products. Amounts of irritants below this threshold value can be overcome by host defenses such as salivary buffering, detoxification, and immune responses. In essence it is based on the *quantity* rather than the *quality* of the plaque flora. In contrast, the specific plaque hypothesis states that only certain plaques cause infections, owing to the presence of specific pathogens and/or a relative increase in the levels of certain indigenous plaque organisms. The diagnosis of infection may be made by bacteriological examination of the plaque flora, but it is usually based on clinical criteria.

Control of dental plaque

Perspectives, problems, and prospects

Because the two most important dental diseases, caries and periodontal disease, are directly caused by dental plaques, there has been a tremendous effort to find some way of either preventing the formation of plaque or effectively removing it from the surface of teeth. In essence, the approaches to controlling plaques can be classified as:

1. Agents acting against the microflora per se
2. Agents interfering with bacterial attachment by:
   a. attacking plaque matrix components
   b. altering the tooth surface
3. Mechanical removal of plaque

These approaches are by no means new. Mechanical methods of plaque removal with chewing sticks and toothpicks are common to many cultures. Caries prevention by the administration of antibacterial substances was already tested by W.D. Miller in 1890,[154] who wrote:

> The fact that decay of the teeth is of parasitic origin having been once established . . . we ought to be able by means of properly chosen antiseptic materials not only to arrest decay, but to prevent its appearance. This is, indeed, the avowed object of the very many antiseptic mouth-washes now on the market.

Unfortunately, the available disinfectants were toxic and had other undesirable side effects, so the concept of chemical control of plaque did not materialize at that time. However, over the years there has been increasing interest in the use of antibacterial agents as a form of plaque control, as well as, of course, in more effective techniques for the mechanical removal of plaque. The literature is extensive, and only the highlights will be covered. Excellent, detailed, and comprehensive reviews are available on the use of antimicrobial agents* and on mechanical plaque control.[8,66,144]

Before consideration of specific chemotherapeutic agents, whether antibacterial or antiadherent, a problem common to all such agents should be mentioned. Effective therapy requires an adequate level of the drug in the infected area for enough time to permit it to exert its maximum therapeutic potential. Yet this principle has largely been ignored by many who have tried to prevent or treat bacterial infections of tooth surfaces with antimicrobial or related agents.[155] Most compounds have been tested as topical agents in such vehicles as mouthrinses, dentifrices, chewing gums, or gels, all requiring repeated application. Usually investigators have performed these studies without knowing the concentration of the drug necessary to inhibit the growth of the odontopathic plaque microorganisms. Such highly empiric modes of administration do not accurately reflect the drug's therapeutic potential.[48,96,169] As might be expected, the results have been variable. Some investigators have reported significant reductions in plaque scores or suppression of specific microorganisms, whereas others have found no significant effect when compared with a placebo. In most instances, positive effects were temporary and the plaque scores or the specific organisms returned to pretreatment levels within hours, days, or weeks. Strålfors[237] has calculated that 99.9% of the bacteria in the oral cavity must be killed to inhibit plaque formation for at least 6 hours, on the assumption that one brushes about every 12 hours.

Drugs placed in the mouth are continuously diluted by the saliva and washed away. Even if the minimal inhibitory concentration of a drug were used initially, rapid clearance from the oral cavity would usually prevent maintenance of an effective concentration. The failure or limited success of many agents in preventing caries or periodontal disease can be attributed to their transitory presence in the mouth. It is not that they cannot kill plaque microflora or hydrolyze plaque matrices; many of them do so in the test tube. It is primarily a problem of effective delivery.

There are some ways around this difficulty. One is the use of an agent with substantivity. Substantivity refers to a prolonged association between a material and a substrate that is greater or more prolonged than would be expected with simple mechanical deposition. It involves mechanisms such as adsorption, ion exchange, or chemical interaction.[250] Agents exhibiting substantivity include the bis-biguanides, alexidine and chlorhexidine, and fluoride; all are capable of adsorption to or chemical

*References 49, 60, 86, 124, 129, 138, 185.

interaction with oral surfaces. The biguanides bind to labial and buccal mucosa, and fluoride binds to the tooth surface. Alternatively, drugs lacking substantivity could be incorporated into a controlled release delivery system to provide uniform and prolonged release in the mouth.[34] A device could be attached to one or more teeth, with the drug embedded in a matrix that permits gradual, local release for days or weeks after insertion. Such depot preparations are a logical extension of present topical delivery methods for use in the oral cavity. However, extensive animal and clinical testing is still required to determine which drugs and concentrations will be most effective.

Agents acting against the microflora

The rationale for selecting a specific chemotherapeutic agent for treating dentogingival plaque infections depends on whether one is following the NSPH or SPH. Treatment of patients under the NSPH is prophylactic and open-ended until adverse effects are caused by the drug. Such prophylactic agents for plaque control need to be extremely safe because of their frequent use over a lifetime in such over-the-counter forms as mouthrinses or dentifrices. In contrast, treatment of patients under the SPH is targeted therapy over a finite period until a clinical cure is effected or until the key organism(s) is eliminated or reduced to an insignificant level(s).

Dental literature is replete with clinical trials of antimicrobial agents, some of which are shown in Table 6-7. Because caries and most forms of periodontal disease are caused by the chronic presence of plaque, many of the clinical trials have used a reduction of plaque scores, which can be demonstrated in days or weeks, rather than reduction of disease, which requires several years of testing. Under the SPH, agents could be screened in a relatively short time for their ability to suppress or eliminate the virulent microorganisms within the plaque. Of course, long-term effectiveness for disease prevention would still need to be proven.

An ideal therapeutic agent against plaque infections must be safe in the form that is used, with no untoward systemic or local side effects, such as irritation, injury, or host sensitization. It must be effective against the specific plaque pathogens and must prevent, or cure, the disease caused by them. Preferably it should be a drug that is not used for the treatment of serious medical problems,[48] although this is by no means an essential restriction.[129] If the drug is to be used topically, it should not be absorbable through the oral or gastrointestinal mucosa. It should have no taste, or if it has an unpleasant taste it must be possible to completely mask it with compatible flavoring agents. It should be stable so that it will act over a prolonged period, either by substantivity or by release from a controlled delivery system. This listing of requirements of an ideal antiplaque agent sounds almost as if it must have the attributes of Caesar's wife: being above all suspicion. No drug has yet been accepted by the Food and Drug Administration as a topical *prophylactic* agent for

Table 6-7 Antimicrobial agents tested for plaque prevention or reduction

Category	Spectrum	Agent
Antibiotics	Broad	Actinobolin*
		Chlortetracycline
		Tetracycline
		Streptomycin*
		Kanamycin*
		Neomycin*
		Niddamycin*
	Gram +	Bacitracin*
		Erythromycin
		Penicillin
		Vancomycin*
		Gramicidin*
		Spiramycin†
	Gram –	Polymyxin B*
Other antibacterial agents	Broad	Benzophenanthridines
		Sanguinarine
		Bis-biguanides*
		Alexidine
		Chlorhexidine
		Bispyridines
		Octenidine
		Phenolic compounds
		Phenol
		β-naphthol
		Hexylresorcinol
		Halogens
		Iodine & iodophors
		Chlorine
		Oxychlorosene
		Chloramine-T
		Fluoride
		Oxygenating agent
		Peroxide
		Perborate
	Broad (only anaerobes)	Metronidazole
	Mostly gram +	Quaternary ammonium compounds
		Cetylpyridinium chloride
		Benzethonium chloride
		Domiphen bromide

*Not absorbed or poorly absorbed across gastrointestinal tract.
†Some gram-negative also.

preventing plaque formation.[249] A major concern in the prophylactic use of antibacterial agents is their tendency to disrupt the normal microbial ecological balance of the host. The Advisory Review Panel on over-the-counter dental products has recommended to the Food and Drug Administration that all mouthrinses claiming to prevent, control, or treat plaque or gingivitis by chemical agents should be categorized as not generally recognized as safe and effective.[249] The Council on Dental Therapeutics of the American Dental Association, on the other hand, has established guidelines for the acceptance of chemotherapeutic products for the control of supragingival dental plaque and gingivitis.[34] Both over-the-counter and prescription-only products must demonstrate statistically significant reductions (as compared with a placebo or a control treatment) at the 95% confidence level for plaque scores as well as for gingivitis in a long-term (minimum of 6 months) clinical trial conducted by two independent investigators. However, in conjunction with mechanical debridement, some drugs may be used *therapeutically,* such as systemic penicillin for treatment of necrotizing ulcerative gingivitis infections or tetracycline for treatment of rapid or juvenile periodontitis infections.

Antibiotics

Penicillin, erythromycin, and tetracycline, when administered in the diet of experimental rodents, can be highly effective in controlling plaque and dental caries.[48] In three of four studies conducted on humans, penicillin used topically in dentifrices has not been shown as beneficial, probably because of insufficient concentrations and duration of the drug in the mouth. Because of the potential problems of resistant bacteria and penicillin sensitivity, its use as a topical agent for prevention of caries is not permitted. It is worth noting that children who receive long-term systemic penicillin for rheumatic fever have distinctly less caries than their untreated siblings.[67,120]

Spiramycin reduces bacterial colonization on rodent teeth when applied topically.[95] Based on subjective clinical impressions, systemically administered spiramycin is reported to have therapeutic effects on human periodontal disease.[71]

Considerable interest has centered on vancomycin, bacitracin, kanamycin, niddamycin, and polymyxin B, topical antibiotics that are not absorbed from the gastrointestinal tract. Vancomycin has been found to improve gingival health and reduce halitosis for short periods when used on patients with periodontal disease.[156,207] It does not reduce total plaque scores in individuals in whom no clinical disease is present.[126,150] Gingivitis developed at the usual rate in humans who stopped toothbrushing and rinsed three times daily with vancomycin. Their plaque flora became almost entirely gram-negative.[83] Children who used 3% vancomycin gel in custom-fitted trays for 5 minutes daily under supervision in school (about 150 treatments a year) averaged one less decayed or filled surface in 1 year. The reduction was significant in fissures and in newly erupting teeth but not on smooth or proximal surfaces or teeth present at baseline.[40] Three daily rinses over a 5-day period with polymyxin B favored proliferation of a gram-positive flora and depressed the gram-negative flora. Similar rinsing with tetracycline markedly suppressed the plaque flora and gave a lower plaque index score.[126] Niddamycin is a nonabsorbable macrolide antibiotic tested as a mouthrinse under the code number CC10232. Reduced calculus and gingivitis scores have been reported after use of such a rinse,[233] but prolonged use is contraindicated because of the possible emergence of drug-resistant organisms that may be resistant to other macrolide antibiotics such as erythromycin.

Kanamycin is a poorly absorbed aminoglycoside antibiotic with a broad spectrum of activity. It has been tested in short-term, intensive treatment (2 to 5 days) every fifth week, according to the concepts of the specific plaque hypothesis.[133,135] Subjects who have moderate to severe gingivitis show improvement under such a regimen, although 5% kanamycin paste does not eliminate the gingivitis. This could be due to the inability of the delivery system to bring the drug into the periodontal pocket. In children with rampant caries, a week of kanamycin gel treatment, before and after the placement of dental restorations, reduces the caries increment for 14 to 37 months after treatment.

In several of these studies the use of antibiotics caused pronounced shifts in the balance of the oral flora. Such alterations of the indigenous flora are potentially hazardous.[11,110]

Bis-biguanides

Other than fluorides, no agent has received as much attention in dentistry as the bis-biguanides, chlorhexidine and alexidine. The literature on their clinical effects, mechanism of action, effect on the oral ecology, toxicology, and side effects is extensive and continually growing[37,124,129] so that only the highlights and principles can be covered here.

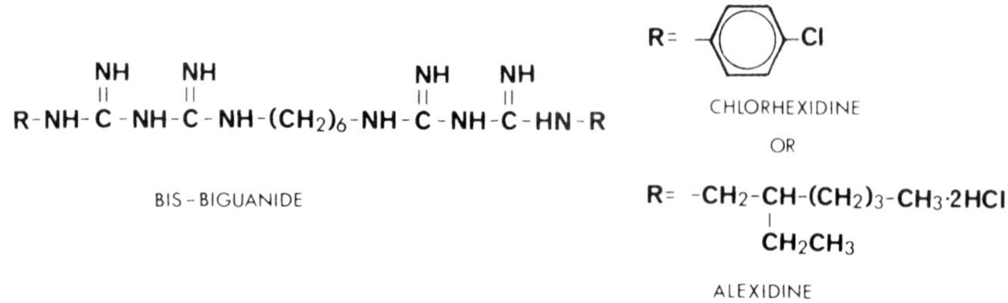

The bis-biguanides are fungicidal and bactericidal against gram-positive and gram-negative organisms.[46] They are cationic agents interacting with microorganisms that have a negative charge at physiological pH. The most important anionic groups on the bacterial surface, to which the bis-biguanides bind, are probably the phosphate groups of teichoic acid in gram-positive bacteria and the phosphate groups of lipopolysaccharides in gram-negative bacteria. When the bis-biguanide binds to the organism, its cell membrane becomes permeable, allowing the cytoplasmic contents to leak. At high concentrations, chlorhexidine causes precipitation of cytoplasmic proteins. By virtue of their cationic properties, the bis-biguanides also bind electrostatically to hydroxyapatite powder, to acquired pellicle, to plaque, and to buccal and labial mucosa.[192] Neither the clean tooth surface nor the tongue is of major importance as receptor sites for chlorhexidine.[255] Nevertheless, this substantivity of the bis-biguanides for the other oral surfaces means that reservoirs of chlorhexidine form in the mouth and subsequently the drug is slowly released, preventing plaque formation for hours.[20]

Chlorhexidine and alexidine have been tested clinically in mouthrinse, gel, paste, and other topical vehicles. They can inhibit the development of plaque, gingivitis, and experimental caries.* In the absence of oral hygiene, heavy accumulations of plaque already present are removed and chronic gingivitis is reduced in humans, dogs, and monkeys following use of these agents. Frequent use gives rise to some undesirable side effects, the most conspicuous being the development of a yellow-brown stain on the teeth and dorsum of the tongue. Although the stain is extrinsic, it cannot be removed by brushing with a normal toothpaste; mechanical polishing is necessary for its removal.[80] A few individuals have experienced mucosal desquamation and soreness. Solutions containing bis-biguanides have a disagreeable bitter taste and require masking by compatible flavoring agents to be palatable. Some patients experience a persistent aftertaste or disturbed salt taste sensation.[180] Extensive studies on the safety of these compounds, including acute and chronic tests, show extremely low levels of toxicity both locally and systemically. No teratologic or reproductive changes have been found.[52] In 1986 the FDA approved, and the ADA Council on Dental Therapeutics accepted, a chlorhexidine mouthrinse for use in prevention and treatment of gingivitis. However, there is no indication that the effect of a chlorhexidine rinse extends beyond 3 mm of sulcular depth, which limits its therapeutic effect on periodontitis.

The bis-biguanides are remarkably effective antiplaque agents. They should be employed not prophylactically but as therapeutic agents for patients with active disease. This requires diagnosis and supervised use until the disease is controlled. Accordingly, these agents should be available by prescription and not as over-the-counter products. As such, the bis-biguanides could be useful adjuncts in the treatment of periodontal disease or rampant caries. They are not a panacea or "magic bullet"; in the absence of conventional therapeutic and preventive measures, the bis-biguanide alone has not been able to cure periodontal disease or prevent caries.

*References 5, 7, 27, 43, 127, 201, 256.

Although bis-biguanides have substantivity, their use has never resulted in the elimination of *S mutans* from all sites in the mouth for longer than a week or two.[47] Recently, chlorhexidine acetate (20%) applied in a varnish (40% Sumatra benzoin in 95% ethanol) and then covered with a layer of polyurethane provided sustained release of the agent for up to 12 days.[4] Professional application of these varnishes to the teeth successfully eliminated *S mutans* for prolonged periods, from 6 to 18 months.[197] Long-term clinical trials will be needed to determine if such therapy is effective in reducing caries.

Other antibacterial agents

The most commonly used antimicrobial agents in commercially available mouthrinses are the quaternary ammonium compounds such as cetylpyridinium chloride, benzethonium chloride, and domiphen bromide, and the phenolic compounds including phenol, beta-naphthol, and hexylresorcinol. These agents kill microorganisms by reacting with their proteins to cause coagulation, precipitation, and denaturation. Essential metabolic enzymes are inactivated, and cell membranes are disrupted. Both the phenols and quarternary ammonium compounds have an unpleasant taste, and their efficacy is substantially reduced in the presence of organic matter. Their bactericidal or bacteriostatic efficacy depends on the concentration and time of contact. These variables have already been discussed. Commercial mouthwashes vary considerably in antimicrobial effectiveness; in general, those containing cationic surfactants (quaternary ammonium compounds, bis-biguanides) and complex organic nitrogenous compounds (hexatidine, bispyridine compounds) are more active than the older formulations based on phenols.

Agents such as peroxides and perborates release molecular oxygen. Organisms vary considerably in their susceptibility to nascent oxygen. Some organisms possess catalase that rapidly breaks down these agents so that their effect is fleeting. Their foaming action may effect a transient mechanical debridement of some plaque, but these compounds have questionable capabilities as antimicrobial agents. Iodine and its organic combinations, such as povidone-iodine, have germicidal activity resulting from the irreversible iodination of bacterial proteins and oxidation. The antiseptic action of oxychlorosene and chloramine-T depends on the liberation of free chlorine. Most of these antimicrobial agents lack substantivity, are rapidly destroyed or inactivated in the presence of organic matter, and have an unpleasant taste. These limit their practical application as effective agents in the control of dental plaque.

The concentration of fluoride used in topical preparations ranges from 225 ppm in a 0.05% sodium fluoride rinse and 1,000 ppm in fluoridated dentifrices, to 12,300 ppm in an acidulated phosphate fluoride (APF) gel or solution. Loesche[129,131] has summarized the data, which show that when high fluoride concentrations are applied to the tooth surface, an immediate bactericidal effect occurs. The proportions of *S mutans* in plaque are reduced specifically. *S sanguis* is not affected because it can readily recolonize.

Organic amine fluorides are hydrofluorides of cationic detergents, having a long aliphatic hydrocarbon chain. The amine fluorides are bacteriostatic and completely inhibit plaque formation in vitro on nichrome wires.[41,210] Following short-term (3 and 4 days) clinical testing of an amine fluoride mouthrinse, a reduction in bacterial plaque populations was found, but the effect on plaque scores was equivocal.[209] On clinical testing of an amine fluoride dentifrice and mouthrinse used daily for 20 weeks, there was no recognizable difference in plaque and gingival scores when compared with placebo treatment.[187]

Metronidazole, a nitroimidazole, is very active against *Trichomonas vaginalis* and obligate anaerobic bacteria. When used systemically, it is effective in the treatment of acute necrotizing ulcerative gingivitis and other dental infections.[80,211] Metronidazole has been shown to be carcinogenic in mice at about 12 times the maximum therapeutic dose in man. At low dosage delivered locally, it could be effective against the anaerobic flora *(F nucleatum, Selenomas sputigena, B melaninogenicus)* but not the facultative bacteria associated with periodontal disease.[174]

Agents interfering with bacterial attachment

Attacking plaque matrix

Insoluble extracellular glucans are important in plaque formation because they enhance cell-to-cell adhesion and intercellular cohesion of certain streptococcal and actinomycetes strains.[170] Investigators have sought to disperse dental plaque by using dextranases (EC 3.2.1.11α-1,6 glucan 6-glucanohydrolase) for enzymatic attack on the polysaccharides of the plaque matrix. Various mold dextranases hydrolyze the streptococcal polysaccharides in vitro.[51,56,168] Dextranase has also been incorporated in the diet and/or drinking water of rats and monkeys in an attempt to therapeutically interfere with plaque formation.* These animal experiments suggested that dextranase could reduce plaque formation provided it was present at the time of sucrose ingestion, but that dextranase was less effective in removing mature plaque. Furthermore, caries reduction by dextranase was significant only in rats kept in relative gnotobiosis and was ineffective in conventional animals.[65]

Dextranase mouthrinses have been tested in clinical trials that used various durations and frequencies of rinsing, ranging from 1 minute, four times per day to 5 minutes, seven times per day (Table 6-8).[26,96,121,178] Rinsing with these enzyme solutions does not prevent the development

*References 19, 22, 50, 64, 65, 101.

Table 6-8 Human clinical trials with glucan hydrolases

Investigators	Agent	Duration (min)	Frequency (per day)	Total time (min)	Results
Caldwell et al, 1971[26]	1→6 glucan hydrolase	1 2	4 4	4 8	No effect on plaque score, dry weight, carbohydrate content, gross bacterial composition
Lobene, 1971[120]	1→6 glucan hydrolase	3	8	24	No change in plaque score; reduction in plaque dry weight
Keyes et al, 1971[93]	1→6 glucan hydrolase	5	7	35	Some plaque dispersion; less plaque accumulation; variable *Streptococcus mutans* counts
Nyman et al, 1972[177]	1→6 glucan hydrolase	3	5	15	No significant reduction in plaque score, gingivitis, or exudate
Kelstrup et al, 1973[89]	1→6 glucan hydrolase	2	7	14	No change in plaque score; reduction in *Streptococcus mutans* counts
Duany et al, 1975[44]	1→6 glucan hydrolase	6	2	12	No significant difference in DMFS* increment between dextranase, placebo, and control groups
Kelstrup et al, 1978[90]	1→3 glucan hydrolase	20–25	6	120–150	Reduction in plaque and gingival exudate; soft tissue side effects

*(*DMFS*) decayed, missing, filled surfaces.

of plaque, although in one study the proportion of *S mutans* in plaque was reduced.[90] A gel containing dextranase has been applied in custom-made trays, twice daily for 6 minutes during the school year. The caries increment at the end of a 2-year period was not significantly different between the dextranase-treated group and a control group.[44] Proteolytic enzymes of bacterial or pancreatic origin have also been used topically in an attempt to disrupt the plaque matrix.

The use of dextranase as a caries control agent represents an attractive concept of disease control in which the therapeutic agent is directed at a specific metabolic product of the causative organism rather than at the organism itself.[50] It is less likely to have adverse effects on the balance of the oral ecosystem than some of the antimicrobial agents. The inefficiency of topical dextranase preparations when tested clinically is due to the brief encounter between enzyme and substrate. Improved delivery modes could make this form of chemotherapy more effective. Chewing gum has been tested as a vehicle for mutanase (α-1.3 glucan glucanhydrolase).[40] Although it is not known for how long the enzyme was released from the gum, reductions in plaque and gingival exudate were found. Unfortunately, a high frequency of soft tissue side effects (sore or bleeding tongue, disturbed taste, oral ulceration) was encountered.

Alteration of surface characteristics

One cannot prevent surface accumulation of integuments. However, the quality of the integument and its biological function may be changed by alteration of the surface characteristics of the tooth. Certain fluoride salts alter the free surface energy[40] but do not prevent plaque formation. Potentially this could influence the quality of plaque through an altered initial deposit of acquired pellicle. Other agents, such as silicone, which also alter surface characteristics have proven unsuccessful clinically in preventing plaque accumulation.

Mechanical removal of plaque

Historical and cultural aspects

Apes and monkeys use wisps of straw or small twigs to dislodge food debris from between teeth. Primitive humans used their fingernails and splinters of wood. The first known formal toothpick, dating back to about 3000 BC, was Sumerian and was made of gold. The Chinese designed gold and silver toilet sets that included stilettolike toothpicks. Greeks, Romans, Hebrews all used toothpicks. In Roman times toothpicks were fashioned from bronze, gold, or silver. Pliny advised against toothpicks cut from vulture feathers, saying they turned the breath sour, but recommended the bones of hares and porcupine quills. Hippocrates (460 BC) recommended a ball of wool soaked in honey for cleaning the teeth. Sponges, shredded ends of certain sticks, lint, and fingers all served as early brushing devices.

The origin of the toothbrush is not definitely known. The earliest records of actual toothbrushes are from China and date back to 1498. These toothbrushes had bone or ivory handles with natural bristles perpendicular to the longitudinal axis of the handle. Commercial development of toothbrushes occurred in Europe in the late eighteenth and early nineteenth centuries, and there has been little change in basic design. Toothbrushes are now accepted all over the world as the main aid to oral hygiene. One relatively recent innovation has been the introduction of electric toothbrushes.

Before toothbrushes, chew sticks made of wood were widely used and still are in parts of Africa and India. The preferred materials are plants of the citrus, ebony, and coffee families. Extracts of some of these plants, such as *Massularia accuminate, Fegara zanthoxyloides, Serindeia warnecki, Prosopsis africana,* and *Anoigeissus schrimperi,* inhibit plaque formation or absorption to salivary-coated hydroxyapatite. The active constituent from *S warnecki* has been isolated and found to have the characteristics of a high molecular weight polyphenolic tannin.[261] Other species, *Garcinia kola* and *Garcinia afzelia,* had little activity and *Pinus* species used in commercial toothpicks had no activity. It has been suggested that the low caries rate in Africa may be associated with these active ingredients; however, it could also be explained by the dietary habits of the population. With very few exceptions, between-meal snacks are not eaten, nor are cakes and candies.

Use of chewing sticks or sponges can bring about a high level of oral hygiene. The chewing stick is a soft wood stick obtained from certain trees *(Terminalia togoensis, Terminalia galucescens).* It is the traditional method of cleaning teeth in West Africa, where the people fashion it from a stick by shredding and rolling the shreds into balls with the fingers. The sponge is chewed 20 to 30 minutes, then held between the fingers and used to scrub the teeth and gums.[142]

Plaque detection

Mechanical plaque removal is more efficient when the plaque is clearly visible to the patient. The first requirement is a mirror and adequate lighting. Dyes or disclosing solutions are helpful in staining the plaque deposits which otherwise are poorly contrasted, resembling the white or off-white color of the teeth.

Mühlemann[165] has described the characteristics of some disclosing agents such as erythrosine, basic fuchsin, mercurochrome, malachite green, tartrazine, proflavine, and fluorescein sodium. Other less commonly used plaque stains include Bismarck brown, methylene blue, and iodine solutions. Erythrosine (FD&C red no. 3) is most commonly used in the United States and is available in tablet, gel, and solution forms. A "two-tone" dye consisting of erythrosine and malachite green causing red and/or blue staining is also commercially available.

In addition to staining plaque, most of these dyes also stain the tongue and oral mucosa, persisting for several hours. This is esthetically undesirable and socially embarrassing. Fluorescein sodium has the advantage that it is not normally visible, absorbing at 200 to 540 nm and therefore it does not discolor the mucosa. The disadvantages of this dye are the additional cost of the tungsten light and filters (Plak-lite) that are required to detect plaque stained with fluorescein and the necessity of a darkened room.

Agents that stain and disclose bacterial plaque in situ are nonspecific, reacting with organic matter whether it be epithelial or bacterial cells, food debris, or plaque matrix. They are thought to enhance patient motivation and efficacy in oral hygiene procedures.

Toothbrushing

Many sizes and shapes of toothbrushes are available.[6] The bristles may be natural (usually hog hairs) or nylon filaments of various arrangements, degrees of hardness, sharpedged or endrounded.[213] No clear-cut differences in the ability to remove plaque can be attributed to any of these properties.[8] However, worn toothbrushes, especially those with matted bristles, are less efficient in removing plaque.[105] Most dentists recommend a multitufted brush with a medium-to-small head to permit access to the posterior regions. Limitations in size and shape are dictated by the curvilinear alignment of the teeth and anatomical structures such as the ramus of the mandible, the cheeks, and the tongue. A straight-trim brush with soft, rounded, and polished bristles is preferable because it is less likely to cause tissue damage or abrasion, although the brushing habits of the individual and the abrasivity of the dentifrice are also important factors.

Many different methods of brushing have been advocated. They can be categorized based on the motion:

1. Horizontal
2. Vertical
3. Roll
4. Vibratory (Charters, Stillman, or Bass)
5. Circular (Fones)
6. Physiological
7. Scrub-brush

Detailed descriptions of these methods are available elsewhere.[66,144] Patients who have not had special instruction most commonly employ a horizontal scrubbing technique with a back-and-forth motion. For the young child, this scrub method of brushing with very short back-and-forth vibratory strokes is the favored procedure.[76] Vertical and roll methods involve either an up-and-down motion of the brush or a sweeping of the bristles across the gingiva and crown in a rolling motion. Provided that these actions are repeated on all buccal and lingual surfaces, that the occlusal surfaces are cleaned by horizontal motions, and that sufficient time and care are used, it is feasible to obtain a high degree of cleanliness of these surfaces.[199] Comparisons of different toothbrushing methods have given conflicting results as to efficacy in plaque removal. However, there is general agreement that toothbrushing alone, even when well performed, does not suffice in removing plaque from interproximal areas. Additional materials such as dental floss, toothpicks, and interproximal brushes are necessary to remove plaque from these sites.[9]

Other oral hygiene procedures

Dental floss and tape can effectively remove plaque from interdental spaces, but their use is time consuming and requires some dexterity. Numerous plastic floss holders are available for patients who have difficulty in manipulating floss with their fingers. Notwithstanding some exaggerated claims, there is no difference in the cleaning ability of waxed and unwaxed floss.[72,89]

Toothpicks are widely used and can effectively remove interproximal plaque from those sites where gingival recession has occurred. Many materials and designs have been used, the most common being wooden, rounded or triangular, tapering to a point. Plastic (Perio-Aid Marquis; D. Plak. R, Dentool Inc) or metal (Proxa-Brush, John O. Butler Co) handles that accommodate the broken end of a round wooden toothpick facilitate their use in the posterior and lingual areas. Other devices for cleaning interproximal spaces include pipe cleaners, wool yarn, and interproximal brushes resembling miniature test-tube cleaners. Their use is limited to adults with wide interdental spaces. Several water-jet devices, which either attach directly to a faucet or have a motor-driven pump, have been touted as oral hygiene aids. These irrigation appliances remove very little bacterial plaque (mostly from the surface) and are not a substitute for other mechanical cleaning procedures.

Mechanical cleaning procedures are considered effective means of controlling plaque in the individual patient who is well motivated and properly instructed and who is willing to invest the time and effort necessary to obtain oral cleanliness. Oral cleanliness is a defined state in which all surfaces of all teeth are plaque-free. Most patients go through the ritual of brushing their teeth once or more a day.[32] The average time spent in brushing is 1 minute, which does not suffice to achieve oral cleanliness. Evidence from clinical practice and group studies indicates that the technical skill, time, effort, and perseverance required to continually maintain oral cleanliness exceed either the ability or the motivation of the average human being.[123]

Chapter review

- Define acquired pellicle, food debris, and dental calculus.
- Define dental plaque, supragingival and subgingival plaque.
- State how acquired pellicle forms. What evidence is there that this process does not require bacteria?

- Compare the chemical composition of acquired pellicle with that of salivary glycoprotein.
- Name the salivary proteins found in acquired pellicle and plaque and tell how they can be identified.
- List the biological functions attributed to acquired pellicle.
- Compare the size of various organisms from plaque. Indicate how this influences the histological appearance of plaque.
- Describe the ultrastructural appearance of supragingival smooth surface plaque.
- List some differences between plaque growing in fissures, on the smooth tooth surface, and in the gingival sulcus associated with chronic periodontitis.
- Describe the "corncob" formations seen in plaque.
- Indicate what is meant by "percent recovery" of dental plaque flora. State what techniques can be used to maximize this percent recovery. State why it is not 100%.
- List the factors that influence the pH of dental plaque.
- Define autogenic succession and give an example from plaque biology.
- Describe the phases of supragingival plaque formation and development.
- Name the extracellular polysaccharides found in plaque and state their function.
- State the nonspecific plaque hypothesis (NSPH) and the specific plaque hypothesis (SPH).
- Identify the major limitation of topical drug therapy in the oral cavity and possible solutions to the problem.
- Define substantivity and give examples of agents exhibiting this property.
- List the properties of an "ideal" therapeutic agent against plaque infections.
- State the danger of prolonged topical antibiotic therapy in the oral cavity.
- List the antimicrobial agents employed in commercial mouthrinses. State the mechanism of their action and on what it depends.
- Explain the rationale of topical application of dextranases and proteases.
- Evaluate the effectiveness of various mechanical means (toothbrushes, chewing fibrous foods, toothpicks, water jets, floss) in removing dental plaque from the different tooth surfaces.

Selected readings

Babb, J.L., and Hamada, S. 1982. Microbiology of dental plaque. In *Dental Microbiology*, J.R. McGhee, S.M. Michalek, G.H. Cassell (eds), Philadelphia: Harper and Row, pp. 663–678.

Bowen, W.H. 1976. Nature of plaque. *Oral Sci Res* 9:3–21.

Carlsson, J. 1983. Microbiology of plaque associated periodontal disease. In *Textbook of Clinical Periodontology*, J. Lindhe (ed), Copenhagen: Munksgaard, pp. 125–147.

Frandsen, A. (ed) 1972. *Oral Hygiene.* Copenhagen: Munksgaard.

Gibbons, R.J., and Van Houte, J. 1975. Bacterial adherence in oral microbial ecology. *Annu Rev Microbiol* 29:19–44.

Hardie, J.M., and Bowden, G.H. 1974. The normal microbial flora of the mouth. In *The Normal Microbial Flora of Man*, F.A. Skinner and J.G. Carr (eds), New York: Academic Press, pp. 47–83.

Leach, S.A. (ed) 1980. *Dental Plaque and Surface Interactions in the Oral Cavity.* London: Information Retrieval, Inc.

Listgarten, M.A. 1976. Structure of surface coatings on teeth. A review. *J Periodontol* 47:139–147.

Loesche, W.J. 1976. Chemotherapy of dental plaque infections. *Oral Sci Rev* 9:65–107.

Mann, W.V. 1977. Oral hygiene technics and home care. In *A Textbook of Preventive Dentistry*, R.C. Caldwell and R.E. Stallard (eds), Philadelphia: W.B. Saunders, pp. 214–239.

McHugh, W.D. (ed) 1970. *Dental Plaque.* Edinburgh: E.S. Livingstone, Ltd.

Newbrun, E. 1989. Anticaries and antiplaque/antigingivitis agents. In *Pharmacology and Therapeutics for Dentistry*, 3rd ed, E.A. Neidle, D.C. Kroeger, and J.A. Yagiela (eds), St. Louis: C.V. Mosby Co. (in press).

Newman, H.N. 1980. *Dental Plaque, the Ecology of the Flora on Human Teeth.* Springfield, Ill.: Charles C Thomas.

Newman, H.N., and Poole, D.F.G. 1974. Structural and ecological aspects of dental plaque. In *The Normal Microbial Flora of Man*, F.A. Skinner and N.B. Carr (eds), New York: Academic Press, pp. 111–134.

Robinovitch, M.R., and Sreebny, L.M. (eds) 1972. *Dental Plaque and Its Relation to Oral Disease.* Seattle: University of Washington Press.

Rowe, W.H. (ed) 1973. *Dental Plaque: Interfaces.* Proceedings of Symposium, Ann Arbor: University of Michigan.

Schluger, S., Yuodelis, R.A., and Page, R.C. 1977. *Periodontal Disease.* Philadelphia: Lea and Febiger, pp. 135–166, 344–369.

Theilade, J. 1978. Development of bacterial plaque in the oral cavity. *J Clin Periodontol* 4:1–12.

Theilade, E., and Theilade, J. 1976. Role of plaque in the etiology of periodontal disease and caries. *Oral Sci Rev* 9:23–63.

Van Houte, J. 1982. Bacterial Adherence and Dental Plaque Formation. *Infection* 10:252–260.

References

1. Armstrong, W.G. 1967. The composition of organic films formed on human teeth. *Caries Res* 1:89–103.
2. Armstrong, W.G. 1968. Origin and nature of the acquired pellicle. *Proc R Soc Med* 61:923–930.
3. Armstrong, W.G., and Hayward, A.F. 1968. Acquired organic integuments of human enamel. *Caries Res* 2:294–305.
4. Balanyk, T.E., and Sandham, H.J. 1985. Development of sustained-release antimicrobial dental varnishes effective against *Streptococcus mutans* in vitro. *J Dent Res* 64:1356–1360.
5. Bassiouny, M.A., and Grant, A.A. 1975. The toothbrush application of chlorhexidine. A clinical trial. *Br Dent J* 139:323–328.
6. Bay, I., Kardel, K.M., and Skougaard, M.R. 1973. Plaque-removing ability of toothbrushes. *R Soc Health J* 93:218–222.
7. Bay, L.M., and Russell, B.G. 1975. Effect of chlorhexidine on dental plaque and

gingivitis in mentally retarded children. *Community Dent Oral Epidemiol* 3:267–270.
8. Bergenholtz, A. 1972. Mechanical cleaning in oral hygiene. In *Oral Hygiene*, A Frandsen (ed), Copenhagen: Munksgaard, pp. 27–62.
9. Bergenholtz, A., and Brithon, J. 1980. Plaque removal by dental floss or toothpicks. *J Clin Periodontol* 7:516–524.
10. Bibby, B.G. 1968. Concerning dental plaque. *Caries Res* 2:97–103.
11. Bibby, B.G. 1970. Antibiotics and dental caries. In *Dietary Chemicals vs. Dental Caries*, R.F. Gould (ed), Adv Chem Series 94:46–54.
12. Birkeland, J.M., and Charlton, G. 1976. Effect of pH on the fluoride into activity of plaque. *Caries Res* 10:72–80.
13. Birkeland, J.M., and Jorkjend, L. 1974. The effect of chewing apples on dental plaque and food debris. *Community Dent Oral Epidemiol* 2:161–162.
14. Birkeland, J.M., and Rölla, G. 1972. In vitro affinity of fluoride to proteins, dextrans, bacteria and salivary components. *Arch Oral Biol* 17:455–463.
15. Birkhed, D., Rosell, K.G., and Bowden, G.H. 1979. Structure of extracellular polysaccharides synthesized from sucrose by Neisseria isolated from human dental plaque. *Arch Oral Biol* 24:63–66.
16. Birkhed, D., Rosell, K.G., and Granath, K. 1979. Structure of extracellular water-soluble polysaccharides synthesized from sucrose by oral strains of *Streptococcus mutans, Streptococcus salivarius, Streptococcus sanguis* and *Actinomyces viscosus*. *Arch Oral Biol* 24:53–51.
17. Björn, H., and Carlsson, J. 1964. Observations on a dental plaque morphogenesis. *Odontol Revy* 15:23–28.
18. Black, G.V. 1898. Dr. Black's conclusions reviewed again. *Dent Cosmos* 40:440.
19. Block, P.L., Dooley, C.L., and Howe, E.E. 1969. The retardation of spontaneous periodontal disease and the prevention of caries in hamsters with dextranase. *J Periodontol* 40:105–110.
20. Bonesvoll, P., and Gjermo, P. 1978. A comparison between chlorhexidine and some quaternary ammonium compounds with regard to retention, salivary concentration and plaque-inhibiting effect in the human mouth after mouth rinses. *Arch Oral Biol* 23:289–294.
21. Bowden, G.H., Hardie, J.M., and Slack, G.L. 1975. Microbial variations in dental plaque. *Caries Res* 9:253–277.
22. Bowen, W.H. 1971. The effect of dextranase on caries activity in monkeys *(Macaca irus)*. *Br Dent J* 131:445–449.
23. Bowen, W.H. 1976. Nature of plaque. *Oral Sciences Rev* 9:3–21.
24. Boyde, A., and Williams, R.A.D. 1971. Estimation of the volumes of bacterial cells by scanning electron microscopy. *Arch Oral Biol* 16:259–267.
25. Burnett, G.W., and Pennel, B.M. 1973. Dental integuments and deposits as etiological factors in periodontal disease and dental caries. In *Surface Chemistry and Dental Integuments*, A. Lasslo and R.P. Quintana (eds), Springfield, Ill.: Charles C Thomas, pp. 3–73.
26. Caldwell, R.C., Sandham, H.J., Mann, W.V., Finn, S.B., and Formicola, A.J. 1971. The effect of dextranase mouthwash on dental plaque in young adults and children. *J Am Dent Assoc* 82:124–131.
27. Carlson, H.C., Porter, K., and Alms, T.H. 1977. The effect of an alexidine mouthwash on dental plaque and gingivitis. *J Periodontol* 48:216–218.
28. Carlsson, J. 1968. A numerical taxonomic study of human streptococci. *Odontol Revy* 19:137–160.
29. Carlsson, J. 1968. Plaque formation and streptococcal colonization on teeth. *Odontol Revy* 19:Suppl. 14.
30. Carlsson, J., and Egelberg, J. 1965. Effect of diet on early plaque formation in man. *Odontol Revy* 16:112–125.
31. Carlsson, J., and Sundström, B. 1968. Variations in composition of early dental plaque following ingestion of sucrose and glucose. *Odontol Revy* 19:161–169.
32. Chen, P., Bochacki, V., Reynolds, H.S., Beanan, J., Tatakis, D.N., Zambon, J.J., and Genco, R.J. 1986. The use of monoclonal antibodies to detect *Bacteroides gingivalis* in biological samples. *Infect Immun* 54:798–803.
33. Cohen, L.K., O'Shea, R.M., and Putnam, W.J. 1967. Toothbrushing. Public opinion and dental research. *J Oral Ther* 4:229–246.
34. Council on Dental Therapeutics, American Dental Association. 1986. Guidelines for acceptance of chemotherapeutic products for the control of supragingival dental plaque and gingivitis. *J Am Dent Assoc* 112:529–532.
35. Cowsar, D.R. 1975. Drug delivery systems. Design criteria. In *Polymer Science and*

Technology, R.L. Kronenthal, Z. Ozer, and E. Martin (eds), vol. 8, New York: Plenum, pp. 237–244.
36. Critchley, P., and Bowen, W.H. 1970. Correlation of the biochemical compositions of plaque with the diet. In *Dental Plaque,* W. McHugh (ed), Edinburgh: E. & S. Livingstone, Ltd, pp. 157–169.
37. Davies, R.M. 1974. Control of oral flora by hibitane and other antibacterial agents. In *The Normal Microbial Flora of Man,* F.A. Skinner and J.G. Carr (eds), New York: Academic Press, pp. 101–110.
38. Dawes, C. 1968. The nature of dental plaque, films and calcareous deposits. *Ann NY Acad Sci* 153:102–119.
39. Dawes, C., Jenkins, G.N., and Tonge, C.H. 1973. The nomenclature of the integuments of the enamel surface of teeth. *Br Dent J* 115:65–68.
40. De Paola, P.F., Jordan, H.V., and Soparkar, P.M. 1977. Inhibition of dental caries in school children by topically applied vancomycin. *Arch Oral Biol* 22:187–191.
41. Dobell, C. 1932. *Antony van Leeuwenhoek and His "Little Animals."* New York: Harcourt, Brace and Co, pp. 237–255.
42. Dolan, M.M., Kavanagh, B.J., and Yankell, S.L. 1972. Artificial plaque prevention with organic fluorides. *J Periodontol* 43:561–563.
43. Duany, L.F., and Zinner, D.D. 1975. Longitudinal effects of an antibacterial oral rinse on gingivitis and dental plaque. *Pharmacol Ther Dent* 2:229–234.
44. Duany, L.F., Zinner, D.D., Mena, J.C., and Gonzalez, J.M. 1975. The effect of dextranase on oral health in children. *J Prev Dent* 2:23–27.
45. Eastcott, A.D., and Stallard, R.E. 1973. Sequential changes in developing human dental plaque as visualized by scanning electron microscopy. *J Periodontol* 44:218–224.
46. Emilson, C.G. 1977. Susceptibility of various microorganisms to chlorhexidine. *Scand J Dent Res* 85:255–265.
47. Emilson, C.G., Lindquist, B., and Wennerholm, K. 1987. Recolonization of human tooth surfaces by *Streptococcus mutans* after suppression by chlorhexidine treatment. *J Dent Res* 66:1503–1508.
48. Fitzgerald, R.J. 1972. Inhibition of experimental dental caries by antibiotics. *Antimicrob Agents Chemother* 1:296–302.
49. Fitzgerald, R.J. 1973. The potential of antibiotics as caries-control agents. *J Am Dent Assoc* 87:1006–1009.
50. Fitzgerald, R.J., Keyes, P.H., Stoudt, T.H., and Spinell, D.M. 1968. The effects of dextranase preparation on plaque and caries in hamsters, a preliminary report. *J Am Dent Assoc* 76:301–304.
51. Fitzgerald, R.J., Spinell, D.M., and Stoudt, T.H. 1968. Enzymatic removal of artificial plaques. *Arch Oral Biol* 13:125–128.
52. Foulkes, D.M. 1973. Some toxicological observations on chlorhexidine. *J Periodont Res* 8(Suppl. 12):55–57.
53. Fox, D.J., and Dawes, C. 1970. The extraction of protein matrix from human dental plaque. *Arch Oral Biol* 15:1069–1077.
54. Frank, R.M. 1973. Microscopie electronique de la carie des sillons chez l'homme. *Arch Oral Biol* 18:9–25.
55. Frank, R.M., and Brendel, A. 1966. Ultrastructure of the approximal dental plaque and the underlying normal and carious enamel. *Arch Oral Biol* 11:883–912.
56. Gibbons, R.J., and Banghart, S.G. 1967. Synthesis of extracellular dextran by cariogenic oral bacteria and its presence in human dental plaque. *Arch Oral Biol* 12:11–24.
57. Gibbons, R.J., Socransky, S.S., deAraujo, W.C., and Van Houte, J. 1964. Studies of the predominant cultivatable microbiota of dental plaque. *Arch Oral Biol* 9:365–370.
58. Gibbons, R.J., and Van Houte, J. 1973. On the formation of dental plaque. *J Periodontol* 44:347–360.
59. Gibbons, R.J., and Van Houte, J. 1975. Bacterial adherence in oral microbial ecology. *Annu Rev Microbiol* 29:19–44.
60. Gjermo, P. 1972. Chemical cleaning of teeth. In *Oral Hygiene,* A. Frandsen (ed), Copenhagen: Munksgaard, pp. 63–88.
61. Glantz, P.O. 1960. On wettability and adhesiveness. *Odontol Revy* 20(Suppl. 17):1–132.
62. Gordon, D., Stutman, M., and Loesche, W.J. 1971. Improved isolation of anaerobic bacteria from the gingival crevice area of man. *Appl Microbiol* 21:1046–1050.
63. Guggenheim, B. 1976. Ultrastructure and some biochemical aspects of dental plaque. A review. In *Microbial Aspects of Dental Caries,* H.M. Stiles, W.J. Loesche, and T.C.

O'Brien (eds), Sp. Suppl. Microbiol. Abstr. 1:89–107.

64. Guggenheim, B., König, D.G., Mühlemann, H.R., and Regolati, B. 1969. Effect of dextranases on caries in rats harbouring an indigenous cariogenic bacterial flora. *Arch Oral Biol* 14:555–558.
65. Guggenheim, B., Regolati, B., and Mühlemann, H.R. 1972. Caries and plaque inhibition by mutanase in rats. *Caries Res* 6:253–254.
66. Hall, W.B., and Douglass, G. 1977. Plaque control. In *Periodontal Disease,* S. Schluger, R.A. Youdelis, and R.C. Page (eds), Philadelphia: Lea & Febiger, pp. 344–369.
67. Handleman, S.L., Mills, J.R., and Hawes, R.R. 1966. Caries incidence in subjects receiving long term antibiotic therapy. *J Oral Ther* 2:338–345.
68. Hardie, J.M., and Bowden, G.H. 1974. The normal microbial flora of the mouth. In *The Normal Microbial Flora of Man,* F.A. Skinner and J.G. Carr (eds), New York: Academic Press, pp. 47–83.
69. Hardie, J.M., and Bowden, G.H. 1975. Bacterial flora of dental plaque. *Br Med Bull* 31:131–136.
70. Hardie, J.M., and Bowden, G.H. 1976. The microbial flora of dental plaque: bacterial succession and isolation considerations. In *Microbial Aspects of Dental Caries,* H.M. Stiles, W.J. Loesche, and T.C. O'Brien (eds), Sp. Suppl. Microbiol. Abstr. 1:63–87.
71. Harvey, R.F. 1961. Clinical impressions of a new antibiotic in periodontics. Spiramycine. *J Can Dent Assoc* 27:576–585.
72. Hill, H.C., Levi, P.A., and Glickman, I. 1973. The effects of waxed and unwaxed dental floss on interdental plaque accumulation and interdental gingival health. *J Periodontol* 44:411–413.
73. Hoeven, J.S. van der. 1974. A slime-producing microorganism in dental plaque of rats, selected by glucose feeding. *Caries Res* 8:193–210.
74. Holt, R.L. 1975. Studies on human dental plaque. III. Variation of protein constituents among individuals. *J Oral Pathol* 4:95–105.
75. Holt, R.L., and Mestecky, J. 1975. Studies on human dental plaque. II. Immunochemical characteristics. *J Oral Pathol* 4:73–85.
76. Hoover, C.I., and Newbrun, E. 1977. Survival of bacteria from human plaque under various transport conditions. *J Clin Microbiol* 6:212–218.
77. Horowitz, A.M. 1980. Oral hygiene measures. *J Can Dent Assoc* 46:43–46.
78. Hotz, P., Guggenheim, B., and Schmid, R. 1972. Carbohydrates in pooled dental plaque. *Caries Res* 6:103–121.
79. Howell, A., Rizzo, A., and Paul, F. 1965. Cultivable bacteria in developing and mature human dental calculus. *Arch Oral Biol* 10:307–313.
80. Hoyos, D.F., Murray, J.J., and Shaw, L. 1977. The effect of chlorhexidine gel on plaque and gingivitis in children. *Br Dent J* 142:366–369.
81. Ingham, H.R., Hood, I.J.C., Bradnum, P., Tharagonnet, D., and Selkon, J.B. 1977. Metronidazole compared with penicillin in the treatment of acute dental infections. *Br J Oral Surg* 14:264–269.
82. Jenkins, G.N., Edgar, W.M., and Ferguson, D.B. 1969. The distribution and metabolic effects of human plaque fluorine. *Arch Oral Biol* 14:105–119.
83. Jensen, S.B., Löe, H., Schiött, C., and Theilade, E. 1968. Vancomycin induced changes in bacterial plaque composition as related to development of gingival inflammation. *J Periodont Res* 3:284–293.
84. Jones, S.J. 1971. Natural plaque on tooth surfaces. A scanning electron micrograph study. Apex, *J Univ College Hosp Dent Soc* 5:95–98.
85. Jones, S.J. 1972. A special relationship between spherical and filamentous microorganisms in mature human dental plaque. *Arch Oral Biol* 17:613–616.
86. Jordan, H.V. 1973. A systematic approach to antibiotic control of dental caries. *J Can Dent Assoc* 39:703–708.
87. Jordan, H.V. 1976. Cariogenic flora. Establishment, localization and transmission. *J Dent Res* 55(Sp. Issue C):C10–C14.
88. Katayama, T., Suzuki, T., and Okada, S. 1975. Clinical observation of dental plaque maturation. Application of oxidation-reduction indicator dyes. *J Periodontol* 46:610–613.
89. Keller, S.E., and Manson-Hing, L.R. 1969. Clearance studies of proximal tooth surfaces. III and IV. In vivo removal of interproximal plaque. *Ala J Med Sci* 6:399–405.
90. Kelstrup, J., Funder-Nielsen, T.D., and Moller, E.N. 1973. Enzymatic reduction of the colonization of *Streptococcus mutans* in human dental plaque. *Acta Odontol Scand* 31:249–253.
91. Kelstrup, J., Holm-Pedersen, P., and Poulsen, S. 1978. Reduction of the formation of dental plaque and gingivitis in humans by crude mutanase. *Scand J Dent Res* 86:93–

102.

92. Kelstrup, J., and Theilade, W. 1974. Microbes and periodontal disease. *J Clin Periodontol* 1:15–35.
93. Kenney, E.B., and Ash, M.M. 1969. Oxidation reduction potential of developing plaque, periodontal pockets and gingival sulci. *J Periodontol* 40:630–632.
94. Keyes, P.H., Hicks, M.A., Goldman, B.M., McCabe, R.M., and Fitzgerald, R.J. 1971. Dispersion of dextranous bacterial plaques on human teeth with dextranase. *J Am Dent Assoc* 82:136–141.
95. Keyes, P.H., Rowberry, S.A., Englander, H.R., and Fitzgerald, R.J. 1966. Bio-assays of medicaments for the control of dentobacterial plaque, dental caries periodontal lesions in Syrian hamsters. *J Oral Ther* 3:157–173.
96. Keyes, P.H., and Schern, R. 1971. Chemical adjuvants for control and prevention of dental plaque disease. *J Am Soc Prevent Dent* 1:18–22.
97. Kleinberg, I. 1974. The role of dental plaque and inflammatory periodontal disease. *J Can Dent Assoc* 40:56–65.
98. Knox, K.W. 1970. Antigens of oral bacteria. *Adv Oral Biol* 4:91–130.
99. Kolenbrander, P.E., and Andersen, R.N. 1984. Cell to cell interactions of *Capnocytophaga* and *Bacteroides* species with other oral bacteria and their potential role in development of plaque. *J Periodont Res* 19:564–569.
100. Kondo, W., Sato, N., Sato, M., and Masaki, H. 1970. Studies of 12 strains of oral iodophilic filamentous organisms. *J Dent Res* 49:671–672.
101. König, K.G., and Guggenheim, B. 1968. In vivo effects of dextranase on plaque and caries. *Helv Odontol Acta* 12:48–55.
102. Krasse, B. 1970. A review of the bacteriology of dental plaque. In *Dental Plaque,* W.D. McHugh (ed), Edinburgh: E. & S. Livingstone, pp. 199–205.
103. Kraus, F.W., and Mestecky, J. 1976. Salivary proteins and the development of dental plaque. *J Dent Res* 55:C149–C152.
104. Kraus, F.W., Orstavik, D., Hurst, D.C., and Cook, C.H. 1973. The acquired pellicle variability and subject-dependence of specific proteins. *J Oral Pathol* 2:165–173.
105. Kreifeldt, J.G., Hill, P.H., and Calisti, L.J.P. 1980. A systematic study of the plaque removal efficiency of worn toothbrushes. *J Dent Res* 59:2047–2055.
106. Krembel, J., Frank, R.M., and Deluzarche, A. 1969. Fractionation of human dental plaque. *Arch Oral Biol* 14:563–565.
107. Lancy, P., Dirienzo, J.M., Appelbaum, B., Rosan, B., and Holt, S.C. 1983. Corncob formation between *Fusobacterium nucleatum* and *Streptococcus sanguis*. *Infect Immun* 40:303–309.
108. Leach, S.A., Critchley, P., Kolendo, A.B., and Saxton, C.A. 1967. Salivary glycoproteins as components of the enamel integuments. *Caries Res* 1:104–111.
109. Leach, S.A., and Saxton, C.A. 1966. An electron microscopic study of the acquired pellicle and plaque formed on the enamel of human incisors. *Arch Oral Biol* 11:1081–1094.
110. Leyden, J.J., and Marples, R.R. 1973. Ecological principles and antibiotic therapy in chronic dermatoses. *Arch Dermatol* 107:208–211.
111. Lie, T. 1977. Scanning and transmission electron microscope study of pellicle morphogenesis. *Scand J Dent Res* 85:217–231.
112. Lindhe, J., Liljenberg, B., and Listgarten, M. 1980. Some microbiological and histopathological features of periodontal disease in man. *J Periodontol* 51:264–269.
113. Lindhe, J., and Wicen, P.O. 1969. The effects on the gingivae of chewing fibrous food. *J Periodont Res* 4:193–201.
114. Listgarten, M.A. 1976. Structure of the microbial flora associated with periodontal disease in man. *J Periodontol* 47:1–18.
115. Listgarten, M.A. 1976. Structure of surface coatings on teeth. A review. *J Periodontol* 47:139–147.
116. Listgarten, M.A., and Hellden, L. 1978. Relative distribution of bacteria at clinically healthy and periodontally diseased sites in humans. *J Clin Periodontol* 5:115–132.
117. Listgarten, M.A., and Heneghan, J.B. 1973. Observations on the periodontium and acquired pellicle of adult germfree dogs. *J Periodontol* 44:85–91.
118. Listgarten, M.A., Mayo, H., and Amsterdam, M. 1973. Ultrastructure of the attachment device between coccal and filamentous microorganisms in "corn cob" formation of dental plaque. *Arch Oral Biol* 18:651–656.
119. Listgarten, M.A., Mayo, H.E., and Tremblay, R. 1975. Development of dental plaque on epoxy resin crowns in man. A light and electron microscopic study. *J Periodontol* 46:10–26.
120. Littleton, N.W., and White, C.L. 1964. Dental findings from a preliminary study of

children receiving extended antibiotic therapy. *J Am Dent Assoc* 68:520–525.
121. Lobene, R.R. 1971. A clinical study of the effect of dextranase on human dental plaque. *J Am Dent Assoc* 82:132–135.
122. Löe, H. 1969. Present day status and direction for future research on the etiology and prevention of periodontal disease. *J Periodontol* 40:678–682.
123. Löe, H. 1970. A review of the prevention and control of plaque. In *Dental Plaque*, W.D. McHugh (ed), Edinburgh: E. & S. Livingstone, pp. 259–270.
124. Löe, H. 1973. Mechanisms for control of dental plaque pathogenicity. In *Dental Plaque: Interfaces,* N.H. Row (ed), Proceedings of a Symposium, Ann Arbor: University of Michigan, pp. 131–152.
125. Löe, H., Theilade, E., and Jensen, S.B. 1965. Experimental gingivitis in man. *J Periodontol* 36:177–187.
126. Löe, H., Theilade, E., Jensen, S.B., and Schiött, C.R. 1967. Experimental gingivitis in man. *J Periodontol* 2:282–289.
127. Löe, H., von der Fehr, C., and Schiött, C.R. 1972. Inhibition of experimental caries by plaque prevention. The effect of chlorhexidine mouthrinses. *Scand J Dent Res* 80:1–9.
128. Loesche, W.J. 1975. Bacterial succession in dental plaque. Role in dental disease. *Microbiology* 44:132–136.
129. Loesche, W.J. 1976. Chemotherapy of dental plaque infections. *Oral Sci Rev* 9:65–107.
130. Loesche, W.J. 1976. Periodontal disease and the treponemes. In *The Biology of Parasitic Spirochetes,* R.C. Johnson (ed), New York: Academic Press, pp. 261–275.
131. Loesche, W.J. 1977. Topical fluorides as an antibacterial agent. *J Prev Dent* 4:21–26.
132. Loesche, W.J., Bradbury, D.R., and Woolfolk, M.T. 1977. Reduction of dental decay in rampant caries individuals following short-term kanamycin treatment. *J Dent Res* 56:254–265.
133. Loesche, W.J., Green, E., Kenney, E.B., and Nafe, D. 1971. Effect of topical kanamycin sulfate on plaque accumulation. *J Am Dent Assoc* 83:1063–1069.
134. Loesche, W.J., Hockett, R.N., and Syed, S. 1972. The predominant cultivable flora of the tooth surface plaque removed from institutionalized subjects. *Arch Oral Biol* 17:1311–1325.
135. Loesche, W.J., and Nafe, D. 1973. Reduction of supragingival plaque accumulations in institutionalized Down's syndrome patients by periodic treatment with topical kanamycin. *Arch Oral Biol* 18:1131–1143.
136. Loesche, W.J., Paunio, K.U., Woolfolk, M.P., and Hockett, R.N. 1974. Collagenolytic activity of dental plaque associated with periodontal pathology. *Infect Immun* 9:329–336.
137. Mandel, I.D. 1966. Dental plaque. Nature, formation and effects. *J Periodontol* 37:357–367.
138. Mandel, I.D. 1972. New approaches to plaque prevention. *Dent Clin North Am* 16:661–671.
139. Mandel, I.D. 1973. Personal communication.
140. Mandel, I.D., Levy, B.M., and Wasserman, D.H. 1957. Histochemistry of plaque formation. *J Periodontol* 28:132–137.
141. Manganiello, A.D., Socransky, S.S., Smith, C., Propas, D., Oram, V., and Dogon, I.L. 1977. Attempts to increase viable count recovery of human supragingival plaque. *J Periodontol Res* 12:107–119.
142. Manley, J.L., Limongelli, W.A., and Williams, A.C. 1975. The chewing stick. Its uses and relationship to oral health. *J Prev Dent* 2:7–9.
143. Manly, R.S. 1943. A structureless recurrent deposit on teeth. *J Dent Res* 22:479–486.
144. Mann, W.V. 1977. Oral hygiene technics and home care. In *A Textbook of Preventive Dentistry,* R.C. Caldwell and R.E. Stallard (eds), Philadelphia: W.B. Saunders, pp. 214–239.
145. Mayhall, C.W. 1970. Concerning the composition and source of the acquired enamel pellicle of human teeth. *Arch Oral Biol* 15:1237–1341.
146. Mayhall, C.W. 1975. Studies on the composition of the enamel pellicle. *Ala J Med Sci* 12:252–271.
147. Mayhall, C.W. 1977. Amino acid composition of experimental salivary pellicles. *J Periodontol* 48:78–91.
148. Mayhall, C.W., and Butler, W.T. 1976. The carbohydrate composition of experimental salivary pellicles. *J Oral Pathol* 5:358–370.
149. McDougall, W.A. 1963. Studies on the dental plaque. I. The histology of the dental plaque and its attachment. *Aust Dent J* 8:261–273.

150. McFall, W.T., Shoulars, H.W., and Carnevale, R.A. 1968. Effect of vancomycin on inhibition of bacterial plaque. *J Dent Res* 47:1195.
151. McHugh, W.D. (ed)1970. *Dental Plaque.* Edinburgh: E. & S. Livingstone, Ltd.
152. Meckel, A.H. 1965. The formation and properties of organic films on teeth. *Arch Oral Biol* 10:585–598.
153. Mettraux, G.R., Gusberti, F.A., and Graf, H. 1984. Oxygen tension (pO_2) in untreated human periodontal pockets. *J Periodontol* 55:516–521.
154. Miller, W.D. 1890. *The Microorganisms of the Human Mouth.* Reprinted by S. Karger, Basel, 1973, pp. 225–237.
155. Mirth, D.B., and Bowen, W.H. 1976. Chemotherapy. Antimicrobials and methods of delivery. In *Microbial Aspects of Dental Caries,* H.M. Stiles, W.J. Loesche, and T.C. O'Brien (eds), Sp. Suppl. Microbiol. Abstr. 1:249–262.
156. Mitchell, D.F., and Holmes, L.A. 1965. Topical antibiotic control of dentogingival plaque. *J Periodontol* 36:202–208.
157. Miyasaki, K., and Newbrun, E. 1981. Effect of pH and some reagents in the sucrose-independent nonspecific sorption of *Streptococcus mutans* to glass. *Arch Oral Biol* 26:735–743.
158. Möller, J.R.A. 1966. Microbiological examination of root canals and periapical tissues of human teeth. *Odont T* 24:1–380.
159. Moreno, E.C., and Zahradnick, R.T. 1974. Chemistry of enamel subsurface demineralization in vitro. *J Dent Res* 53:226–234.
160. Mouton, C., Nisengard, R.J., Mahima, P.A., Evans, R.T., and Genco, R.J. 1977. Immunofluorescent identification of the "corn cob" configuration in supragingival human plaque. *J Dent Res* 56(Sp. Issue B, Abstr. 286):B123.
161. Mouton, C., Reynolds, H.S., Gasiecki, E.A., and Genco, R.J. 1979. In vitro adhesion of tufted oral streptococci to *Bacterionema matruchotii. Curr Microbiol* 3:181–186.
162. Mouton, C., Reynolds, H.S., and Genco, R.J. 1977. Combined micromanipulation, culture and immunofluorescent techniques for isolation of the coccal organisms comprising the "corn cob" configuration of human dental plaque. *J Biol Buccale* 5:321–332.
163. Mouton, C., Reynolds, H.S., and Genco, R.J. 1980. Characterization of tufted streptococci isolated from the "corn cob" configuration of human dental plaque. *Infect Immun* 27:235–245.
164. Mühlemann, H.R. 1970. International conference on gingival dental plaque. Introduction. The purpose of the conference. *Int Dent J* 20:351–352.
165. Mühlemann, H.R. 1976. *Introduction to Oral Preventive Medicine.* Berlin: Die Quintessenz, pp. 138–142.
166. Mühlemann, H.R., and Schroeder, H.E. 1964. Dynamics of supragingival calculus formation. *Arch Oral Biol* 1:175–203.
167. Nesbitt, W.E., Doyle, R.J., and Taylor, K.G. 1982. Hydrophobic interactions in the adherence of *Streptococcus sanguis* to hydroxylapatite. *Infect Immun* 38:637–644.
168. Newbrun, E. 1972. Extracellular polysaccharides synthesized by glucosyltransferases of oral streptococci. *Caries Res* 6:132–147.
169. Newbrun, E., Felton, R.A., and Bulkacz, J. 1976. Susceptibility of some plaque microorganisms to chemotherapeutic agents. *J Dent Res* 55:574–579.
170. Newbrun, E., Finzen, F., and Sharma, M. 1977. Inhibition of adherence of *Streptococcus mutans* to glass surfaces. *Caries Res* 11:153–159.
171. Newman, H.N. 1973. The organic films on enamel surface. II. The dental plaque. *Br Dent J* 135:101–106.
172. Newman, H.N. 1976. The apical border of plaque in chronic inflammatory periodontal disease. *Br Dent J* 144:105–113.
173. Newman, H.N., Seymour, G.J., and Challacombe, S.J. 1979. Immunoglobulins in human dental plaque. *J Periodontol Res* 14:1–9.
174. Newman, M.G., Hulem, C., Colgate, J., and Anselmo, C. 1979. Antibacterial susceptibility of plaque bacteria. *J Dent Res* 58:1722–1732.
175. Newman, M.G., and Socransky, S.S. 1977. Predominant microbiota in periodontosis. *J Periodontol Res* 12:120–128.
176. Newman, M.G., Socransky, S.S., Savitt, E.D., Propas, D.A., and Crawford, A. 1976. Studies of the microbiology of periodontosis. *J Periodontol* 47:373–379.
177. Nord, C.E., and Söder, P.O. 1972. Hyaluronidase activity of dental plaque material from children with healthy and diseased gingiva. *Odontol Revy* 23:55–61.
178. Nyman, S., Lindhe, J., and Janson, J.C. 1972. The effect of a bacterial dextranase on human dental plaque formation and gingivitis development. *Odontol Revy* 23:243–252.

179. Olsson, J., and Krasse, B. 1976. A method for studying adherence of oral streptococci to solid surfaces. *Scand J Dent Res* 84:20–28.
180. O'Neil, T.C.A. 1976. The use of chlorhexidine mouthwash in the control of gingival inflammation. *Br Dent J* 141:276–280.
181. Orstavik, D., and Kraus, F.W. 1973. The acquired pellicle. Immunofluorescent demonstration of specific proteins. *J Oral Pathol* 2:68–76.
182. Orstavik, D., and Kraus, F.W. 1974. The acquired pellicle. Enzyme and antibody activities. *Scand J Dent Res* 82:202–205.
183. Orstavik, D., and Orstavik, J. 1976. In vitro attachment of *Streptococcus sanguis* to dental crown and bridge cements. *J Oral Rehabil* 3:139–144.
184. Parker, R.B. 1971. Our common enemy. *J Am Soc Prev Dent* 1:14–17, 28–29.
185. Parsons, J.C. 1974. Chemotherapy of dental plaque. A review. *J Periodontol* 45:177–186.
186. Poole, A.E., and Gilmour, M.N. 1971. The variability of unstandardized plaques obtained from single or multiple subjects. *Arch Oral Biol* 16:681–687.
187. Ringelberg, M.L., and Webster, D.B. 1977. Effects of an amine fluoride mouthrinse and dentifrice on the gingival health and the extent of plaque of school children. *J Periodontol* 48:350–353.
188. Ritz, H.L. 1967. Microbial population shifts in developing human dental plaque. *Arch Oral Biol* 12:1561–1568.
189. Robinovitch, M.R., and Sreebny, L.M. (eds) 1972. *Dental Plaque and Its Relation to Oral Disease.* Seattle: University of Washington Press.
190. Robrish, S.A., Grove, S.B., Bernstein, R.S., Marucha, P.T., Socransky, S.S., and Amdur, B. 1976. Effect of sonic treatment on pure cultures and aggregates of bacteria. *J Clin Microbiol* 3:474–479.
191. Rölla, G., Iverson, O.J., and Bonesvoll, P. 1978. Lipoteichoic acid—the key to the adhesiveness of sucrose grown *Streptococcus mutans*. In *Secretory Immunity and Infection,* J.R. McGhee, J. Mestecky, and J.L. Babb (eds), New York: Plenum, pp. 607–618.
192. Rölla, G., and Melsen, B. 1975. On the mechanism of the plaque inhibition by chlorhexidine. *J Dent Res* 54(Sp. Issue B):B57–B62.
193. Rölla, G., Scheie, A.A., and Ciardi, J.E. 1985. Role of sucrose in plaque formation. *Scand J Dent Res* 93:105–111.
194. Rosan, B., and Hammond, B.F. 1974. Extracellular polysaccharides of *Actinomyces viscosus Infect Immun* 10:304–308.
195. Rowe, W.H. (ed) 1973. *Dental Plaque Interfaces.* Proceedings of Symposium, Ann Arbor: University of Michigan.
196. Ruby, J.D., Shirey, R.E., Gerencser, V.F., and Stelzig, D.A. 1982. Extracellular iodophilic polysaccharide synthesized by *Neisseria* in human dental plaque. *J Dent Res* 61:627–631.
197. Russell, C., and Coulter, W.A. 1975. Continuous monitoring of pH and Eh in bacterial plaque grown on an artificial mouth. *Appl Microbiol* 29:141–144.
198. Sandham, H.J., Brown, J., Phillips, H.I., and Chan, K.H. 1988. A preliminary report of long-term elimination of detectable mutans streptococci in man. *J Dent Res* 67:9–14.
199. Saxton, C.A. 1971. Scanning electron microscope study of bacterial colonization on the tooth surface. In *Tooth Enamel II,* F.W. Fearnhead and M.V. Stack (eds), Bristol: John Wright & Sons, Ltd, pp. 218–221.
200. Saxton, C.A. 1973. Scanning electron microscopic study of formation of dental plaque. *Caries Res* 7:102–119.
201. Schiött, R.C., Löe, H., Jensen, S.B., Kilien, M.J., Davies, R.M., and Glavind, K. 1970. The effect of chlorhexidine mouthrinses on the human oral flora. *J Periodontol Res* 5:84–89.
202. Schluger, S., Yuodelis, R.A., and Page, R.C. (eds) 1977. *Periodontal Disease.* Philadelphia: Lea & Febiger, pp. 135–166.
203. Schroeder, H.E. 1970. The structure and relationship of plaque to hard and soft tissues. Electron microscopic interpretation. *Int Dent J* 20:353–381.
204. Schroeder, H.E., and De Boever, J. 1970. The structure of microbial dental plaque. In *Dental Plaque,* W.D. McHugh (ed), Edinburgh: E. & S. Livingstone, Ltd, pp. 49–74.
205. Schroeder, H.E., and Hirzel, H.C. 1969. A method of studying dental soft plaque morphology. *Helv Odontol Acta* 13:22–27.
206. Schwartz, R.S., and Massler, M. 1969. Tooth accumulated materials. A review and classification. *J Periodontol* 40:407–413.
207. Scopp, I.W., Gillette, W., Kumar, V., and Larato, D. 1967. Treatment of oral lesions

with topically applied vancomycin hydrochloride. *Oral Surg* 24:703–706.
208. Sharma, M.L., and Newbrun, E. 1975. Chemical composition of the washed cells of *Streptococcus sanguis* (804) and *Streptococcus mutans* (B-14). *J Dent Res* 54:482–486.
209. Shern, R.J., Rundell, B.B., and Defever, C.J. 1974. Effects of an amine fluoride mouthrinse on the formation and microbial content of plaque. *Helv Odontol Acta* 8(Suppl. 8):57–62.
210. Shern, R., Swing, K.W., and Crawford, J.J. 1970. Prevention of plaque formation by organic fluorides. *J Oral Med* 25:93–97.
211. Shinn, D.L.S. 1962. Metronidazole in acute ulcerative gingivitis. *Lancet* 1:1191.
212. Silverman, G., and Kleinberg, I. 1967. Fractionation of human dental plaque and the characterization of its cellular and acellular components. *Arch Oral Biol* 12:1387–1405.
213. Silverstone, L.M., and Featherstone, M.J. 1988. A scanning electron microscope study of the end rounding of bristles in eight toothbrush types. *Quintessence Int* 19:87–107.
214. Singer, L., Jarvey, B.A., Venkateswarlu, P., and Armstrong, W.C. 1970. Fluoride in plaque. *J Dent Res* 49:455.
215. Slomiany, B.L., Murty, V.L., Zdebska, E., Slomiany, A., Gwozdzinski, K., and Mandel, I.D. 1986. Tooth surface-pellicle lipids and their role in the protection of dental enamel against lactic acid diffusion in man. *Arch Oral Biol* 31:187–191.
216. Slots, J. 1975. Comparisons of five growth media and two anaerobic techniques for isolating bacteria from dental plaque. *Scand J Dent Res* 83:274–278.
217. Slots, J. 1976. The predominant cultivable organisms in juvenile periodontitis. *Scand J Dent Res* 84:1–10.
218. Slots, J. 1977. Microflora in the healthy gingival sulcus in man. *Scand J Dent Res* 85:247–254.
219. Slots, J., Reynolds, H.S., and Genco, R.J. 1980. *Actinobacillus actinomycetemcomitans* in human periodontal disease: a cross-sectional microbiological investigation. *Infect Immun* 29:1013–1020.
220. Soames, J.V., and Davies, R.M. 1975. The structure of subgingival plaque in a beagle dog. *J Periodontol Res* 9:333–341.
221. Socransky, S.S. 1974. Personal communication.
222. Socransky, S.S., and Manganiello, A.D. 1971. The oral microbiota of man from birth to senility. *J Periodontol* 42:485–496.
223. Socransky, S.S., and Manganiello, A.D. 1975. Mechanism of Eh reduction in dental plaque. *J Dent Res* 54(Sp. Issue A, Abstr. 118):74.
224. Socransky, S.S., Manganiello, A.D., Propas, D., Oram, V., and van Houte, J. 1977. Bacteriological studies of developing supragingival dental plaque. *J Periodontol Res* 12:90–106.
225. Söder, P.O. 1972. Proteolytic activity in the oral cavity. Proteolytic enzymes from human saliva and dental plaque material. *J Dent Res* 51:389–393.
226. Sönju, T., Christensen, T.B., Kornstad, L., and Rölla, G. 1974. Electron microscopy, carbohydrate analyses and biological activities of the proteins adsorbed in two hours to tooth surfaces in vivo. *Caries Res* 8:113–122.
227. Sönju, T., and Glantz, P.O. 1975. Chemical composition of salivary integuments formed in vivo on solids with some established surface characteristics. *Arch Oral Biol* 20:687–691.
228. Sönju, T., and Rölla, G. 1972. Chemical analysis of pellicle formed in two hours on cleaned human teeth in vivo. Rate of formation and amino acid analysis. *Caries Res* 7:30–35.
229. Sönju, T., and Rölla, G. 1973. Chemical analysis of the acquired pellicle formed in two hours on cleaned teeth in vivo. Caries Res 7:30–38.
230. Sönju, T., and Skjörland, K. 1976. Pellicle composition and initial bacterial colonization on composite and amalgam in vivo. In *Microbial Aspects of Dental Caries,* H.M. Stiles, W.J. Loesche, and T.C. O'Brien (eds), Sp. Suppl. Microbiol. Abstr. 1:133–141.
231. Staat, R.H., Langley, S.D., and Doyle, R.J. 1980. *Streptococcus mutans* adherence; presumptive evidence for protein-mediated attachment followed by glucan-dependent cellular accumulation. *Infect Immun* 27:675–681.
232. Staat, R.H., and Peyton, J.C. 1984. Adherence of oral streptococci: evidence for nonspecific absorption to saliva-coated hydroxlapatite surfaces. *Infect Immun* 44:653–659.
233. Stallard, R.E., Volpe, A.R. Orban, J.E., and King, W.J. 1969. The effect of an antimicrobial mouth rinse on dental plaque, calculus and gingivitis. *J Periodontol* 40:683–694.
234. Stiles, H.M., Loesche, W.J., and O'Brien, T.C. (eds) 1976. *Microbial Aspects of Dental*

Caries. Sp. Suppl. Microbiol. Abstr. vol 2. Washington, D.C.: Information Retrieval, Inc.

235. Strålfors, A. 1950. Investigations into the bacterial chemistry of dental plaques. *Odont T* 58:155.
236. Strålfors, A. 1961. Disinfection of dental plaques in man. In *Caries Symposium, Zurich. Proc. Int. Symp.*, H.R. Mühlemann and G. König (eds), Berne: Hans Huber, pp. 154–161.
237. Strålfors, A. 1962. Disinfection of dental plaques in man. *Odont T* 70:182–203.
238. Syed, S.A., Loesche, W.J., and Löe, H. 1975. Bacteriology of dental plaque in experimental gingivitis. II. Relationship between time, plaque score and flora. *J Dent Res* 54(Sp. Issue A, Abstr. 109):72.
239. Takazoe, I., Matsukubo, T., and Katow, T. 1978. Experimental confirmation of "corn cob" in vitro. *J Dent Res* 57:384–387.
240. Tanner, A.C.R., Haffer, C., Bratthall, G.T., Visconti, R.A., and Socransky, S.S. 1979. A study of the bacteria associated with advancing periodontitis in man. *J Clin Periodontol* 6:278–307.
241. Tanzer, J.M. 1977. Microbiology of periodontal disease. In *International Workshop on Research in Biology of Periodontal Disease*, E. Barrington et al (eds), Chicago: University of Illinois Press, pp. 153–182.
242. Tanzer, J.M., Freedman, M.L., Woodiel, F.N., Eifert, R.L., and Rinehimer, L.A. 1976. Association of *Streptococcus mutans* virulence with synthesis of intracellular polysaccharide. In *Microbial Aspects of Dental Caries*, H.M. Stiles, W.J. Loesche, and T.C. O'Brien (eds), Sp. Suppl. Microbiol. Abstr. 3:597–616.
243. Taubman, M. 1974. Immunoglobulins of human dental plaque. *Arch Oral Biol* 19:439–446.
244. Theilade, E., and Theilade, J. 1976. Role of plaque in the etiology of periodontal disease and caries. *Oral Sci Rev* 9:23–63.
245. Theilade, J., Fejerskov, O., and Horsted, M. 1976. A transmission electron microscopic study of 7-day old bacterial plaque in human tooth fissures. *Arch Oral Biol* 21:587–598.
246. Thomson, L.A., Little, W.A., Bowen, W.H., Sierra, L.I., Aguirrer, M., and Gillespie, G. 1980. Prevalence of *Streptococcus mutans* serotypes, *Actinomyces*, and other bacteria in the plaque of children. *J Dent Res* 59:1581–1589.
247. Tinanoff, N. 1976. The significance of the acquired pellicle in the practice of dentistry. *J Dent Child* 43:20–25.
248. Tonzetich, J. 1977. Production and origin of oral malodor. A review of mechanisms and methods of analysis. *J Periodontol* 48:13–20.
249. U.S. Department of Health, Education and Welfare, Food and Drug Administration. 1979. Oral mucosal injury drug products for over-the-counter human use. *Fed Register* 44:63270–63290.
250. Van Abbe, N.J. 1974. The substantivity of cosmetic ingredients to the skin, hair and teeth. *J Soc Cosmet Chem* 25:23–31.
251. van Houte, J. 1967. Iodophilic polysaccharide in bacteria from dental plaque. Thesis, The Netherlands: University of Utrecht.
252. van Houte, J., de Moor, C.E., and Jansen, H.M. 1970. Synthesis of iodophilic polysaccharide by human oral streptococci. *Arch Oral Biol* 15:262–266.
253. van Houte, J., and Green, D.B. 1974. Relationship between the concentration of bacteria in saliva and the colonization of teeth in humans. *Infect Immun* 9:624–630.
254. van Houte, J., and Saxton, A.C. 1971. Cell wall thickening and intracellular polysaccharide in microorganisms of the dental plaque. *Caries Res* 5:30–43.
255. Waaler, S.M., and Rölla, G. 1985. Importance of teeth and tongue as possible receptor sites for chlorhexidine in relation to its clinical effect. *Scand J Dent Res* 93:222–226.
256. Weatherford, T.W., Finn, S.B., and Jamison, H.C. 1977. Effects of an alexidine mouthwash on dental plaque and gingivitis in humans over a 6-month period. *J Am Dent Assoc* 94:528–536.
257. Williams, B.L., Pantalone, R.M., and Sherris, J.C. 1976. Subgingival microflora periodontitis. *J Periodontol Res* 11:1–18.
258. Williams, J.L. 1897. A contribution to the study of pathology of enamel. *Dent Cosmos* 39:169–196.
259. Winkler, K.C., and Backer Dirks, O. 1958. The mechanism of dental plaque. *Int Dent J* 8:561–585.
260. Wolinsky, L.E., and Sote, E.O. 1984. Isolation of natural plaque-inhibiting substances from Nigerian chewing sticks. *Caries Res* 18:216–225.

Chapter 7

Histopathology of Dental Caries

For there was never yet philosopher
That could endure the toothache patiently.

Much Ado About Nothing, Act 5

A knowledge of the macroscopic appearance and location of carious lesions is useful clinically in detecting and diagnosing caries. Familiarity with the shape of the lesion in different locations is of fundamental importance in understanding the design of cavity preparations.

Despite the problems of working with hard tissues, the morphological changes associated with caries have been studied extensively. It is difficult to prepare satisfactory thin histological sections of enamel because it is so highly mineralized, hard, and brittle. Techniques for making demineralized sections have been developed, but because the carious process is largely one of demineralization, these methods can provide only limited information. Many workers have preferred to study ground enamel sections that are relatively thick, usually between 60 and 100 μm. Valuable information has been obtained by examining such sections by transmitted, reflected, and polarized light, but the findings obtained by these methods are often inconclusive and open to variable interpretation.

Microradiography is a process for studying the degree of mineralization and demineralization of a tissue. Thin ground sections are placed in contact with a glass slide bearing a fine-grained emulsion capable of high resolution. The section is then exposed to "soft" x-rays produced at low voltage from a diffraction tube with a copper target (Kα radiation, $\lambda = 15.4$ nm). The 1:1 size x-ray absorption image thereby produced can be examined under a microscope and photographed. Microradiography of carious lesions offers the distinct advantage that the photodensity of the image on the film is directly related to the amount of mineral. Microdensitometric tracings of this image permit quantitative measurement of the degree of demineralization. However, this technique still uses thick sections and the magnification is limited. With the advent of transmission and scanning electron microscopy, a more logical explanation of the histological changes observed in caries has been forthcoming.

Dental plaque is essential for the development of the carious lesion and has an intimate relationship to the underlying affected enamel. Because the layer of plaque is usually lost during the preparation of ground sections, the older histological descriptions commonly emphasized alterations seen in enamel and dentin and omitted the plaque-enamel relationship. The biological and ultrastructural features of dental plaque are discussed elsewhere (see chapter 6).

Time factors in caries development

Speed of lesion formation

Caries is commonly considered to be a chronic disease in man because lesions develop over a period of months or years. In children estimates vary widely on the speed at which an incipient lesion (diagnosed by "a catch of the probe") develops into a clinical cavity. The average time from the stage of incipient caries to clinical caries is 18 ± 6 months. This conclusion was based on a 5-year longitudinal survey of institutionalized children presumably using normal oral hygiene.[42] Children residing in institutions generally eat more regular meals and have less opportunity for between-meal eating than other children. Caries progression may be even more rapid.

Omitting oral hygiene procedures and deliberately rinsing the mouth nine times daily with a sucrose solution can greatly accelerate the caries process. Such frequency of sucrose exposure is not farfetched; children living at home may actually ingest sucrose-containing foods and beverages this often. Microscopic observation in vivo revealed new lesions ranging from hardly recognizable changes in the optical properties of the enamel to greyish-white spots and accentuation of perikymata within

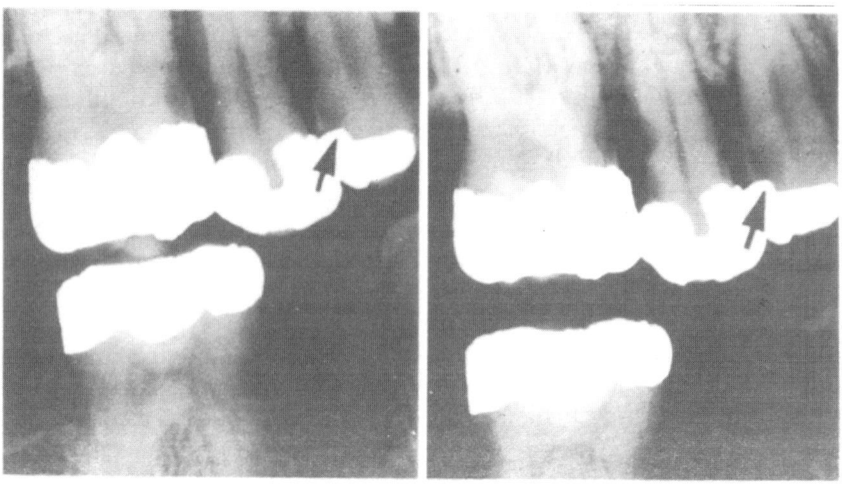

Fig 7-1 Bitewing radiographs taken on 3/19/73 *(left)* and 10/8/73 *(right)* of patient who underwent radiation therapy during May 1973. Note the rapid spread of the carious lesion in the first premolar *(arrow)*.

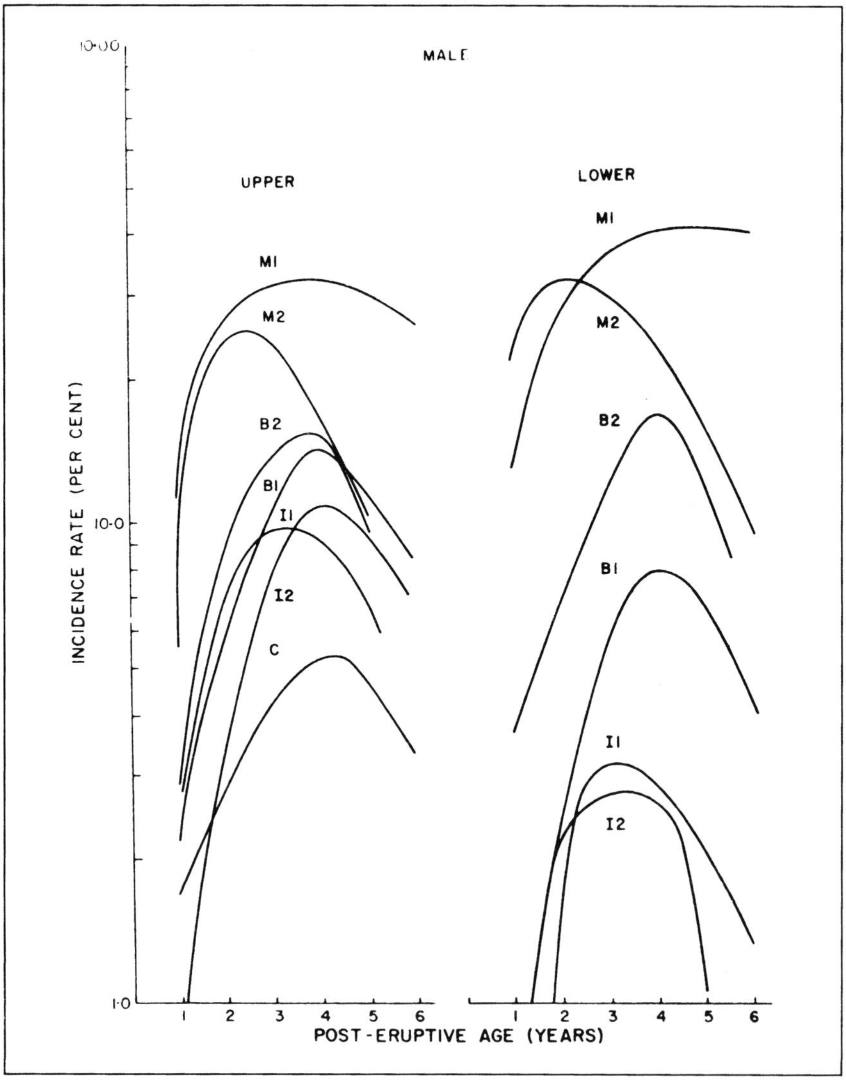

Fig 7-2 Curves showing annual probability of caries attack of the permanent teeth of male children in Kingston, New York. Semilogarithmic scale. *(M2),* Second molars; *(M1),* first molars; *(B2),* second premolars; *(B1),* first premolars; *(C),* canines; *(I2),* lateral incisors; *(I1),* central incisors. (Courtesy of Carlos and Gittelsohn.[5])

3 weeks in humans on such a regimen.[11] Changes resembling early caries can also be detected clinically by the naked eye and in color photographs.[10] These incipient changes can be reversed upon reinstitution of good oral hygiene practice and regular application of fluoride.

In some patients with xerostomia following radiation therapy, caries can be detected clinically within 3 months; total destruction of the teeth may follow unless stringent preventive measures are imposed.[4] The bitewing radiographs in Fig 7-1 were taken 7 months apart. Two months after the first radiograph the patient received radiation therapy and later exhibited mucositis, dryness of the mouth, and loss of taste. Note the rapidity of advance of the secondary caries in this case.

Careful epidemiological observation on longitudinal rates and patterns of caries incidence in a large group of children has revealed that all teeth exhibit surprisingly similar patterns of annual attack curves (Fig 7-2). In general, the annual probability of caries attack reaches a peak 2 to 4 years following eruption and declines thereafter, possibly reflecting a posteruptive "maturation" of the enamel surface.[5] Mineralization of plaque in some fissures[50] would tend to seal them and might explain why fissures that remain caries-free for the first few years posteruption are subsequently less susceptible to caries.

The 2-year time interval between eruption and maximum caries incidence is related to the time required for detectable lesions to develop. Thus, studies on the effectiveness of any therapeutic procedure to prevent caries must extend over a minimum of 2 years. Once an enamel lesion has occurred, it takes about 3 years to progress to the dentin. The rate of progress of the carious lesion depends on posteruptive age of the tooth, location of the lesion, and diet of the individual.

Caries of enamel

Macroscopic changes of enamel

On smooth enamel surfaces, the earliest visible changes are usually manifested as a loss of transparency, resulting in an opaque chalky region ("white spot"). There may also be an accentuation of the perikymata, which are the external termini of the striae of Retzius, appearing as grooved structures on the enamel surface (Fig 7-3). In locations where caries has progressed more slowly or become arrested, brown or yellow pigmentation of the enamel may be seen. Smooth surface lesions, when sectioned longitudinally, are cone-shaped with the apex directed toward the dentin. What determines the shape of the lesion is still not known.

Occlusal fissures are deep invaginations of enamel; they can be extremely diverse in shape and have been described as broad or narrow funnels, constricted hourglasses, multiple invaginations with inverted Y-shaped divisions, and irregularly shaped.[8,21,33,34] A classification of fissure morphology with percent distribution of types has been reported:[38]

1. V type, wide at the top and gradually narrowing toward the bottom (34%)
2. U type, almost the same width from top to bottom (14%)
3. I type, an extremely narrow slit (19%)

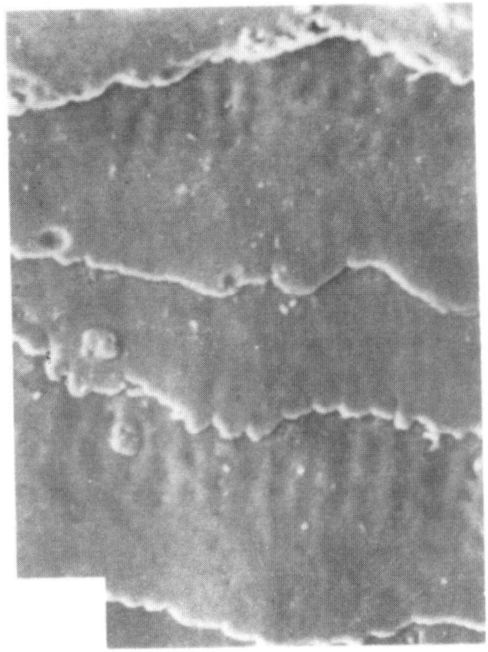

Fig 7-3 Outer surface of enamel showing perikymata and indentations relating to enamel prisms (SEM, original magnification ×700). (Courtesy of D. Scott.)

4. IK type, extremely narrow slit associated with a larger space at the bottom (26%)
5. Other types (7%)

These types are shown diagrammatically in Fig 7-4. Several morphological variations may be found along the length of an individual occlusal fissure, so that it is not always possible to categorize a tooth as having a particular type of occlusal morphology.[12] Scanning electron micrographs of replicas of occlusal fissures reveal the variable shapes that may occur.[20] Frequently, fissures having a broad base give rise to several pits, which when sectioned appear as inverted Ys. Many teeth have areas at the base of fissures where scant enamel covers the dentin.

The carious lesion more often starts at both sides of the fissure wall rather than at the base, penetrating nearly perpendicularly toward the dentinoenamel junction. Visual changes such as chalkiness or yellow, brown, or black discoloration may be seen. In newly erupted teeth, brown stain is indicative of underlying decay, while in teeth of older individuals it may be due to arrested or remineralized lesions. The lesion is commonly described as cone-shaped with the base directed toward the dentin and apex toward the enamel surface (Figs 7-5 and 7-6). Increasing severity of alteration is found with increasing narrowness and depth of the fissure. These macroscopic alterations of the enamel in initial caries precede cavitation and occur without apparent break in the enamel surface.

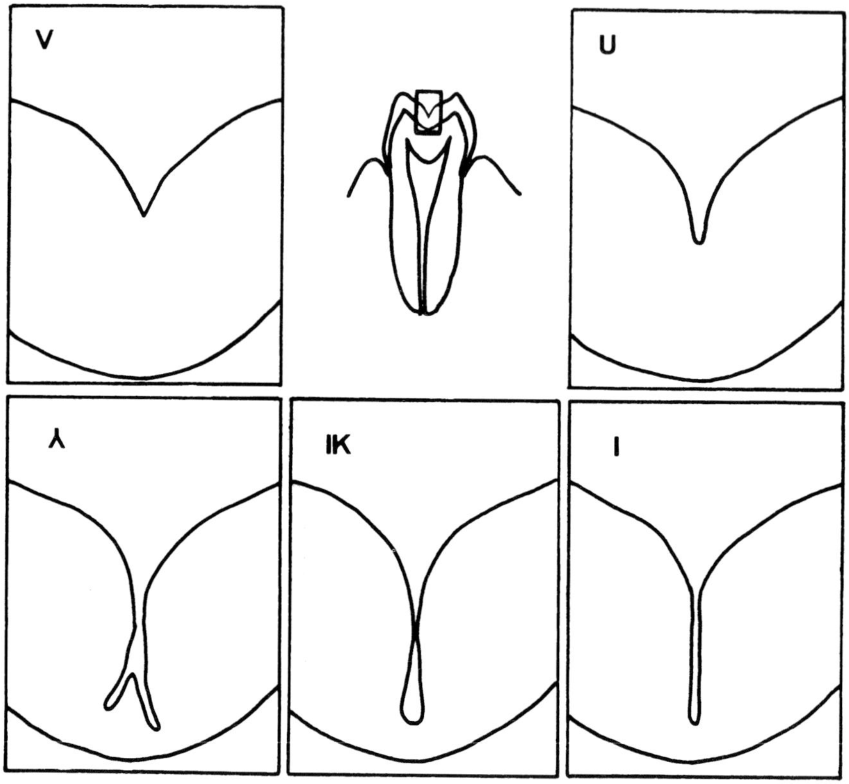

Fig 7-4 Diagram of various morphological types of occlusal fissures. *(V),* Wide at top and gradually narrowing toward the bottom; *(U),* almost same width from top to bottom; *(ʎ),* inverted Y, bifurcating at the bottom; *(IK),* hourglass, extremely narrow slit associated with a large space at the bottom; *(I),* extremely narrow slit.

Microscopic changes of enamel

Abundant evidence supports the concept that, in its early stages, caries causes minimal damage to the outer smooth surface but considerable demineralization below the surface.[2,9,39,47] The histological features of typical smooth surface lesions have been divided for descriptive purposes into a number of different zones, ranging from three to seven.[9,22] Four zones are clearly distinguishable (Fig 7-7). Starting from the inner advancing front of the lesion, these are *(1)* a *translucent zone, (2)* a *dark zone* separating *(3)* the *body of the lesion* from the translucent zone, and finally *(4)* the *surface layer,* which remains relatively unaffected. One should realize, however, that there is no sudden or dramatic change from zone to zone, but rather a gradual series of changes within the lesion. Furthermore, all zones may not be visible by polarized light microscopy

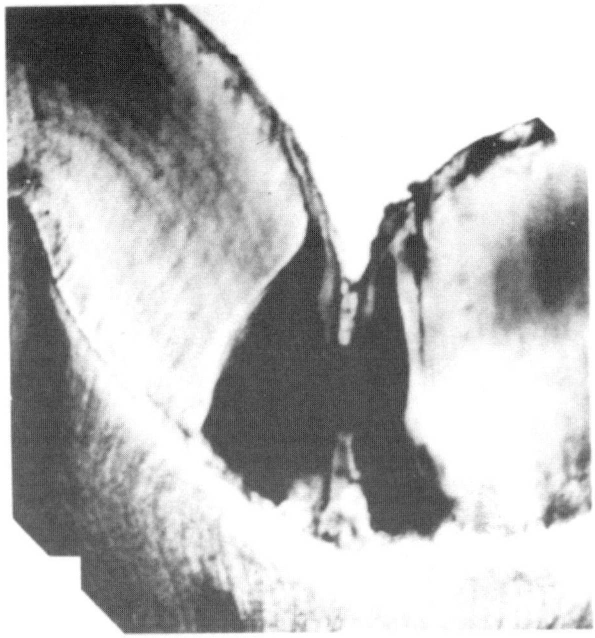

Fig 7-5 Carious occlusal fissure showing dark staining starting at sides as well as base of the fissure (transmitted light, original magnification ×15).

unless several imbibition media (at least two), with different refractive indices, are used to examine the lesion.

The translucent zone is only seen when longitudinal ground sections are examined in a clearing agent having a refractive index similar to that of enamel. The formation of a translucent zone appears to be the earliest change in enamel at the advancing front of the lesion. It is detected in about half of the lesions, appears structureless, and is characterized by approximately 1.2% loss of mineral.[23]

The dark zone is a common feature of the carious lesion, varying considerably in width.[6] It shows positive birefringence in polarized light, whereas normal enamel has a negative intrinsic birefringence relative to the prism direction. Birefringence is the property of resolving a beam of plane polarized light into two rays at different velocities. As a result of caries, "spaces" or pores devoid of mineral develop in enamel. These spaces give rise to form birefringence, which may alter the observed birefringence. An average reduction of 6% of mineral per unit volume has been reported for enamel sampled from the dark zone.

The body of the lesion, the largest zone, is positively birefringent. The striae of Retzius are enhanced within this region and the prism structure is also well marked, showing a pattern of cross-striations. Microchemical analyses indicate a reduction of 24% in mineral per unit volume compared with sound enamel. There is a corresponding increase in unbound water and organic content due to the ingress of bacteria and saliva.[27]

The surface layer ranges between 20 and 100 μm thick; it is thinner

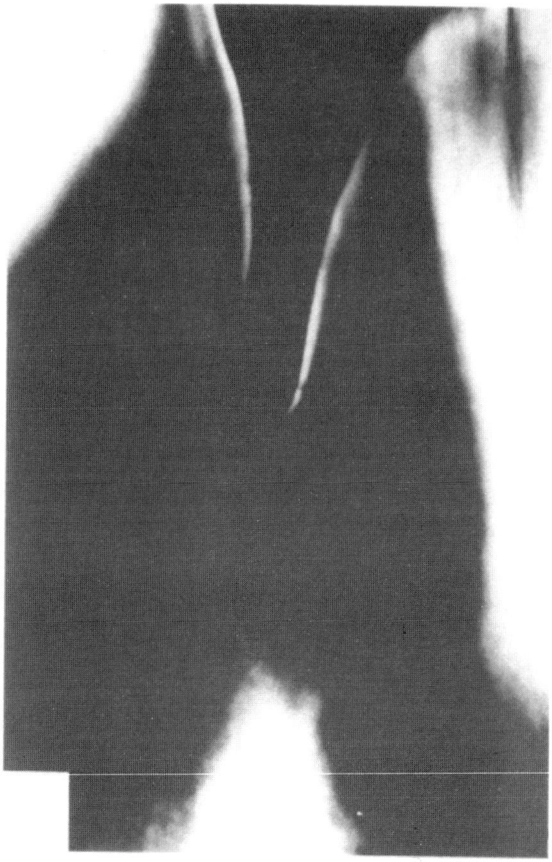

Fig 7-6 Carious occlusal fissure from Fig 7-5, showing pathway of demineralization with radiopaque surface layer (microradiograph, original magnification ×40).

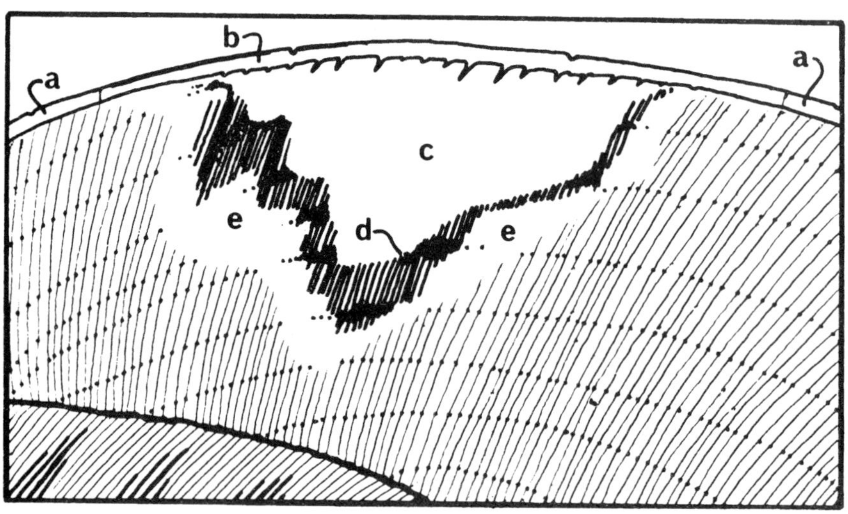

Fig 7-7 Schematic representation of smooth surface carious lesion showing the four major zones: *(a)*, normal enamel surface; *(b)*, surface layer, slightly demineralized; *(c)*, body of the lesion; *(d)*, dark zone; *(e)*, translucent zone.

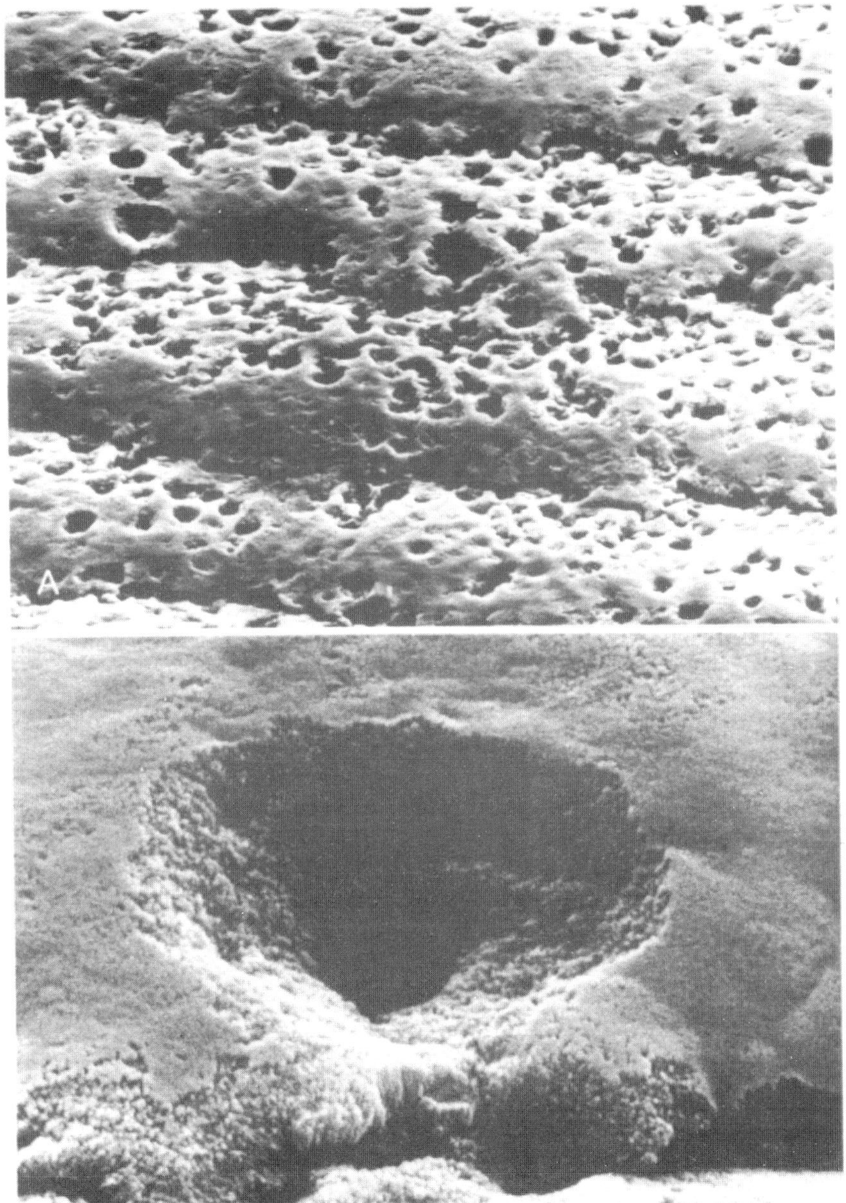

Fig 7-8 *(A)* Initial carious lesion of enamel on approximal surface. Numerous pits due to the Tomes' process. Overlapping perikymata are also seen. Focal holes larger than the Tomes' processes are marked with arrows (SEM, original magnification ×416). *(B)* Detailed appearance of eroded focal hole (SEM, original magnification ×3,690). (Courtesy of A. Thylstrup and O. Fejerskov.)

in active lesions and thicker in inactive ones.[32] This surface layer appears relatively unaffected in the initial lesion as compared with the subsurface zones. It retains a negative birefringence in polarized light. In microradiographs, it is radiopaque and sharply demarcated from the underlying radiolucent areas. However, examination of initial carious lesions at approximal surfaces by scanning electron microscopy reveals funnel-shaped focal holes (Fig 7-8) at some sites on the surface layer.[23,51] A more characteristic finding is a broadening of the prism sheaths.[23] These observations imply that minute pathways exist in the surface layer but are not detectable by light microscopy.

Photodensity tracings of the roentgenograms of incipient carious lesions reveal, however, that partial demineralization (about 8% loss by volume) has taken place[3,39,47] (Fig 7-9). This is in good agreement with chemical analyses, by which an average of 9.9% less mineral was found in this layer. The appearance under polarized light and in microradiographs and the chemical alterations found in the major zones of a smooth surface lesion are summarized in Table 7-1.

Carious breakdown of enamel used to be considered dependent on enamel structure. Thus the process has been described as following the striae of Retzius, attacking prism "sheaths" and the cross-striations of the prisms before affecting the prism cores. Unquestionably the prism structure is accentuated in microradiographs of carious enamel (Fig 7-10), but there has been disagreement regarding the demineralization pattern. Some authors explain this as a preferential loss of "interprismatic substance," while others maintain that demineralization progresses more rapidly within the prisms. In the former case, the dark parallel lines on the microradiographs would correspond to loss of interprismatic mineral; in the latter case, each dark line would correspond to the demineralized prism core. Alternate radiolucent and radiopaque bands, parallel to the striae, can readily be found in microradiographs of ground sections of carious lesions.[7,39] This appearance gives the impression of demineralization spreading along the striae of Retzius.

At one time, the onset of caries was thought to be related to the presence of lamellae (proteolytic theory), which were considered pathways of primary invasion. The supporting evidence for this hypothesis was not convincing. Since lamellae are present in all teeth, inevitably some of them are involved in carious lesions. However, the association between lamellae and lesions is random and does not suggest a cause-and-effect relationship.[44]

Histochemical staining of early lesions of enamel has shown them to be more permeable (penetrable by methyl green) and to contain free calcium ions detected with Alizarin red S.[48] Normal enamel remains uncolored by these dyes. Some lesions also react with periodic acid-Schiff reagent or reveal increased metachromasia (indicative of available polysaccharides)[2,49] in the demineralized zones. These latter reactions are probably due to the well-documented ingress of exogenous organic material rather than the release of endogenous "mucoprotein" in the enamel.

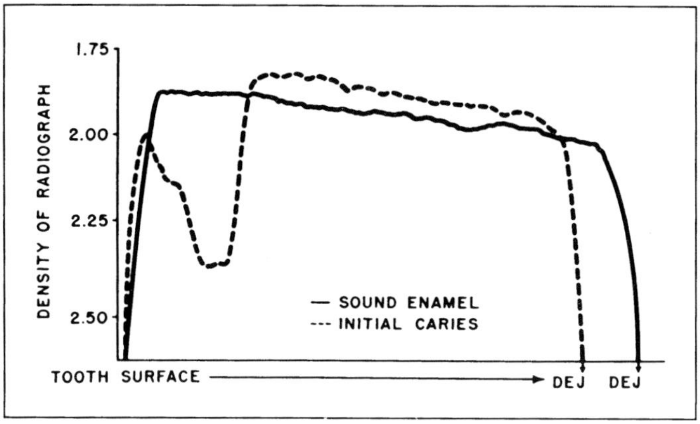

Fig 7-9 Photodensity tracings of microradiographs of sound enamel (———) and initial enamel caries (- - -).

Table 7-1 Smooth surface carious lesion in enamel

Zone	Birefringence	X-ray	Mineral loss (%)
Translucent	–	Opaque	1.2
Dark	+	Opaque	6
Body of lesion	+	Lucent	24
Surface layer	–	Opaque	10

Ultrastructural changes in enamel

The first alteration found in enamel is the scattered destruction of individual apatite crystals both within the enamel prisms and at their borders. The progressive dissolution of the crystals results in broadening of the intercrystalline spaces so that small areas become filled with amorphous material. Some of the amorphous material gives a positive histochemical reaction of carbohydrates, which is not seen in normal enamel.[29]

Peripheral arcadelike clefts (transverse section) or channels (longitudinal section), bounded by rows of resistant crystals, can readily be observed in regions of incipient damage (Fig 7-11). The crystals remaining at the prism junction appear larger, more isodiametric and electron-dense than elsewhere (Fig 7-12). This has been interpreted as evidence for some recrystallization taking place during the carious process. More advanced dissolution has been seen of the crystals that are directed vertically into the demineralizing zone in the center of heads of the prisms. There is a lesser degree of damage to the crystals in the tails of the prisms that are distributed at an angle or lengthwise to the demineralizing zone.

Central defects in individual crystals have been described and are particularly obvious in transverse sections.[26,28] High-resolution electron microscopy clearly shows that carious dissolution starts in the center of one end of the crystal and develops anisotropically along the *c*-axis. The central hole thus formed extends along the entire crystal length (Fig 7-

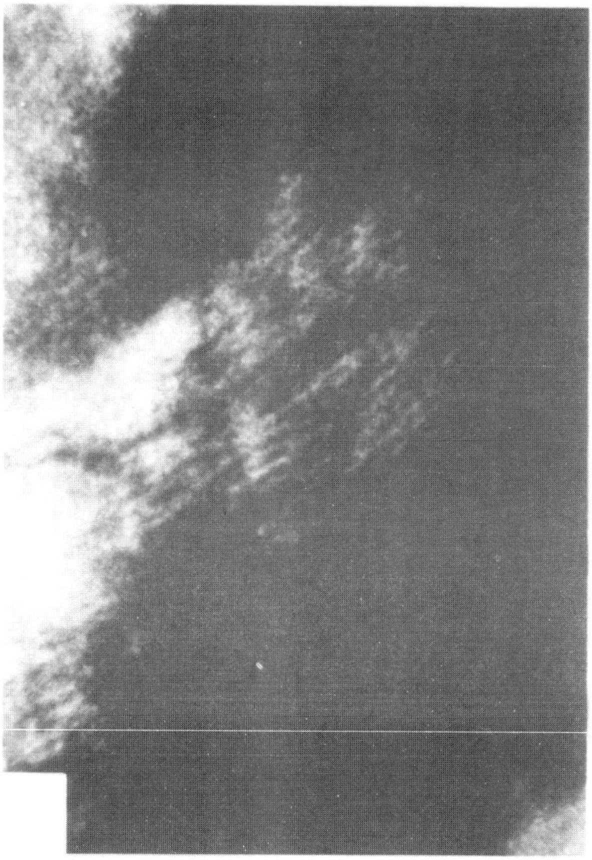

Fig 7-10 Accentuated prism structure at the bottom of the carious fissure shown in Fig 7-5 (microradiograph, original magnification ×540.)

13). The central dissolution parallels the lateral external crystal surface, resulting in hollow hexagons or rectangles. After formation of the central hole, the dissolution extends as lateral localized destruction toward the external surface.[14,52,53] Usual descriptions of the structure of a crystal imply that the lattice structure is perfect. In fact, no real crystals are perfect. All contain a variety of lattice defects, such as dislocation points or point defects, which affect the chemical and physical properties of the crystals. The central core of enamel crystallites could have formed more rapidly during mineralization, and, therefore, less perfectly than the more slowly crystallized exterior. If dislocations are more numerous in the core of the crystallite, this would allow faster transport and diffusion along the dislocation line and account for the observed demineralization.[1] These steps in the dissolution of a hydroxyapatite crystallite are shown in Fig 7-14.

As the number of dissolved crystals increases, the densely calcified tissue becomes progressively more porous (Fig 7-15). Initially, the remaining apatite crystals preserve their preferential orientation, but at the more advanced stage, disorganization of the crystal arrangement is

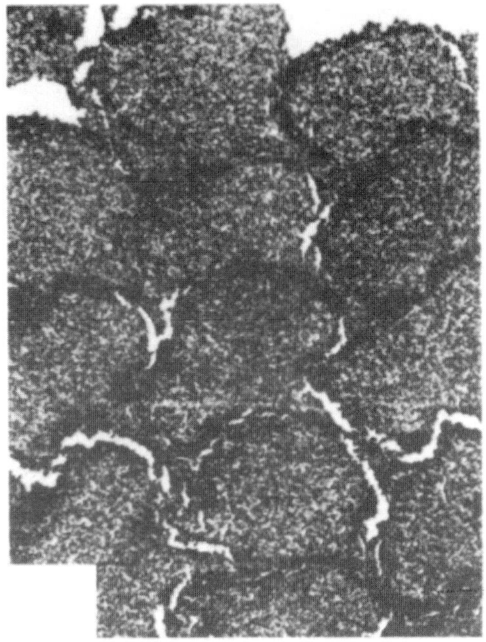

Fig 7-11 Human enamel with caries. Slight gaps have developed between rows of crystals (TEM, original magnification ×6,500). (Courtesy of D. Scott.)

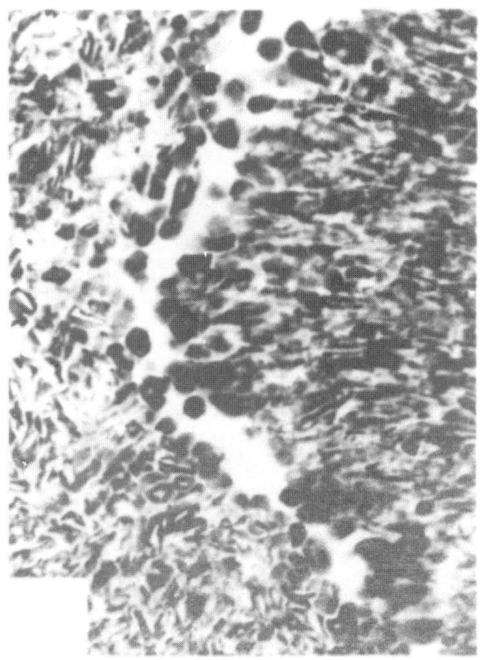

Fig 7-12 Human enamel with caries. Higher magnification of junction between prisms reveals a slight cleft bordered by larger, more resistant crystals (TEM, original magnification ×30,000). (Courtesy of D. Scott.)

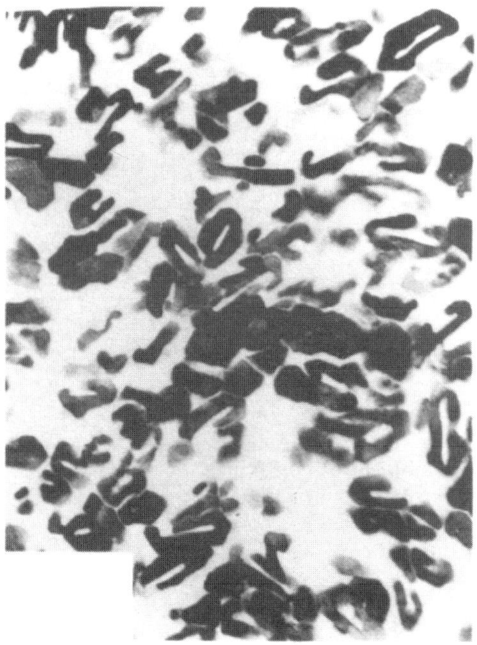

Fig 7-13 Human enamel with caries. Central areas of cross-sectioned crystals are dissolved (TEM, original magnification × 120,000). (Courtesy of D. Scott.)

seen. Eventually, with diffuse destruction of the apatite crystals, numerous bacteria can be observed invading the enamel lesion.[13]

Bacterial penetration into enamel and even dentin without clinically visible loss of tooth substance has been observed.[45,46] Bacteria formed colonies within the prism structure and also between enamel prisms. The colonies, as observed by scanning electron microscopy, consisted predominantly of rod-shaped and, occasionally, filamentous microorganisms.

Caries of coronal dentin

Macroscopic changes of dentin

On reaching the dentin, the carious lesion spreads laterally along the dentinoenamel junction, often undermining the enamel. As the lesion invades the dentin, it proceeds along a saucer-shaped front and follows the direction of the dentinal tubules. The resulting lesion is cone-shaped with the base at the dentinoenamel junction and the apex pointing toward the pulp. The affected dentin displays different degrees of discoloration from brown to dark brown or almost black.

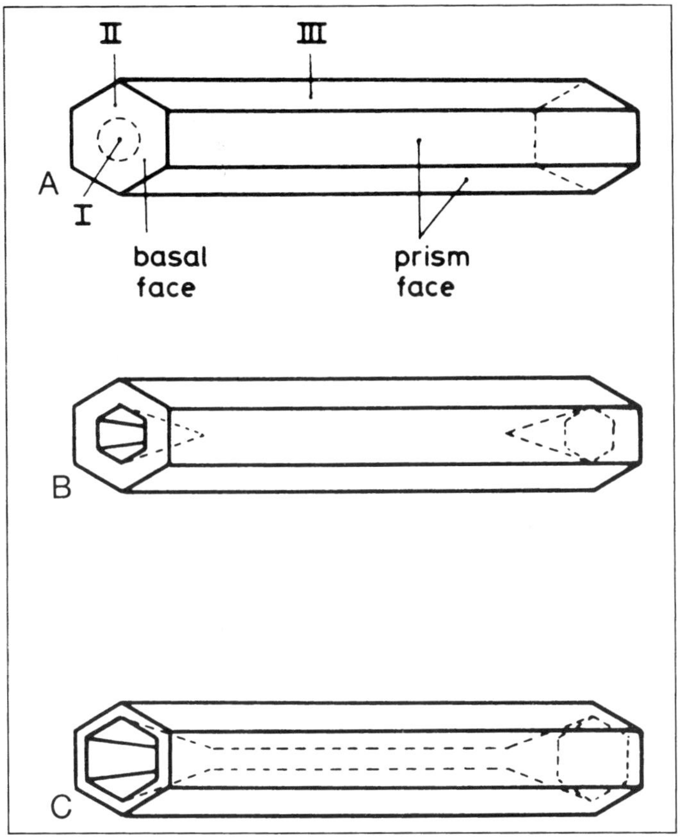

Fig 7-14 Schematic representation of the initial dissolution of a hexagonal hydroxyapatite crystallite. *(A)* The prism and basal planes are indicated. The active sites are denoted by *I, II,* and *III,* respectively. The reactivity I > II > III. *(B)* Initial etchpit formation. *(C)* Later state; the center of the crystal has been removed parallel to the *c* axis. (Courtesy of J. Arends.)

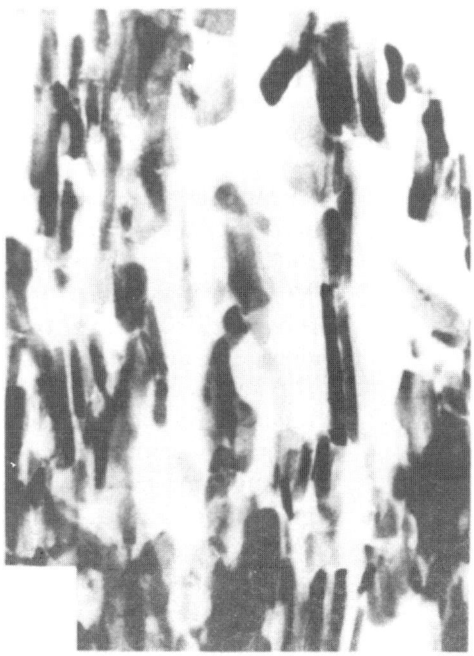

Fig 7-15 Human enamel with caries. In areas of longitudinally sectioned crystals, void areas can be seen (TEM, original magnification ×100,000). (Courtesy of D. Scott.)

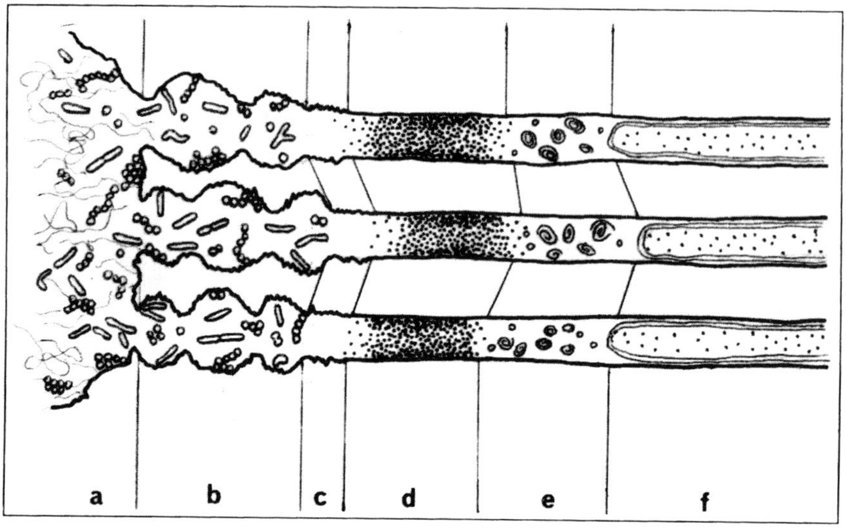

Fig 7-16 Schematic drawing of the zones seen in transmitted light of slowly progressing dentinal caries. *(a)*, Zone of decomposed dentin; *(b)*, zone of bacterial invasion showing dilations of tubules; *(c)*, demineralized zone; *(d)*, zone of dentinal sclerosis, showing occlusion of lumen with mineral deposits; *(e)*, zone of fatty degeneration; *(f)*, retreating odontoblastic processes.

Microscopic changes of dentin

As the carious lesion invades the dentin, the dentinal tubules become involved. For descriptive purposes, the pathological changes have been divided into five zones. Proceeding from the lesion inward to normal dentin, these zones are *(1)* zone of *decomposed dentin, (2)* zone of *bacterial invasion, (3)* zone of *demineralization, (4)* zone of *dentinal sclerosis,* and *(5)* zone of *fatty degeneration,* shown schematically in Fig 7-16. These zones are only discrete and distinguishable as separate entities in slowly advancing carious lesions (chronic); they tend to merge into a continuum in more rapidly progressing lesions (acute). The zones are probably passive changes imparted on the dentin by the invading microorganisms, including their indirect effect due to demineralization. The *acute* carious lesion is characterized by rapid decomposition and demineralization. The *chronic* type, on the other hand, exhibits typical changes in the degree of mineralization subjacent to the demineralized zone.

After specific staining, lipid has been seen in active (but not in arrested) lesions in both ground and decalcified sections. Fatty degeneration is frequently said to precede dentinal sclerosis, although no systematic findings support this statement. In fact, the use of the term "fatty degeneration" has been challenged, since it is not a degenerative process. Two types of lipid staining have been seen, one of which is more superficial and probably of bacterial origin. The other type may be due to unmasking of lipids present in peritubular dentin, by demineralization.[37] The altered tubules acquire a refractive index similar to the adjacent

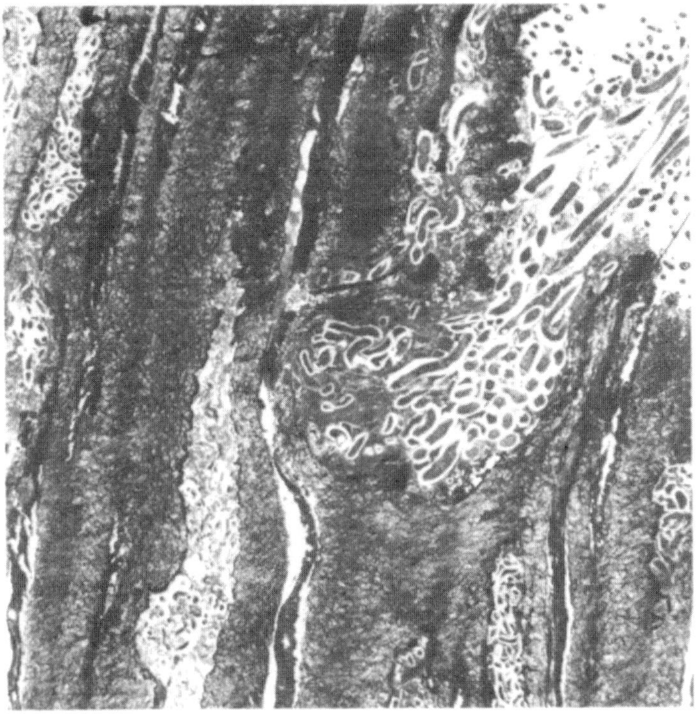

Fig 7-17 Carious dentin, illustrating bacterial invasion and dilations of dentinal tubules. A zone of decomposed dentin is shown in the upper right field. (Undecalcified ultrathin section, original magnification ×3,400). (Courtesy of P. Schüpbach.)

matrix, consequently presenting a homogeneous transparent or translucent appearance in transmitted light, that is, the "translucent zone" of dentinal caries. This translucent zone is identical to the sclerosed dentin (zone 4) and makes the dentin impermeable to vital stains such as methylene blue. Presumably the sclerosis is an attempt to block the advancing carious lesion. Next to the sclerosed dentin is a narrow zone of demineralization, affecting the intertubular matrix. Occlusion of dentinal tubules observed in this zone and in the sclerotic dentin is probably due to a reprecipitation of crystalline material that had dissolved during the carious process.

The most noticeable change in carious dentin is the zone of bacterial invasion (Fig 7-17). Frequently the lumen of the tubule is distended, giving a ballooned or dilated appearance variously described as beadings, varicosities, moth-eaten, or rosary patterns. In older literature, these dilations are referred to as "liquefaction foci," an imprecise term because these distentions are filled with bacteria and debris, not liquid. These dilations eventually coalesce, forming the outermost zone of decomposed dentin.

Additional changes that may occur in carious dentin are the formation

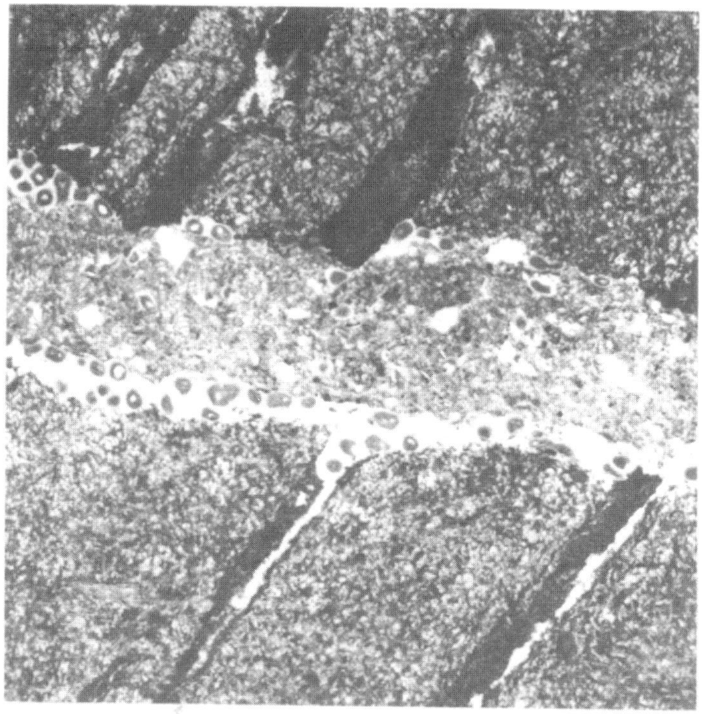

Fig 7-18 Carious dentin, showing a cleft at approximately right angles to the dentinal tubules, which are obliterated (sclerosed). The cleft contains many microorganisms. (Undecalcified ultrathin section, original magnification ×7,600). (Courtesy of P. Schüpbach.)

of clefts and of dead tracts. Cracks or clefts occur at right angles to the tubules (Fig 7-18). These cleavages follow the contour lines of Owen. Dead tracts are opaque zones, appearing black in transmitted light, formed by a sealing off of the affected dentinal tubules in response to irritation (Fig 7-19).

Caries of enamel and dentin invariably result in inflammation of the pulp. The degree of inflammatory response depends on the rapidity of the caries attack. If dentinal sclerosis occurs, injurious agents will have reduced or no access to the pulp.

Severe pulpal inflammation subjacent to the carious lesion may result in destruction of the odontoblasts in the corresponding area. If healing occurs, new odontoblasts form from undifferentiated mesenchymal cells in the dental pulp. The tubules in the subsequently formed irregular secondary dentin (reparative dentin) are then no longer contiguous with those in the primary dentin. This lack of continuity between the tubules of the primary and secondary dentin is important clinically because a "barrier effect" is established, walling off further irritation. If the caries attack is chronic in nature, at least some odontoblasts survive and continuity is maintained.

As in the case of carious enamel, histochemical staining consistently

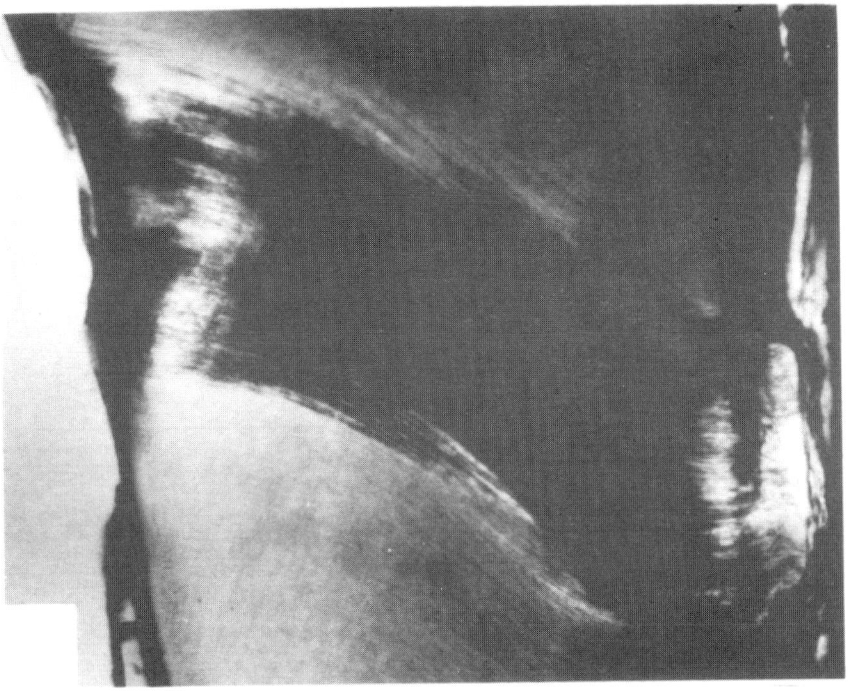

Fig 7-19 Dead tract in cervical dentin. Note secondary dentin formation (ground section, original magnification ×25).

discloses free calcium ions in carious dentin, well demarcated from the unreacting sound dentin. This is interpreted as evidence of demineralization playing an important part in carious destruction of dentin.[31]

In cavity preparation, the dentist attempts to remove the infected dentin before restoring the lesion, using the clinical criteria of softening and discoloration in judging how much of the dentin should be removed. In chronic carious lesions these are valid criteria because softening, discoloration, and bacterial invasion parallel one another. Softening (demineralization) of the dentin precedes discoloration and is always ahead of the bacterial front.[19] In acute carious lesions, there is more softening and it extends further ahead of the bacteria than in the chronic lesion. Discoloration of the dentin is not marked and is not a reliable guide for clinical removal of infected dentin in acute lesions.

Fusuyama and co-workers have proposed a simplified classification of carious dentin into two zones, based on brief (10-second) staining with a 0.5% solution of basic fuchsin in propylene glycol.[18,41,43] The outer or first carious layer, corresponding to the zones of decomposed dentin and bacterial invasion, stains red with fuchsin. The inner or second carious layer does not take up the fuchsin stain on short exposure, but will if the dye is left in the cavity too long. More recently, a

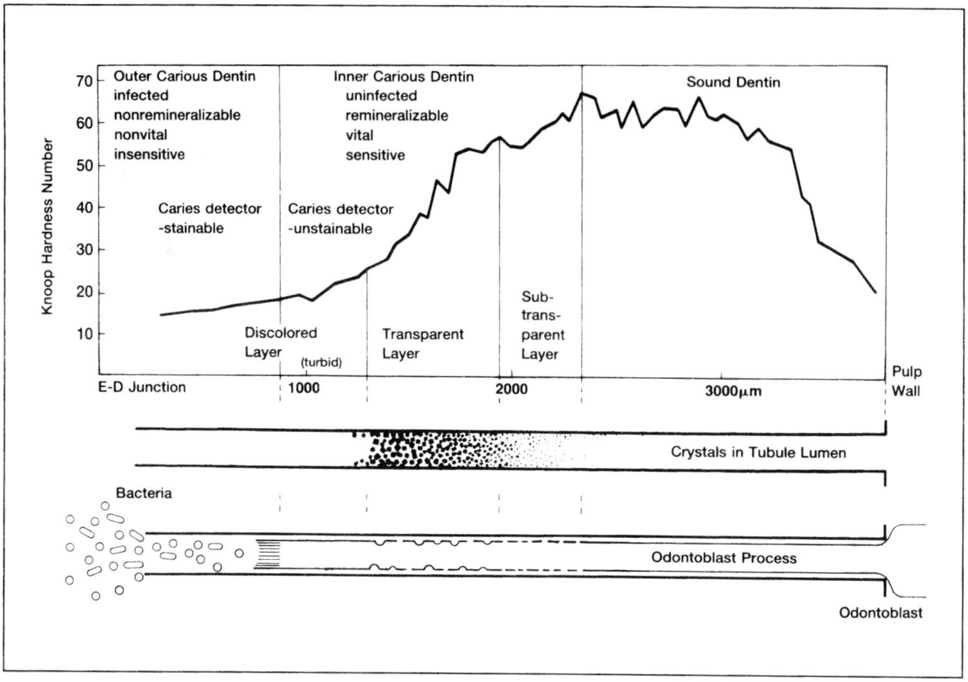

Fig 7-20 Intratubular crystal deposition and morphological changes of the odontoblast processes in various dentin layers of a carious tooth in relation to the hardness curve. (Courtesy of H. Hosuda and T. Fusayama.)

1% acid red (9-[2′-sulfonium-4′-sulfophenyl]-6-diethylamino-3-[N,N-diethyl-amino]-3 isoxanthene-sodium salt) solution in propylene glycol has been introduced because it is noncarcinogenic. It is marketed as Caries Detector (Kurarey Co). The portion of the carious dentin reacting with the dye and the nonstaining dentin are shown schematically, together with the corresponding Knoop Hardness measurements and morphological changes observed in the dentinal tubules, in Fig 7-20.[25] The zone of decomposed dentin (outer carious dentin) in soft, infected dentin, cannot be remineralized and must be removed during cavity preparation. The acid red dye reacts with dentinal collagen that has been treated by lactic acid, but not with intact dentinal collagen or dentinal collagen demineralized by EDTA.[35] Histochemical techniques using the Mallory-Azan stain also distinguish between the outer layer, which stains red, and the inner layer, which stains blue.[40] This is interpreted as evidence that the collagen fibers in the outer layer are irreversibly denatured and is supported by chemical analyses[36] and ultrastructural observations.[41] In the outer carious dentin, the cross-links (dihydroxynorleucine and hydroxynorleucine) decrease markedly. These biochemical findings suggest that remineralization (eg, dentinal bridges) can occur only in the inner carious dentin where the collagen denaturation is reversible, depending on pH. Collagen fibers are believed to be important in the remineralization of carious dentin.[30] The inner layer of carious dentin, although partially softened by demineralization, contains few if any bacteria and, because it can be remineralized, should be preserved.

Ultrastructural changes in dentin

Replacement of odontoblastic processes by amorphous material has been detected by electron microscopy at the front of the lesion. The odontoblastic processes, which are rich in microfilaments and microtubules in the inner layer of human carious dentin, show no sign of degeneration prior to sclerosis. The cell process does not retract during the mineralization of the periodontoblastic space, and can be completely surrounded by minerals. The odontoblastic process, as well as the nerve fibril found in the tubule, provide intracellular matrix for mineralization.[15] More superficially, crystals appear in the amorphous material, eventually occluding the tubule with mineral. Two types of crystals have been observed in this zone of dentinal sclerosis: platelike hydroxyapatite crystals and large, isodiametric rhombohedral crystals, "caries crystals." These latter do not occlude the tubule completely and are not part of a defensive response.[30] They have been identified as whitlockite by electron diffraction. It is likely that these crystals result from reprecipitation of ions dissolved from the dentin during carious destruction or from calcium of extrinsic origin. As in the case of light microscopy, the most striking feature of carious dentin is the penetration of the tubules by microorganisms, packing their lumen. As these areas are demineralized, the collagen fibers become exposed. In the outer carious layer there are few collagen fibers, and those remaining have lost their cross-bands and interbands.[41] The peritubular dentin disappears, and the intertubular dentin is markedly demineralized with only scattered leaflike crystals remaining. In the inner carious layer the intertubular dentin is partially demineralized, and apatite crystals are bound to collagen fibers that retain their distinct cross-bands and interbands. The peritubular dentin is reduced in thickness from inside, but the network of organic matrix and the odontoblastic process remains distinct.

Root caries

Root caries, involving both cementum and dentin, typically appears as a slowly progressing, chronic lesion. The histopathological changes seen in root dentin are similar to those seen in slowly advancing coronal caries, namely sclerosis with occlusion of the tubules. Secondary dentin formation may occur (see Fig 7-19).

Caries of cementum alone cannot be detected clinically. The exposed cementum is usually only from 20 to 50 μm thick near the cementoenamel junction, so that by the time root caries is diagnosed, dentinal

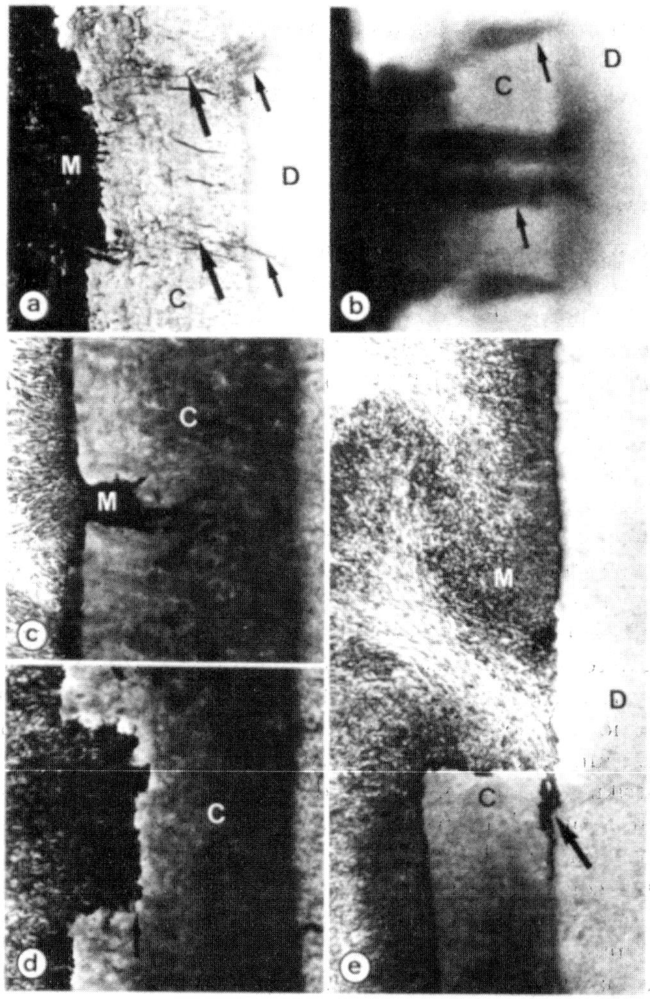

Fig 7-21 Initial lesions of exposed cementum and root dentin.

a: Photomicrograph of an undecalcified semithin section of cementum *(C)* and the underlying dentin *(D)*. Note the exposed cementum covered by microorganisms *(M)* and the small clefts *(large arrows)* traversing the cementum and reaching the peripheral dentin *(small arrows)*. Toluidine blue stain; original magnification ×260.

b: Microradiograph from an area in **a.** Note the local demineralization of the cementum *(C)* and of the peripheral dentin *(D)* in defined halolike areas and along the clefts *(arrows)*. Original magnification ×260.

c: Photomicrograph of a decalcified semithin section showing penetration of microorganisms *(M)* probably along demineralized clefts. PAS and methylene blue/azure II stain; original magnification ×360.

d: Photomicrograph of a decalcified semithin section showing stepwise destruction of cementum *(C)* along an incremental line *(arrow)*. PAS and methylene blue/azure II stain; original magnification ×360.

e: Photomicrograph of a decalcified semithin section showing exposed dentin *(D)* under a mat of microorganisms *(M)* and the typical fracture of cementum *(C)*. Sound cementum is undermined by microorganisms *(arrow)*. Note that there is no evidence of bacterial penetration into tubule-free peripheral dentin. PAS and methylene blue/azure II stain; original magnification ×180.

(Printed with permission from P. Schüpbach and B. Guggenheim, unpublished results.)

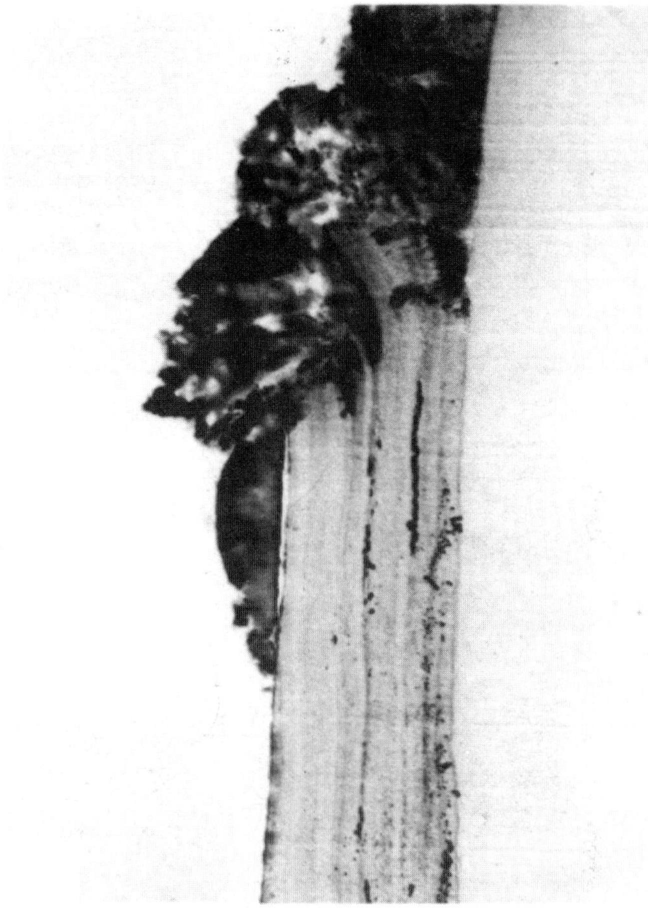

Fig 7-22 Caries of cementum, labial surface of maxillary premolar. Dental plaque covers exposed cementum and dentin. Cementum appears to be delaminating (decalcified frozen section; toluidine blue stain; original magnification ×90). (Courtesy of G. Armitage.)

involvement has occurred. Carious cementum is, of course, also covered by a layer of plaque (Fig 7-21). Brown discoloration with softening of the tooth structure may be found. In the initial lesion clefts in the cementum are seen both by light microscopy and microradiography. Microorganisms eventually penetrate along demineralized clefts, leading to stepwise destruction of the cementum (see Fig 7-21). Later damage to the cementum is seen along a broad front, sometimes manifesting as a "delamination" along the incremental lines (Fig 7-22). The lesion may penetrate along the course of Sharpey's fibers, which are oriented at right angles to the surface of the root. In microradiographs, regional differences in mineral distribution may give rise to a brushlike appearance in carious cementum due to alternating radiolucent and radiodense areas.[17] A radiopaque surface layer covering subsurface demineralized

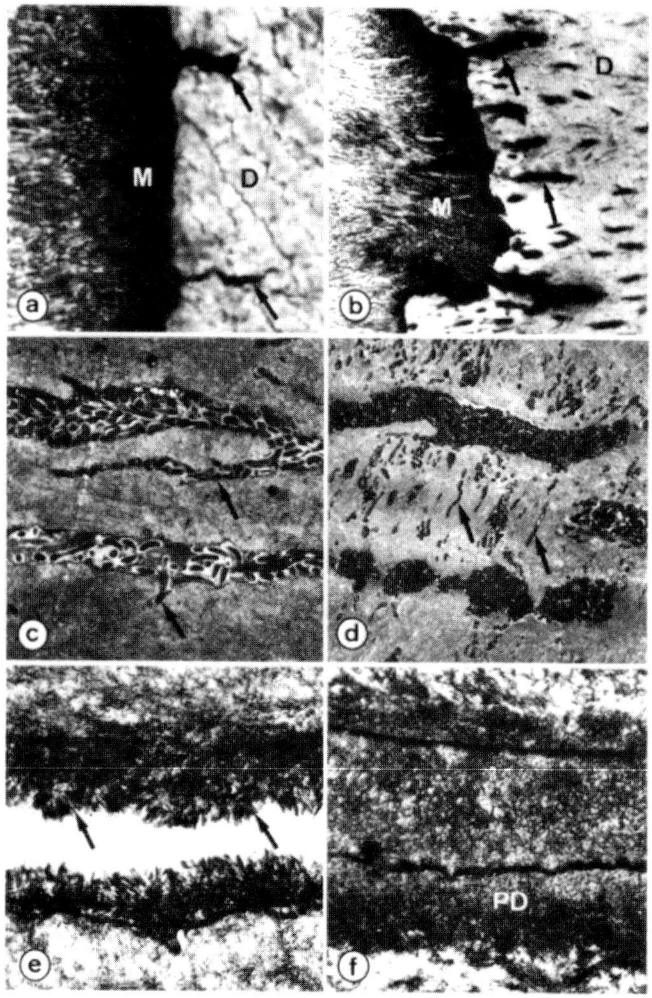

Fig 7-23 Advanced lesions of root dentin.
a: Photomicrograph of a decalcified semithin section showing the first bacterial penetration along small clefts into the peripheral tubule-free dentin *(arrows)*. *(M)* Microorganisms; *(D)* dentin. PAS and methylene blue/azure II stain; original magnification ×500.
b: Photomicrograph of a decalcified semithin section. Note spreading of the lesion toward dentinal tubules and infecting of the latter *(arrows)*. *(M)* Microorganisms; *(D)* dentin. PAS and methylene blue/azure II stain; original magnification ×200.
c: Electron micrograph of an undecalcified ultrathin section showing widened dentinal tubules and their side branches containing bacteria *(arrows)*. Original magnification ×3,200.
d: Electron micrograph of an undecalcified ultrathin section showing bacterial spreading perpendicular to the widened dentinal tubules along the incremental lines of dentin *(arrows)*. Original magnification ×2,800.
e: Electron micrograph of an undecalcified section showing the sclerotic defense response of dentin. Note the dentinal tubule partly closed with mineralized crystals that grow from the periphery inward *(arrows)*. Original magnification ×18,000.
f: Electron micrograph of an undecalcified section showing a completely occluded dentinal tubule and thickened peritubular dentin *(PD)*. Original magnification ×18,000.
(Printed with permission from P. Schüpbach and G. Guggenheim, unpublished results.)

cementum is a common finding. About a third of specimens with root caries show dentinal tubular reactions (dead tracts, translucent dentin).[54] Examination of the ultrastructure reveals tablet-shaped crystals of hydroxyapatite, some areas of marked depletion of the crystals, and small areas devoid of crystals, with bacterial indentations at the surface or lacunae in the subsurface of the cementum.[16]

In the advanced lesion involving root dentin, the dentinal tubules become infected with bacteria both along the main tubules and their side-branches (Fig 7-23, *c* and *d*). As was noted in caries of coronal dentin, there may be a sclerotic response, either partially or completely occluding the tubule with mineral crystals (Fig 7-23, *e* and *f*).

Caries of cementum appears to be a stepwise process, initially involving dissolution of the mineral phase and possibly some collagen degradation seen as longitudinal splitting of the fibers. Periods of tissue destruction may alternate with periods of reprecipitation of mineral crystals.

Chapter review

- Indicate at what stage a tooth is most caries-susceptible. Offer an explanation.
- State how long it normally takes for an intact tooth surface to develop into a clinically detectable carious lesion.
- Indicate why clinical trials of effectiveness of an anticaries agent should extend over a minimum of 2 years.
- Draw the different morphological types of occlusal fissures.
- List and describe the characteristics of the four zones usually distinguishable in ground sections of smooth surface carious lesions of enamel examined by polarized light.
- State the alterations seen in hydroxyapatite crystals undergoing carious dissolutions.
- Describe the ultrastructural alterations seen in carious enamel, indicating their locations.
- Describe the vital responses seen in dentin due to caries.
- List and describe the nonvital changes seen by light microscopy in carious dentin.
- State the chemical alterations that take place in carious enamel and dentin.
- Define dead tracts and "caries crystals."
- State the macroscopic changes detectable in early carious lesions.

Selected readings

Fejerskov, O., and Thylstrup, A. 1986. Pathology of dental caries. In *Textbook of Cariology*, O. Fejerskov and A. Thylstrup (eds), Copenhagen: Munksgaard, pp. 204–234.

Johnson, A.R. 1975. The early carious lesion of enamel. *J Oral Pathol* 4:128–157.

Pindborg, J.J. 1970. *Pathology of the Dental Hard Tissues*. Philadelphia: W.B. Saunders, pp. 256–276.

Scott, D.B., Simmerlink, J.W., and Nygaard, V. 1974. Structural aspects of dental caries. *J Dent Res* 53:165–178.

Silverstone, L.M. 1973. Structure of carious enamel, including the early lesion. In *Dental Enamel, Development, Structure and Caries*, A.H. Melcher and G.A. Zarb (eds), Oral Science Rev 3:100–160.

Silverstone, L.M. 1977. Structural alterations of human dental enamel during incipient carious lesion development. In *Incipient Caries of Enamel*, N.H. Rowe (ed), Ann Arbor: University of Michigan.

References

1. Arends, J. 1973. Dislocation and dissolution of enamel. *Caries Res* 1:261–268.
2. Bergman, G., Brännström, M., and Lind, P.O. 1961. Schmelzkaries. Eine kombinierte lichtmikroskopische, microradiographische und histochemische Untersuchung. *Arch Oral Biol* 4:147–150.
3. Bergman, G., and Lind, P.O. 1966. A quantitative microradiographic study of incipient enamel caries. *J Dent Res* 45:1477–1484.
4. Brown, L.R., Dreizen, S., and Handler, S. 1976. Effect of selected caries preventive regimens on microbial changes following irradiation-induced xerostomia in cancer patients. In *Microbial Aspects of Dental Caries*, H.M. Stiles, W.J. Loesche, and R.C. O'Brien (eds), Sp. Suppl. Microbiol. Abstr. 1:275–290.
5. Carlos, J.P., and Gittelsohn, A.M. 1965. Longitudinal studies of the natural history of caries. II. *Arch Oral Biol* 10:739–751.
6. Crabb, H.S.M. 1966. Enamel caries. *Br Dent J* 121:115–129, 167–174.
7. Crabb, H.S.M. 1974. Incremental bands in microradiographs of ground sections of a carious lesion in enamel. *Caries Res* 6:169–182.
8. Crabb, H.S.M. 1976. Fissures at risk. *Br Dent J* 140:303–307.
9. Darling, A.I. 1956. Studies of the early lesion of enamel caries with transmitted light, polarized light and microradiography. *Br Dent J* 101:289–297, 329–341.
10. Edgar, W.M., Rugg-Gunn, A.J., Jenkins, G.N., and Geddes, D.A.M. 1978. Photographic and direct visual recording of experimental caries-like changes in human dental enamel. *Arch Oral Biol* 23:667–673.
11. Fehr, F.R. von der, Loe, H., and Theilade, E. 1970. Experimental caries in man. *Caries Res* 4:131–148.
12. Fejerskov, D., Melsen, B., and Karring, T. 1973. Morphometric analysis of occlusal fissures in human premolars. *Scand J Dent Res* 81:505–509.
13. Frank, R.M. 1965. The ultrastructure of caries-resistant teeth. In *Caries-resistant Teeth*, Ciba Symposium, G.E.W. Wolstenholme, and M. O'Connor (eds), London: G. and A. Churchill, Ltd, pp. 169–184.
14. Frank, R.M., and Voegel, J.C. 1978. Dissolution mechanisms of the apatite crystals during dental caries and bone resorption. In *Molecular Basis of Biological Degradative Processes*, R.D. Berlin, H. Hermann, I.H. Lepow, and J.M. Tanzer (eds), New York: Academic Press, pp. 277–311.
15. Frank, R.M., and Voegel, J.C. 1980. Ultrastructure of the human odontoblast process and its mineralization during caries. *Caries Res* 14:367–380.
16. Furseth, R. 1971. Further observations on the fine structure of orally-exposed and carious human dental cementum. *Arch Oral Biol* 16:71–85.
17. Furseth, R., and Johansen, E. 1968. A microradiographic comparison of sound and carious human dental cementum. *Arch Oral Biol* 13:1197–1206.
18. Fusayama, T. 1979. Two layers of carious dentin. Diagnosis and treatment. *Oper Dent* 4:63–70.
19. Fusayama, T., Okuse, K., and Hosada, H. 1966. Relationship between hardness, dis-

coloration, and microbial invasion in carious dentin. *J Dent Res* 45:1033–1046.

20. Galil, K.A., and Gwinett, A.J. 1975. Three dimensional replicas of pits and fissures in human teeth. Scanning electron microscopic study. *Arch Oral Biol* 20:493–495.
21. Gillings, B., and Buonocore, M. 1961. Thickness of enamel at the base of the pits and fissures in human molars and bicuspids. *J Dent Res* 40:119–133.
22. Gustafson, G. 1957. The histopathology of caries of human enamel. *Acta Odontol Scand* 15:13–55.
23. Haikel, Y., Frank, R.M., and Voegel, J.C. 1983. Scanning electron microscopy of the human enamel surface layer of incipient carious lesions. *Caries Res* 17:1–13.
24. Hallsworth, A.S., Robinson, C., and Weatherell, J.A. 1972. Mineral and magnesium distribution within the approximal carious lesion of dental enamel. *Caries Res* 6:156–168.
25. Hosuda, H., and Fusayama, T. 1984. A tooth substance saving restorative technique. *Int Dent J* 34:1–12.
26. Johansen, E. 1962. The nature of the carious lesion. *Dent Clin North Am* July, pp. 304–320.
27. Johansen, E. 1965. Electron microscope and chemical studies of carious lesions with reference to the organic phase of affected tissues. *Ann NY Acad Sci* 131:776–785.
28. Johnson, N.W. 1967. Some aspects of the ultrastructure of early human enamel caries seen with the electron microscope. *Arch Oral Biol* 12:1505–1521.
29. Johnson, N.W. 1967. Transmission electron microscopy of early carious enamel. *Caries Res* 1:356–369.
30. Johnson, N.W., Taylor, B.R., and Berman, D.B. 1969. The response of deciduous dentine to caries studied by correlated light and electron microscopy. *Caries Res* 3:348–368.
31. Jolly, M., and Sullivan, H.R. 1960. The pathology of carious human dentine. *Aust Dent J* 5:157–164.
32. Kidd, E.A. 1983. The histopathology of enamel caries in young and old permanent teeth. *Br Dent J* 155:196–198.
33. König, K.G. 1963. Dental morphology in relation to caries resistance with special reference to fissures as susceptible areas. *J Dent Res* 42:461–476.
34. König, K.G. 1965. Findings in serially sectioned teeth showing early fissure lesions. *Adv Fluor Res Dent Caries Prevent* 4:73–79.
35. Kuboki, Y., Liu, C.F., and Fusayama, T. 1983. Mechanism of differential staining in carious dentin. *J Dent Res* 62:713–714.
36. Kuboki, Y., Ohgushi, K., and Fusayama, T. 1977. Collagen biochemistry of the two layers of carious dentin. *J Dent Res* 56:1233–1237.
37. Miller, W.A. 1969. Fat staining in carious dentin. *J Dent Res* 48:109–113.
38. Nagano, T. 1960. The form of pit fissure and the primary lesion of caries. *Dent Abstr* 6:426.
39. Newbrun, E., Brudevold, F., and Mermagen, H. 1959. A microroentgenographic study of demineralized enamel, comparing natural and artificial lesions. *Oral Surg* 12:576–584.
40. Ohgushi, K. 1973. Collagen fibers in the two layers of carious dentin. I. Histochemical study. *J Jpn Stomatol Soc* 40:65–74.
41. Ohgushi, K., and Fusayama, T. 1975. Electron microscopic structure of the two layers of carious dentin. *J Dent Res* 54:1019–1026.
42. Parfitt, G.J. 1956. The speed of development of the carious cavity. *Br Dent J* 100:204–207.
43. Sato, Y., and Fusayama, T. 1976. Removal of dentin by fuchsin staining. *J Dent Res* 55:678–683.
44. Scott, D.B., and Wyckoff, R.W. 1949. Studies of tooth surface structure by optical and electron microscopy. *J Am Dent Assoc* 39:275–282.
45. Seppa, L. 1984. A scanning electron microscopic study of early subsurface bacterial penetration of human molar-fissure enamel. *Arch Oral Biol* 29:503–506.
46. Seppa, L., Alkuijala, P., and Karvonen, I. 1985. A scanning electron microscopic study of bacterial penetration of human enamel in incipient caries. *Arch Oral Biol* 30:595–598.
47. Soni, N.N., and Brudevold, F. 1959. Microradiographic and polarized light studies of initial carious lesions. *J Dent Res* 38:1187–1194.
48. Sullivan, H.R. 1954. The formation of early carious lesions in dental enamel. *J Dent Res* 33:218–230.
49. Sullivan, H.R. 1955. Investigations into the pathogenesis of dental caries. *Oral Surg* 8:168–181.

50. Theilade, J., Fejerskov, O., and Hørsted, M. 1976. A transmission electron microscopic study of 7-day-old bacterial plaque in human tooth fissures. *Arch Oral Biol* 21:587–598.
51. Thylstrup, A., and Fejerskov, O. 1981. Some surface features of early carious enamel at various stages of activity. In *Tooth Surface Interactions and Preventive Dentistry*, G. Rolla, T. Sonju, and G. Emberg (eds), London: Information Retrieval, Inc, pp. 193–205.
52. Voegel, J.C., and Frank, R.M. 1976. The different dissolution steps of a human carious apatite enamel crystal. *J Dent Res* 55(Sp. Issue):D154.
53. Voegel, J.C., and Frank, R.M. 1977. Stages in the dissolution of human enamel crystals in dental caries. *Calcif Tissue Res* 24:19–27.
54. Wefel, J.S., Clarkson, B.H., and Heilman, J.R. 1985. Natural root caries: a histologic and microradiographic evaluation. *J Oral Pathol* 14:615–623.

Chapter 8

Caries Activity Tests

For assessment of the actual caries risk, facts from the case history, the clinical and radiographic examination, the dietary history, and the supplementary laboratory examinations all have to be considered.

Bo Krasse, *Caries Risk,* 1985

Caries activity tests have been used in dental research for many years, and some tests have been adapted for routine use in the dental office. There is no ideal test in existence at the present time, although caries activity tests are a valuable adjunct for patient motivation in a plaque control program.[9]

A multiplicity of caries activity tests have been described in the literature.[13,47,48] Innumerable tests have been devised by investigators in attempting to predict an individual's susceptibility; this suggests two things. First, that there is a very definite need for a good test. Second, that none of the currently available methods are completely satisfactory. Some of the proposed uses of an accurate caries-susceptibility test[47] are as follows.

For the clinician:
1. To determine the need for caries control measures
2. As an indicator of patient cooperation
3. To act as an aid in timing of recall appointments
4. As a guide to insertion of expensive restorations
5. To aid in the determination of prognosis
6. As a precautionary signal to the orthodontist in placing bands

For the research worker:
1. As an aid in the selection of patients for caries study
2. To help in the screening of potential therapeutic agents
3. To serve as an indicator of periods of exacerbation and remission

Snyder[46] has suggested that a suitable caries activity test should:
1. Have a sound theoretical basis
2. Show maximal correlation with clinical status
3. Be accurate with respect to duplication of results
4. Be simple
5. Be inexpensive
6. Take little time

In addition, a good caries-predictive test should possess at least three characteristics: validity, reliability, and feasibility. *Validity* implies predictive validity, so that a child, if placed in a high-caries-activity (positive) category and followed for 2 years, should demonstrate high caries increments. Conversely, a child in a low-caries-activity (negative) category should have minimal or no caries increments. Good predictive validity requires that there be a minimum of false positive or false negative test results. *Reliability* implies that when the test is performed on different occasions, it will give reproducible results. The most *feasible* caries activity tests are those that lend themselves to use in public health programs or for large clinical trials because they are inexpensive, noninvasive, and easy to use by semiskilled personnel.

Current knowledge of the carious process indicates that it is influenced by three major variables: the bacterial flora (specifically, of the dental plaque), the substrate, and the susceptibility of the host (the tooth and the saliva). It is best if one considers the caries activity tests with these factors in mind. Some of the more widely used tests are described in detail on the following pages.

Lactobacillus colony count (Table 8-1)

Action: This test, first introduced by Hadley in 1933, estimates the number of acidogenic and aciduric bacteria in the patient's saliva by counting the number of colonies appearing on tomato peptone agar plates (pH 5.0) after inoculation with a sample of saliva. LBS agar (Rogosa) is more selective; it is acidic, has a high content of acetate and other salts, and has a low surface tension. The selectivity of LBS agar is not complete, however, because other organisms besides lactobacilli will grow. The total number of colonies on this medium reflects the proportion of the aciduric flora in the saliva.

Equipment: The necessary equipment includes saliva-collecting bottles, paraffin, two 9-ml tubes of saline, two agar plates, two bent glass rods, facilities for incubating, and a Quebec Counter and pipettes.

Procedure: Saliva is collected by having the subject chew paraffin before breakfast and then collecting the saliva in a bottle. The specimen is shaken to mix it. A 1:10 dilution is prepared by pipetting 1 ml of the saliva sample into a 9-ml tube of sterile saline solution. This is shaken, and a 1 : 100 dilution is made by pipetting 1 ml of the 1 : 10 dilution into another 9-ml tube of sterile salt solution. The 1 : 100

dilution is mixed thoroughly, and 0.4 ml of each dilution is spread on the surface of an agar plate with a bent glass rod. The plates are labeled and incubated at 37°C for 3 to 4 days. A count of the number of colonies is then made by using the Quebec Counter.

Table 8-1 Results of *Lactobacillus* count

No. lactobacilli per ml saliva	Caries activity
0-1000	Little or none
1000-5000	Slight
5000-10,000	Moderate
>10,000	Marked

It takes only a few minutes to do the test, but the results are not available for several days and the counting of the colonies is a very tedious process. This test is not simple, for it requires relatively complex equipment and personnel with bacteriological training. The cost is relatively high.

The customary procedure of quantitating lactobacilli in paraffin-stimulated saliva can give highly variable counts for the same subject. For example, eating cheese can elevate the *Lactobacillus* counts in patients with no recent caries activity. This variability limits the usefulness of a single count of salivary lactobacilli as a quantitative check of caries activity.[15] Therefore, repeated sampling is recommended.

The *Lactobacillus* plate count is one of the oldest caries activity tests. Its correlation with clinical caries activity has been demonstrated in numerous studies, particularly in comparisons between caries-active and caries-inactive patients, but this has been challenged in other studies. The *Lactobacillus* test has been generally accepted in the past, and it is still used as a reference test for new caries activity tests.

A highly practical and greatly simplified method of estimating lactobacilli is now available (Dentocult, Orion Diagnostica). Undiluted paraffin-stimulated saliva is poured over a plastic slide that is coated with LBS agar. Excess saliva is allowed to drain off, and the slide is placed into a sterile tube, which is tightly closed and incubated at 35° to 37°C for 4 days. The colony density on the slide is not counted but is compared with a model chart and classified as about 1,000, 10,000, 100,000, or 1,000,000 aciduric organisms per ml of saliva. This method gives a highly significant correlation with the conventional lactobacilli count[4,28] and a statistically significant correlation with caries activity.[12] Because the technique is simple, the cost reasonable, and the results easy to read, it offers a practical office test.

Snyder test (Table 8-2)

Action: The Snyder test measures the rapidity of acid formation when a sample of stimulated saliva is inoculated into glucose agar adjusted to pH 4.7 to 5 and with bromcresol green as color indicator. Indirectly the test is also a measure of acidogenic and aciduric bacteria.

Equipment: The equipment includes saliva-collecting bottles, paraffin, a tube of Snyder glucose agar containing bromcresol green and adjusted to pH 4.7 to 5, pipettes, and incubating facilities.

Procedure: Saliva is collected before breakfast by having the subject chew paraffin. A tube of Snyder glucose agar is melted and then cooled to 50°C. The saliva specimen is shaken vigorously for 3 minutes. Then 0.2 ml of saliva is pipetted into the tube of agar and immediately mixed by rotating the tube. The agar is allowed to solidify in the tube and is incubated at 37°C. The color change of the indicator is observed after 24, 48, and 72 hours of incubation by comparison with an uninoculated tube against a white background.

Table 8-2 Results of Snyder test

	Time (hr)		
	24	48	72
Color	Yellow	Yellow	Yellow
Caries activity	Marked	Definite	Limited
Color	Green	Green	Green
Caries activity	Continue test	Continue test	Inactive

The Snyder test is simple, takes 24 to 48 hours, and requires only simple equipment; some training is needed and the cost is moderate. This test meets some of the "ideal test" characteristics. Snyder and others have found a high correlation between the Snyder acid production test and the *Lactobacillus* plate count. Also, Snyder and others have found a high correlation between clinical caries activity and positive Snyder test results on a group basis. The best agreement was between a negative Snyder test and the absence of caries activity. Some researchers have refuted both claims. Neither the Snyder test nor the *Lactobacillus* count can predict the extent of expectancy of caries with any reliability for *one individual.*

Several modifications of the Snyder test have been proposed in order to further simplify the method for use in the private dental office. In one case a much smaller volume (0.2 ml) of culture medium is inoculated with saliva using a calibrated wire loop. This avoids the use of pipettes and saves medium and space. Alban's[1] method uses less agar in the medium so that the tubes do not require melting. There is no attempt to quantitate the salivary inoculum, which is "drooled" directly into the tube. In another modification, the buccal tooth surfaces are swabbed and the cotton applicator incubated in a semifluid Snyder medium.[17] This has the advantage of culturing directly from the plaque.

Reductase test (Table 8-3)

Action: The test measures the rate at which an indicator molecule, diazoresorcinol, changes from blue to red to colorless or leukoform on reduction by the mixed salivary flora. Rapp[37] claims the test "measures the activity of a single enzyme, reductase. This enzyme is involved in some very definite and limiting reactions in the formation of products dangerous to the tooth surface."

Equipment: The reductase test comes in a kit (Treatex, C.W. Erwin & Co) that includes calibrated saliva collection tubes with the reagent on the inside of the tube's cap, plus flavored paraffin.

Procedure: Saliva is collected by chewing a special flavored paraffin and expectorating directly into the collection tube. When the saliva reaches the calibration mark (5 ml) the reagent cap is replaced. The sample is mixed with a fixed amount of diazoresorcinol, the reagent upon which the reductase enzyme is to react. The change in color after 30 seconds and after 15 minutes is taken as a measure of caries activity.

Table 8-3 Results of the reductase test

Color	Time	Score	Caries activity
Blue	15 min	1	Nonconducive
Orchid	15 min	2	Slightly conducive
Red	15 min	3	Moderately conducive
Red	Immediately	4	Highly conducive
Pink or white	Immediately	5	Extremely conducive

Rapp[37] has claimed a good correlation of the results of this test with clinical caries experience. Other investigators[38,41,43] concluded that this test did not give accurate results and was not of diagnostic value, but a correlation between reductase activity and the numbers of salivary anaerobes has been reported. Caries-free adults exhibit low or negative scores on the reductase test. It has been proposed that this test is rather a measure of the oral hygiene status of the individual. Test results vary with time after food intake and after brushing.

Buffer capacity test

Action: Buffer capacity can be quantitated using either a pH meter or color indicators. The test measures the number of milliliters of acid required to lower the pH of saliva through an arbitrary pH interval, such as from pH 7.0 to 6.0, or the amount of acid or base necessary to bring color indicators to their end point.

Equipment: Needed equipment includes a pH meter and titration equipment, 0.05 N lactic acid, 0.05 N base, paraffin, and sterile glass jars containing a small amount of oil.

Procedure: Ten milliliters of stimulated saliva are collected under oil at least 1 hour after eating; 5 ml of this are measured into a beaker. After correcting the pH meter to room temperature, the pH of the saliva is adjusted to 7.0 by addition of lactic acid or base. The level of lactic acid in the graduated cylinder is re-recorded. Lactic acid is then added to the sample until a pH of 6.0 is reached. The number of milliliters of lactic acid needed to reduce pH from 7.0 to 6.0 is a measure of buffer capacity. This number can be converted to milliequivalents per liter.

There is a trend of an inverse relationship between buffering capacity of saliva and caries activity. The saliva of individuals whose mouths contain a considerable number of carious lesions frequently has a lower acid-buffering capacity than the saliva of those who are relatively caries-free. This test, however, does not correlate adequately with caries activity.

Fosdick calcium dissolution test

Action: The test measures the milligrams of powdered enamel

dissolved in 4 hours by acid formed when the patient's saliva is mixed with glucose and powdered enamel.

Equipment: Powdered human enamel, saliva collection bottles, sterile test tubes, test tube agitation equipment, and equipment for determining the calcium content of the saliva. Saliva is stimulated by having the subject chew gum or paraffin, in which case a 5% solution of glucose is needed.

Procedure: Twenty-five milliliters of gum-stimulated saliva are collected. Part of this is analyzed for calcium content. The rest is placed in an 8-inch sterile test tube with about 0.1 g of powdered human enamel. The tube is sealed and shaken for 4 hours at body temperature, after which it is again analyzed for calcium content. The chewing of gum to stimulate the saliva produces sugar; if the paraffin is used, a concentration of about 5% glucose is added. The amount of enamel dissolution increases as the caries activity increases.

In limited studies, the correlation is reported to be good. The time required is 4 hours. However, this test is not simple, the equipment is complex, personnel must be trained, and the cost is high.

Dewar test

Action: This test is similar to the Fosdick calcium dissolution test except that the final pH after 4 hours is measured instead of the amount of calcium dissolved.

This procedure has not been adequately tested for clinical correlation.

Mutans group of streptococci screening tests (Table 8-4)

Plaque/toothpick method

Action: The test involves a simple screening of a diluted plaque sample streaked on a selective culture medium.

Equipment: Sterile toothpicks, sterile Ringer's solution (5 ml), platinum loop, mitis-salivarius agar plates containing sulphadimetine[10] (1 g/L), incubator.

Procedure: Plaque samples are collected from the gingival third of buccal tooth surfaces (one from each quadrant) and placed in Ringer's solution. The sample is shaken until homogenized. The plaque suspension is streaked across a mitis-salivarius agar plate. After aerobic incubation at 37°C for 72 hours, the cultures are examined under a low-power microscope and the total colonies in ten fields are recorded.

Table 8-4 Results of the *Streptococcus mutans* screening test*

			Dental caries experience‡	
Grade	Colonies/10 fields	No. cases†	No. cases with new lesions	New lesions/yr/100 teeth
1	None	21	4	0–8.34
2	<8	11	5	0–8.64
3	≥8	12	12	8.34–21.40

*From Woods.[52]
†Patients aged 6 to 15 years.
‡After 11 to 13 months.

This test is an attempt to semiquantitatively screen the dental plaque for a specific group of caries-inducing streptococci, *Streptococcus mutans.* A pilot study conducted in a private practice on a small group of children over a 1-year period has shown some relationship between the presence of *S mutans* in plaque and subsequent dental caries experience. The relationship seems to hold up best for patients in grade 3, that is, with large numbers of colonies.

Saliva/tongue blade method

Action: The test estimates the numbers of *S mutans* in mixed paraffin-stimulated saliva when cultured on mitis-salivarius bacitracin (MSB) agar (see page 77).

Equipment: Paraffin wax, sterile tongue blades, disposable contact petri dish (RODAC) containing MSB agar, incubator.

Procedure: The subjects chew paraffin wax for 1 minute to displace plaque microorganisms, thereby increasing the proportions of plaque microorganisms in the saliva. The subjects are then given a sterile tongue blade, which they rotate in their mouth ten times, so that both sides of the tongue blade are thoroughly inoculated by the subject's flora. Excess saliva is removed by withdrawing the tongue blade through closed lips. Both sides of the tongue blade are

> then pressed onto an MSB agar in a disposable contact petri dish (RODAC, Falcon), which is then incubated at 37°C for 48 hours. For field studies the plates can be placed into plastic bags containing expired air, which are then sealed (Seal-a-Meal) and incubated at 37°C. Counts of more than 100 colony-forming units (CFU) by this method are proportional to greater than 10^6 CFU of *S mutans* per milliliter of saliva by conventional methods. This simplified and practical method for field studies requires no transport media or dilution steps.[26]

This test was developed for use with large numbers of school children and avoids the necessity of collecting saliva.

An updated and simpler version of this method, Strip mutans (Orion Diagnostica), uses a liquid medium with a long shelf life, to which the bacitracin is added just before incubation. A plastic spatula with a roughened surface is used instead of a wooden tongue blade. Colonies of mutans group streptococci grow directly on the spatula, which is then removed from the liquid medium, drained, and placed under the microscope for counting. The spatula with its attached colonies can be stored for a long time.[8]

S mutans adherence method

Action: The test categorizes salivary samples based on the ability of *S mutans* to adhere to glass surfaces when grown in sucrose-containing broth.

Equipment: Tubes to collect saliva, rack to hold culture tubes, disposable pipettes, incubator. MSB broth is available commercially (Showa Yakuhin Kako Co Ltd) in a form that permits storage without deterioration. The broth is marketed in a sealed vial, to which is added a strip of paper bearing bacitracin, tellurite, and crystal violet. These ingredients elute within 10 minutes, after which the broth is ready for use.

Procedure: Unstimulated saliva (0.1 ml) is inoculated in MSB broth. Inoculated tubes are set at 60° angle and incubated aerobically at 37°C for 24 hours. After growth has been observed, the supernatant medium is removed and the cells adhering to the glass surface are examined macroscopically and scored as follows: − (no growth expressed), + (a few deposits ranging from 1 to 10), + + (scattered deposits of smaller size), + + + (numerous minute deposits with more than 20 large size deposits). When the adherence score is + + +, *S mutans* is present at a level higher than 10^5 CFU/ml of whole saliva. If adherence is scored – or +, *S mutans* is present at less than 10^4 CFU/ml of saliva.[34]

This method is potentially useful for handling many samples in preventive practice and epidemiological studies because of its simplicity.

S mutans dip-slide methods

Action:	These tests (Dentocult SM, Orion Diagnostica; Cariescreen SM, Apo Diagnostics) classify salivary samples according to estimates of *S mutans* colonies growing on modified mitis-salivarius agar.
Equipment:	Paraffin wax, plastic slides coated with MS agar, CO_2 tablets, bacitracin disks or tablets, and buffered diluent.
Procedure A: (Dentocult SM)	The subject chews the paraffin wax, and stimulated saliva is collected for 5 minutes. The saliva is poured over the agar-coated slide, totally wetting the surface, and the excess is allowed to drain off. After the slide dries for 10 to 15 minutes, the bacitracin disks are placed in the middle of the inoculated agar about 1 cm from each other. A CO_2 tablet is inserted in the tube containing the slide, which is then incubated for 48 hours. A zone of inhibition 10 to 20 mm in diameter is formed around each bacitracin disk. If present, *S mutans* appears as small blue colonies growing within the zone of inhibition. The colony density is compared with a model chart and classified as 0 (negligible), 1 (less than 100,000), 2 (100,000 to 1,000,000), and 3 (more than 1,000,000) *S mutans* CFU/ml of saliva.
Procedure B: (Cariescreen SM)	A bacitracin tablet is placed in the buffered diluent and allowed to dissolve completely. Meanwhile, the subject chews paraffin wax for 15 to 20 seconds, swallowing the saliva. While continuing to chew the wax, the subject expectorates approximately 1 to 2 ml of stimulated saliva directly into the diluent vial, which is then capped and gently mixed by repeated inversion. The dip-slide, coated on both sides with MSB agar (without bacitracin), is then immersed for a few seconds in the buffered diluent containing bacitracin and the patient's saliva. A CO_2 tablet is placed in the empty dip-slide vial, and two drops of water are added. The dip-slide is replaced in its vial and the cap securely tightened. The vial is placed upright for 48 hours at 37°C in an incubator and then read or allowed to stand at room temperature overnight.

The colony density on the agar is compared with a reference colony density chart that shows the equivalent of 10,000, 50,000, 100,000, 250,000, 500,000, or 1,000,000 CFU/ml of saliva. This simple, semiquantitative method correlates strongly with actual laboratory methods of quantifying *S mutans* by standard culturing to an upper limit of 10^5 to 10^6 CFU/ml.[21] *S mutans* colonies can be recognized, when viewed through a magnifying lens, by their opaque, highly convex appearance and irregular shape. When the test is used on adults, larger flat gray colonies may grow. These are likely to be *Streptococcus faecalis* and should be disregarded.

S mutans replicate technique

Action: This method localizes *S mutans* colonies on tooth surfaces, using a solid impression matrix comprised primarily of sucrose and a commercial gum base.[39]

Equipment: Impression matrix and liquid culture medium composed of tryptose, trypan blue, gentian violet, potassium tellurite and bacitracin (ie, similar to MSB but omitting fermentable substrate, which is in the solid matrix).

Procedure: An imprint of the tooth surfaces to be sampled is obtained by pressing the matrix against it, after which the matrix is washed for several seconds in water to remove nonadherent cells and saliva. The matrices are placed in the liquid broth, incubated at 37°C overnight, then removed and examined directly for overgrowth of *S mutans* colonies at specific sites (eg, occlusal or root surfaces).

Prediction of future caries activity based on previous caries experience (Table 8-5)

Action: As an alternative to chemical or bacteriological tests for determining caries activity, previous caries experience can be a reasonable indication of future trends. However, it is better to omit occlusal surfaces in such estimates.

Equipment: Dental light, mirror, explorer, radiographs.

Procedure: Koch[23] grouped 9- to 10-year-old children into a high caries-active group and a low caries-active group on the basis of restored:

1. Proximal surfaces of incisors and first permanent molars
2. Buccal surfaces of maxillary first permanent molars
3. Lingual surfaces of mandibular first permanent molars

Addition of these restored surfaces in each individual provided a type of caries index for that child. Those who had a score of four or more were considered high caries-active, whereas those who had a zero score were considered low caries-active. After 1 year the high caries-active group had developed 9.5 new carious tooth surfaces, compared with 5.3 in the low caries-active group. This difference was statistically significant.

Table 8-5 Results of the prediction based on past caries experience*

Caries activity	No. of selected restored surfaces	New carious surfaces
Low	0	5.30
High	>4	9.52

*After 1 year in 9- to 10-year-old children. From Koch.[24]

This method is a practical means of identifying children with high and low caries activity and can be useful in screening children to be used in clinical therapeutic trials or in practice for those who require intensive preventive therapy. Caries increments in the test period were significantly different in the two groups. It is worth noting that about one third of the population sample fell between these two extremes and no prediction concerning the caries increment could be made for this group. When all filled surfaces were used to identify "low" and "high" risk groups, about 75% of the children fell in between.[5] In other words, individual prognosis of future caries based on past caries experience is possible only for about 25% of subjects.

The one characteristic most consistently correlated with caries increments has been the initial DMFS score.[5,19,23] If the past caries experience is considered on a hierarchical basis, is can be an even more effective predictor of future caries activity.[36] However, there are serious drawbacks to using this method as a means of identifying and selecting high-risk populations for preventive treatment. The most obvious disadvantage is that considerable caries will have already occurred in this population. Second, this method is not applicable to the very young, when preventive intervention is desirable. Finally, this method of identification requires professional dental examination.

Relationship between tests and cariogenic factors (Table 8-6)

There is a distinct variation in the distribution of specific organisms in various sites in the oral cavity, and the microbiota are not homogeneously distributed. Most tests utilize saliva as the source of the cariogenic flora, whereas a plaque sample would be more rational. The bacteria found in saliva represent the wash-off from plaque, mucosa, and tongue and most resemble the tongue flora. The cariogenic streptococci first described by Fitzgerald and Keyes,[14] and others resembling them isolated subsequently, have been grouped under the name *S mutans* on the basis

Table 8-6 Caries activity tests—their basis, method, and clinical correlation

Test	Basis	Method	Clinical correlation
Lactobacillus count	Aciduric organisms (salivary)	Quantitative (count/ml) Plate culture	Group correlation, unsatisfactory for individuals
Snyder	Aciduric organisms (salivary)	Qualitative (rate > pH 3.8) Colorimetric tube culture	Group correlation, unsatisfactory for individuals
Swab	Aciduric organisms (plaque)	Qualitative (pH) Colorimetric tube culture	Unsatisfactory
Fosdick	Total organisms (salivary) Buffering capacity	Quantitative Ca dissolved from enamel powder	Not established
Dewar	Total organisms (salivary) Buffering capacity	Quantitative (pH) Modified Fosdick	Unsatisfactory
Rickles	Total organisms (salivary) Buffering capacity	Quantitative (pH)	Unsatisfactory
Reductase	Total organisms (salivary) Oxidation-reduction potential	Qualitative Dye color change	Group correlation, unsatisfactory for individuals
Amylase	Ability to hydrolyze starch	Qualitative or quantitative Reducing sugar or starch 12 color	Unsatisfactory
Buffer capacity	Buffer capacity	Quantitative titration	Correlation of extreme deviation
Streptococcus mutans screening	*S mutans* (plaque)	Semiquantitative (size of plaque sample uncontrolled Uses a selective medium	Best correlation for low caries-activity group

of common physiological and morphological characteristics. *S mutans* and *Streptococcus sanguis* are among the ecological dominants in the early bacterial aggregations on tooth surfaces (both natural and artificial) and constitute a higher percentage of the streptococcal flora in plaque than in saliva.

S mutans will form acid from a number of different sugars but is not aciduric. Yet the two most frequently used caries activity tests, the lactobacillus count and the Snyder test, employ a medium of pH 5.5 or less, which is not likely to foster the growth of these caries-inducing streptococci. In fact, these tests were designed at a time when *Lactobacillus acidophilus*, an aciduric organism, was considered to be the cause of caries. Therefore, the media employed were at least partially selective for lactobacilli but suppressed the oral streptococci.

It has been argued that, although lactobacilli are not the specific cause of caries, the acid conditions that produce caries also favor growth of lactobacilli,[45] and, therefore, a general correlation exists between such tests and subsequent caries incidence. Nevertheless, the relationship between lactobacilli and initial caries can only be an indirect one, and it would seem more logical to develop more direct tests of the cariogenic flora. No correlation has been found between lactobacillus counts and plaque scores.[32] Another feature of the Snyder test and its modifications is that they use an indicator, bromcresol green, which is blue-green at pH 5.4 or above and turns yellow at pH 3.8 or less. The so-called "critical pH" at which a significant amount of enamel dissolves is pH 5.4 to 5.5. It would seem more appropriate, therefore, to use an indicator such as bromcresol purple, which is purple at pH 6.8 and yellow at pH 5.2. This indicator has, in fact, been used in the Rickles test.

The principle of either counting the cariogenic organisms or quantitating their ability to form acid appears to be a valid one. Preferably the test should sample bacteria from plaque and not whole saliva. Furthermore, the medium should be able to sustain the cariogenic flora. Several broth media containing a pH indicator are currently being evaluated for their ability to reflect the levels of *S mutans* in plaque or saliva.

Qualitative tests for the presence or absence of *S mutans* within the plaque show a positive correlation between early detectable lesions and *S mutans*.[18] However, this may not suffice as there is mounting evidence that *S mutans* is pandemic throughout the world.[7] Quantitative counts of this organism in plaque samples show some correlation with caries increments.[52] In selected groups of caries-active and caries-inactive populations, there is a clear-cut correlation between caries activity and the number of "caries-inducing" streptococci.[27] *S mutans* is either absent or constitutes a low proportion (about 1% to 3%) of plaque samples obtained in New Guinea and Morocco from subjects who were either caries-free or had low caries activity.[22,40] It has further been shown that plaque from recently developed or unrestored carious lesions contains a higher proportion of *S mutans* than plaque from caries-free surfaces.[29–31,49] On the other hand, Hoerman et al[18] reported the mean percent of *S mutans* in the total streptococcal population was 8.9% with initial caries present and 9.2% with caries absent. These values are certainly low when compared with more advanced lesions. From the lesion itself *S mutans* constituted 30.9% of total streptococci; near the lesion, 20.4%; and distant from the lesion, 11.6%.[42]

Relationship between tests and cariogenic substrate

Let us now turn to the substrate. There is no question that this is an important variable influencing the carious process. Furthermore, there is overwhelming evidence implicating sucrose as the principal dietary component involved. Several studies have shown that a strict reduction of dietary intake of carbohydrates results in a lowering of the salivary lactobacillus count. However, in addition to restricting dietary intake, there has often been operative intervention by restoration of carious lesions and modification of oral hygiene habits. It is, therefore, not clear whether the fall in the lactobacillus count is due to a change in the dietary habits alone or the combined effect. There is evidence that lactobacilli increase with the appearance of carious lesions. This does not mean that there is a causal relationship; in fact, the bulk of recent gnotobiotic and plaque studies indicate the contrary. A better interpretation is that the cariogenic streptococci can establish themselves on smooth surfaces, given the necessary substrate, and that once a defect has occurred in the enamel, the lactobacilli can multiply there. A comprehensive dietary survey is, therefore, a better way of testing the caries "inducIveness" of the substrate component. There is general agreement that the currently available caries activity tests serve as a check of patient cooperation as regards both dietary regime and oral hygiene procedures. They serve as a practical visual aid in persuading patients to undertake preventive measures.

The following case histories illustrate the usefulness of bacteriological caries activity tests in determining the success of dietary counseling.[10]

Case 1

This was an 18-year-old woman with 24 decayed, missing, or filled teeth and extensive active caries. She worked in a bakery, had poor oral hygiene, a high and often-repeated intake of sugar-containing foods, and high bacterial counts.

After instruction and dietary counseling, both the *Lactobacillus* count and the relative frequency of *S mutans* dropped considerably. The prognosis was considered good, and comprehensive restorative therapy was undertaken. Two years later the counts were still low, and the results of the dental treatment were considered excellent (Table 8-7).

Table 8-7 Bacterial counts of lactobacilli and *Streptococcus mutans*

	Before counseling	After counseling
No. lactobacilli/ml saliva	1.7 million	80,000
% *S mutans* in plaque material	25	2

Case 2

This was a 25-year-old truck driver with 28 decayed, missing, or filled teeth and extensive active caries. Due to irregular working hours he had great difficulty in altering his dietary habits.

The patient was considered uncooperative, and the prognosis was poor for control of his active disease. Therefore, a full maxillary and a partial mandibular denture were made after extraction of a number of carious teeth. After 1 year the bacterial counts were still high. Had extensive restorative therapy been instituted for this patient, it is extremely doubtful that it would have been successful (Table 8-8).

Thus, the evaluation of the success of dietary counseling by bacterial examination gives an objective indication of the cooperation of the patient. A change of dietary habits is reflected in the microflora within several weeks, and the patient is encouraged and motivated to continue his efforts. Furthermore, it affords the practitioner some basis for selection of a restorative treatment plan that is likely to maintain optimum oral health conditions for the individual patient.

Table 8-8 Bacterial counts of lactobacilli and *Streptococcus mutans*

	Before counseling	After counseling
No. lactobacilli/ml saliva	19.3 million	16.6 million
% *S mutans* in plaque material	6	16

Relationship between tests and resistance of the host: tooth and saliva

The third major component affecting the caries process is the host—the enamel and the saliva. None of the tests has attempted to use an individual's enamel, although the Fosdick test has used pooled enamel powder. Difference in fluoride content can significantly alter the solubility of enamel, and a test using pooled enamel other than the patient's cannot be justified. Recently developed techniques of enamel biopsy permit the sampling of an individual patient's tooth; however, biopsy techniques have not yet been adapted for susceptibility tests.

Numerous tests based on biochemical or physiological properties of the saliva have been related to patients' caries prevalence. Only a few of these tests will be considered here.

Salivary pH is notoriously variable, partly because of the loss of CO_2 during storage. It is not surprising, therefore, that there are no clear-cut differences in salivary pH between patients with high and low caries prevalence. Salivary acid buffering capacity has shown some correlation with caries prevalence. It is also known to be related to the flow rate, bicarbonate, and sodium content. However, the correlation of buffering capacity with caries is not adequate for predicting individual caries incidence. Measurements of salivary amylase content have been related to dental caries experience. Some authors have claimed a positive association, some a negative, and many no relation at all. The theoretical premise of such a test is that starches, if rapidly hydrolyzed to maltose, would be utilized more readily by oral flora. However, the conclusions derived from human epidemiological and case studies as well as controlled animal feeding experiments indicate that starch is not significantly cariogenic.

Value of laboratory tests for control of dental disease

The broader title of "dental disease" not just "dental caries" is deliberate, because careful oral hygiene procedures affect not only caries but also periodontal disease. The foregoing discussion suggests that none of the currently used caries activity tests has been shown to satisfactorily predict caries activity. However, this does not mean that such tests have no place in private practice. It has been suggested that the bacteriological tests are a measure of "oral pollution" analogous to an *Escherichia coli* count used by health officers in determining pollution of the water supply.[19] They can and are being used as part of a preventive dentistry program. For example, in one office a modified Snyder test is performed on the first visit. During the second and third visits the patient is instructed in oral hygiene and dietary control. During the fourth visit (3 weeks later), the modified Snyder test is repeated. Most patients show a negative or improved test. This is in contrast to observations on the general population where only about 15% have a negative Snyder test[44] (Table 8-9).

Table 8-9 Results of the Snyder test on 400 salivary samples*

Time (hr)	Result†	Distribution of samples
24	+	20
48	+	40
72	+	25
72	−	15

*From Sims.[44]
†(+) Yellow; color change; (−) green; no change.

The pressing need for triage (selection) in the delivery of preventive dentistry regimens to those patients who are most in need of such intervention is well recognized. Although caries prevalence has been falling in the last decade in the United States and elsewhere,[16,33,51] a pronounced variation in caries activity remains. For example, in a large-scale study to determine costs and effectiveness of combinations of school-based preventive procedures involving approximately 25,000 children, about 20% of the children required about 60% of the caries treatment.[6] Similarly, 20% of Danish children used 50% of dental treatment services,[3] and in a survey in Sweden, 20% of school children were found to be highly infected with *S mutans* and therefore at high risk.[50]

If this high-need population could be identified early, before the development of carious lesions, the cost-efficacy ratio of preventive treatment would be most favorable because it could be directed to those children at greatest risk.

Currently available screening methods based on *S mutans* are very good in identifying populations with low caries increments, but they are less satisfactory in identifying caries-active persons because some who have positive scores develop little caries.[35] Assessing the risk of caries in clinical practice may not be possible by any single test but may instead require repeated samplings and integration of information from a variety of sources, including laboratory tests, clinical examination, and the patient history. For example, when nine factors were assessed—namely sex, race, past caries experience (DMFS and defs scores), number of permanent teeth, indices of fissure retentiveness and occlusal morphology, and levels of *S mutans* and lactobacilli—few of these factors showed any statistically significant difference between children with high versus those with low caries increments.[2] *S mutans* scores, past caries experience, and fissure retentiveness scores were related to high caries increments, but individually they were not reliable predictors. When these same factors were combined in a multiple discriminant model for statistical analysis, using commercially available computer software, prediction performance to identify the children with the greatest caries risk greatly improved.

Other measurements, such as lactobacillus counts, salivary buffer capacity, and toothbrushing frequency, were also not reliable individually for predicting caries risk.[19] However, when several variables were combined mathematically, namely social class, toothbrushing frequency, lactobacillus count, and plaque index (all of which can be recorded by a paraprofessional), the predictability for a high-risk population was correct 50% of the time. Nevertheless, past caries experience in this same population was an even better predictor (correct 60% of the time).[25] By combining past caries experience with these other factors, relatively good predictions should be attainable.

Chapter review

- List the requirements for an "ideal" caries activity test.

- List some of the caries activity tests; indicate what they measure and their limitations.
- State the value of a caries activity test in clinical practice.
- Indicate how accurate these tests are for predicting future caries for an individual patient.
- List the circumstances that could account for high salivary *Lactobacillus* counts.

Selected readings

Bibby, B.G., and Shern, R.J. (eds) 1978. *Methods of Caries Prediction.* Sp. Suppl. Microbiol. Abstr. Washington, D.C.: Information Retrieval, Inc.

Ellen, R.P. 1976. Microbiological assays for dental caries and periodontal disease susceptibility. *Oral Sci Rev* 8:3–23.

Krasse, B. 1985. *Caries Risk.* Chicago: Quintessence Publ Co.

Krasse, B., and Carlos, J.P. (eds) 1986. Microbiologic diagnosis in dental caries and periodontal disease. *Oral Microbiol Immunol* 1:1–91.

Krasse, B., and Newbrun, E. 1982. Objective methods for evaluating caries activity and their application. In *Pediatric Dentistry,* R.E. Stewart, T.K. Barber, K.C. Troutman, and S.H.Y. Wei (eds), St. Louis: C.V. Mosby, pp. 610–616.

Socransky, S. 1968. Caries susceptibility tests. *Ann NY Acad Sci* 153:137–146.

Stolpe, J.R. 1970. Chemical and bacteriological tests for determining susceptibility to, and activity of dental caries: a review. *J Public Health Dent* 30:141–155.

References

1. Alban, A. 1970. An improved Snyder test. *J Dent Res* 49:641.
2. Bader, J.D., Graves, R.C., Disney, J.A., Bohannan, H.M., Stamm, J.W., Abernathy, J.R., and Lindahl, R.L. 1986. Identifying children who will experience high caries increments. *Community Dent Oral Epidemiol* 14:129–201.
3. Bay, I., and Ainamo, J. 1974. Caries experience among children in Copenhagen. *Community Dent Oral Epidemiol* 2:75–79.
4. Birkhed, D., Edwardsson, S., and Andersson, H. 1981. Comparison among a dip-slide test (Dentocult), plate count, and Snyder test for estimating number of lactobacilli in human saliva. *J Dent Res* 60:1832–1841.
5. Birkeland, J.M., Broch, L., and Jorkjend, L. 1976. Caries experience as a predictor for caries incidence. *Community Dent Oral Epidemiol.* 4:66–69.
6. Bohannan, H. 1982. Personal communication.
7. Bratthall, D. 1972. Demonstration of *Streptococcus mutans* strains in some selected areas of the world. *Odontol Revy* 23:401–410.
8. Bratthall, D., and Jensen, B. 1988. Strip mutans for determination of *Strep mutans. J Dent Res* 67 (Sp. Issue Abstr. 73):122.
9. Burnett, F., Scherp, H., and Schuster, G.S. 1976. *Oral Microbiology and Infectious Disease.* 4th ed. Baltimore: Williams & Wilkins, pp. 304–309.
10. Carlos, J.P. (ed) 1974. *Prevention and Oral Health.* DHEW Publication No. (NIH) 74-707. Washington, D.C.: U.S. Government Printing Office; Prev. Med. 1:36–37.
11. Carlsson, J. 1967. A medium for isolation of *Streptococcus mutans. Arch Oral Biol* 12:1657–1658.
12. Crossner, C.G. 1981. Salivary lactobacillus counts in the prediction of caries activity.

Community Dent Oral Epidemiol 9:182–190.
13. Finn, S. 1973. Caries susceptibility tests. In *Clinical Pedodontics*, 4th ed, Philadelphia: W.B. Saunders, pp. 530–534.
14. Fitzgerald, R.J., and Keyes, P.H. 1960. Demonstration of the etiological role of streptococci in experimental caries in the hamster. *J Am Dent Assoc* 61:9–19.
15. Gilmour, M.N., and Zahn, L. 1974. Intra-subject variability of *Lactobacillus* counts. 52nd General Meeting, International Association for Dental Research, Abstr. 273. *J Dent Res* 52 (Sp. Issue):123.
16. Glass, R.L. 1981. Secular changes in caries prevalence in two Massachusetts towns. *Caries Res* 15:445–450.
17. Grainger, R.M., Jarrett, T.M., and Honey, F.S.L. 1965. Swab test for dental caries activity. An epidemiological survey. *J Can Dent Assoc* 31:515–526.
18. Hoerman, K.C., Keene, H.J., Shklair, I.L., and Burmeister, J.A. 1972. The association of *Streptococcus mutans* with early carious lesions in human teeth. *J Am Dent Assoc* 85:1349–1352.
19. Honkala, E., Nyyssönen, V., Kolmakow, S., and Lammi, S. 1984. Factors predicting caries risk in children. *Scand J Dent Res* 92:134–140.
20. Howell, F.V., and Abrams, A.M. 1966. The scope and rationale of laboratory procedures in dental practice. *J South Cal St Dent Assoc* 34:539–545.
21. Jordan, H.V., Laraway, R., Snirch, R., and Marmel, M. 1987. A simplified diagnostic system for cultural detection and enumeration of *Streptococcus mutans*. *J Dent Res* 66: 57–61.
22. Kelstrup, J., Theilade, J., Poulsen, S., and Møller, I.J. 1974. Bacteriological, electron microscopical and biochemical studies on dento-gingival plaque of Moroccan children from an area of low caries prevalence. *Caries Res* 8:61–83.
23. Kingman, A. 1979. A method of utilizing the subjects' initial caries experience to increase efficiency in caries clinical trials. *Community Dent Oral Epidemiol* 7:87–90.
24. Koch, G. 1970. Selection and caries prophylaxis of children with high caries activity. *Odontol Revy* 21:71–82.
25. Kolehmainen, L., Heinonen, O.P., and Haapakoski, J. 1985. Caries prediction and its evaluation in 13- to 15-year-old schoolchildren. *Community Dent Health* 2:15–21.
26. Köhler, B., and Bratthall, D. 1979. Practical method to facilitate estimation of *Streptococcus mutans* levels in saliva. *J Clin Microbiol* 9:584–588.
27. Krasse, B., Jordan, H.V., Edwardsson, S., Svensson, O., and Trell, L. 1968. The occurrence of certain "caries-inducing" streptococci in human dental plaque material. *Arch Oral Biol* 13:911–918.
28. Larmas, M. 1975. A new dip-slide method for the counting of salivary lactobacilli. *Proc Finn Dent Soc* 71:31–35.
29. Littleton, N.W., Kakehashi, S., and Fitzgerald, R.J. 1970. Recovery of specific "caries-inducing" streptococci from carious lesions in teeth of children. *J Dent Res* 49:742–751.
30. Littleton, N.W., Kakehashi, S., and Fitzgerald, R.J. 1970. Study of differences in the occurrence of dental caries in Caucasian and Negro children. *J Dent Res* 49:742–751.
31. Loesche, W.J., Rowan, J., Straffon, L.H., and Loos, P.J. 1975. Association of *Streptococcus mutans* with human dental decay. *Infect Immun* 11:1252–1260.
32. Lynch, M., Crowley, M.C., and Ash, M.S. 1969. Correlation between plaque and bacterial flora. *J Periodontol* 40:634–635.
33. Marthaler, T. 1980. Organisation und Resultate verschiedener Vorbeugungsprogramme in den Schulen. *Schweiz Monatsschr Zahnheilkd* 90:773–784.
34. Matsukubo, T., Ohta, K., Maki, Y., Takeuchi, M., and Takazoe, I. 1981. A semi-quantitative determination of *Streptococcus mutans* using its adherent ability in selective medium. *Caries Res* 15:40–45.
35. Newbrun, E., Matsukubo, T., Hoover, C.I., Graves, R.C., Brown, A.T., Disney, J.A., and Bohannan, H.M. 1984. Comparison of two screening tests for *Streptococcus mutans* and evaluation of their suitability for mass screenings in private practice. *Community Dent Oral Epidemiol* 12:325–331.
36. Poulsen, S., and Horowitz, H.S. 1974. An evaluation of a hierarchical method of describing the pattern of dental caries attack. *Community Dent Oral Epidemiol* 2:7–11.
37. Rapp, G.W. 1962. Fifteen minute caries test. *Ill Dent J* 31:290–295.
38. Rosen, S., and Weinstein, P.R. 1963. Interrelationships among salivary reductase activity of certain oral bacteria and caries in man. *J Am Dent Assoc* 67:876–878.
39. Rosenberg, M., Weis, E., and Eli, I. 1988. A novel replicate technique for localization of caries-associated bacteria on tooth surfaces: development and initial experience. *Caries* 22:42–44.

40. Schamschula, R.G., and Barmes, D.E. 1970. A study of the streptococcal flora of plaque in caries free and caries active primitive peoples. *Aust Dent J* 5:377–382.
41. Shannon, I.L., Gibson, W.A., and Chauncey, H.H. 1964. Reductase activity of human whole saliva as related to dental caries experience. Tech. Document Report, SAM-TDR-64-22, USAF School of Aerospace Medicine.
42. Shklair, I.L., Keene, H.J., and Simonson, L.S. 1972. Distribution and frequency of *Streptococcus mutans* in caries-active individuals. *J Dent Res* 51:882.
43. Shory, N.L. 1966. Comprehensive field evaluation of the Treatex test. *J Am Med Assoc* 72:899–903.
44. Sims, W. 1968. A modified Snyder test for caries activity in humans. *Arch Oral Biol* 13:853–856.
45. Sims, W. 1970. The interpretation and use of Snyder tests and *Lactobacillus* count. *J Am Dent Assoc* 80:1315–1319.
46. Snyder, N.L. 1951. Laboratory methods in the clinical evaluation of caries activity. *J Am Dent Assoc* 42:400–413.
47. Socransky, S. 1968. Caries susceptibility tests. *Ann NY Acad Sci* 153:137–146.
48. Stolpe, J.R. 1970. Chemical and bacteriological tests for determining susceptibility to, and activity of dental caries; a review. *J Public Health Dent* 30:141–155.
49. Stoppelaar, J.D., van de Houte, J., and Backer Dirks, O. 1969. The relationship between extracellular polysaccharide-producing streptococci and smooth surface caries in 13-year-old children. *Caries Res* 3:190–199.
50. Togelius, J., and Bratthall, D. 1982. Frequency of the bacterium *Streptococcus mutans* in the saliva of selected human populations. *Arch Oral Biol* 27:113–116.
51. U.S. Department of Health and Human Services 1981. The prevalence of dental caries in United States children. National Dental Caries Prevalence Survey 1979–1980. NIH Publication #82-2245. Washington, D.C.: U.S. Government Printing Office.
52. Woods, R. 1971. A dental caries susceptibility test based on the occurrence of *Strep mutans* in plaque material. *Aust Dent J* 16:116–121.

Chapter 9

Dentifrices

It is necessary to clean the teeth frequently, more especially after meals, but not on any account with a pin, or the point of a pen-knife, and it must never be done at table.

St. John Baptist de la Salle, *The Rules of Christian Manners and Civility,* I. 1695.

At some time or other in his or her professional career every dentist will be confronted with the question: "Doctor, which toothpaste do you recommend?" There is no pat answer to this question because it will very much depend upon the individual patient's needs (eg, high caries susceptibility, erosion, tobacco staining, halitosis, etc). In order to respond adequately to such a question the dentist needs to know what the components of a dentifrice are and what purpose or function each ingredient serves. He or she must be able to evaluate the current literature in this field and not rely on the information provided by commercial advertisements on television and radio.

Functions of a dentifrice

The primary purpose of a dentifrice (Latin: dens = tooth; fricare = to rub) is to clean and polish the accessible surfaces of the teeth when used in conjunction with a toothbrush.[18] A dentifrice should provide maximum cleaning with a minimum of abrasion to the dental tissues. The amount of cleaning power a dentifrice must have to prevent accumulation of stains will depend on several factors, such as the patient's susceptibility to forming stained pellicle, diet, and toothbrushing habits.[5,31]

In addition to this function, recent developments in formulation have attempted to provide a therapeutic benefit as well as a cosmetic one.[38] The cosmetic effectiveness of a dentifrice in cleaning and polishing teeth can readily be assessed by "before" and "after" intraoral photography or reflectometry to measure changes in lustre. Dentifrices will vary in this regard depending on the type of abrasive or organic solvent they contain. Brushing teeth with a cleaning dentifrice removes some of the plaque accumulation, therefore retarding the development of objectionable mouth odors.

Table 9-1 Composition of dentifrices

Component	Concentration (%)
Abrasive	20–50
Humectant	20–40
Water	20–35
Binder	1–2
Detergent	1–3
Flavor	1–2
Preservative	0.05–0.5
Therapeutic	0.4–1.0

Table 9-2 Abrasives arranged in decreasing order

Name	Formula
Zirconium silicate	$ZrSiO_4$
Flour of pumice	
Levigated alumina	Al_2O_3
Calcium carbonate	$CaCO_3$
Dicalcium phosphate anhydrous	$CaHPO_4$
Calcium pyrophosphate	$Ca_2P_2O_7$
Insoluble sodium metaphosphate	$(NaPO_3)_x$
Dicalcium phosphate dihydrate	$CaHPO_4 \cdot 2H_2O$

Composition

Dentifrices have been prepared in several physical forms, such as paste, powder, liquid, and block form. In the United States, the most popular form is the paste. The exact composition of a particular toothpaste varies with each manufacturer; however, a typical formulation is shown in Table 9-1.

Abrasives

By volume the single largest component of a dentifrice is the polishing agent, comprising 20% to 50% of the final product. The abrasion of a surface involves wearing off, whereas polishing implies the placing of successively finer scratches until a smooth clean surface is attained. The two terms are not necessarily synonymous. An abraded surface is not always polished; however, polishing does require some wearing off of the surface.

The abrasion that occurs during the use of any dentifrice polishing agent is a function of:

1. Inherent hardness of the abrasive material

2. Particle size and shape of the milled product
3. Properties of the abrasive slurry (pH, viscosity, heat conductivity)
4. Hardness of the bristles
5. Stress applied during brushing
6. Properties of the abraded surface (eg, enamel versus dentin)

The harder the abrasive, the sharper the particles; the lower the pH of the slurry, the more the wear of the tooth surface. Injudicious toothbrushing with a hard-bristle toothbrush and excessive pressure may cause extreme wear of tooth substance, creating wedge-shaped notches usually near the gingival margin. In extreme cases pulpal pathosis and periapical lesions may result.[36]

The wear of acrylic, like that of enamel and dentin, depends on the factors stated in the previous paragraph and on the type of bristles used in a brush. There are differences in the irregularities created on a test surface by using "hard" and "soft" nylon bristles.[56]

Certain abrasives commonly used in dentifrices or prophylaxis pastes, arranged in decreasing order of abrasive level, are shown in Table 9-2. The most commonly used agents are silica gels, phosphate salts (dicalcium phosphate, insoluble sodium metaphosphate, calcium pyrophosphate), calcium and magnesium carbonate, aluminum oxide, and other silicate compounds. A substantial proportion of the population requires some degree of abrasivity in their dentifrice to prevent stain accumulation. The least abrasive product that will accomplish this is indicated.[43] In patients having exposed cementum or dentin, highly abrasive dentifrices are definitely contraindicated.

It must be kept in mind that other dentifrice ingredients may modify the abrasiveness. It is possible to have toothpastes containing the same polishing agent but with different abrasive levels[50]; the surface active ingredients and the particle size are of importance in this process. The degree of abrasivity of dentifrices has been of considerable concern to the profession and has often been the basis of advertising claims of low abrasion yet efficacy in cleaning.

Abrasiveness can be measured in the laboratory in several ways: *(1)* by changes in tooth thickness or weight, *(2)* by alteration in surface profile or contour, and *(3)* by removal of radioactivity after brushing with the particular dentifrice.[7,12,49,57] A laser light reflection method, using a high intensity, monochromatic parallel laser beam, measures the surface finish after brushing.[41] Although these various methods measure different properties of the abraded surface, a certain correlation exists, so that relative rankings of the abrasivity of dentifrices are quite similar.[42] The radioactivity method is both sensitive and precise and is the technique routinely used by the Council of Dental Therapeutics of the American Dental Association, by consumer groups, and by industry.[8,9,23] The procedure involves the quantitative determination of dentin removed by brushing roots of extracted teeth that have been irradiated by neutron bombardment to make them radioactive. The relative dentinal abrasivity (RDA) is based on the ratio of dentin removed by the test dentifrice

Table 9-3 Abrasivity of dentifrices

Product	Manufacturer	Abrasive ingredient	Relative dentinal abrasivity MAL*	Relative dentinal abrasivity OHRI†
ADA Standard	—	$Ca_2P_2O_7$	100	100
Aim	Chesebrough-Pond's	SiO_2	94	114
Aim Extra Strength	Chesebrough-Pond's	SiO_2	96	—
Aqua-Fresh	Beecham	SiO_2; $CaCO_3$; HO-$CH_2 \cdot CHOH \cdot CH_2OPO_3Ca$	110	115
Check Up (gel)	Rydelle-Lion	SiO_2	62	—
Check Up (paste)	Rydelle-Lion	SiO_2	89	92
Close-Up	Chesebrough-Pond's	SiO_2	83	90
Colgate (gel)	Colgate-Palmolive	$CaHPO_4 \cdot 2H_2O$	86	—
Colgate (MFP)	Colgate-Palmolive	$CaHPO_4 \cdot 2H_2O$	64	75
Colgate Tartar Control	Colgate-Palmolive	$CaHPO_4 \cdot 2H_2O$	94	85
Crest AF	Procter & Gamble	SiO_2	84	103
Crest Tartar Control	Procter & Gamble	SiO_2	109	125
Denquel	Vicks	$CaCO_3$; SiO_2; $MgAl_2(SiO_4)_2 \cdot 2H_2O$	81	—
Dentagard	Colgate-Palmolive	SiO_2	57	—
Dental Care (paste)	Church & Dwight	$NaHCO_3$	55	—
Dental Care (powder)	Church & Dwight	$NaHCO_3$	37	—
Gleem	Procter & Gamble	$Ca_2P_2O_7$	—	148
Macleans	Beecham	$CaCO_3$; $MgAl_2(SiO_4)_2 \cdot 2H_2O$	—	122
Pearl Drops Fluoride	Carter	Al_2O_3; SiO_2; $CaHPO_4 \cdot 2H_2O$	108	128
Pepsodent	Chesebrough-Pond's	Al_2O_3; SiO_2; $CaHPO_4 \cdot 2H_2O$	106	—
Promise	Block	$CaHPO_4$; $CaHPO_4 \cdot 2H_2O$; SiO_2	49	—
Sensodyne	Block	Diatomaceous earth; SiO_2	94	—
Topical Fluoride (paste)	Jeffrey Martin	$(NaPO_3)_x$; $CaHPO_4$; $MgAL_2(SiO_4)_2 \cdot 2H_2O$	84	136
Topol (gel)	Jeffrey Martin	$CaHPO_4$; $MgAl_2(SiO_4)_2 \cdot 2H_2O$	—	187
Topol (paste)	Jeffrey Martin	$CaHPO_4$; $MgAl_2(SiO_4)_2 \cdot 2H_2O$	109	171
Ultra Brite	Colgate-Palmolive	SiO_2	106	—
Viadent	Vipont	$CaHPO_4$	52	—
Zact Fluoride Paste	Rydelle-Lion	$CaHPO_4 \cdot 2H_2O$; $CaHPO_4$	—	174
Zact (gel)	Rydelle-Lion	$CaHPO_4 \cdot 2H_2O$; $CaHPO_4$	—	176
Zact (paste)	Rydelle-Lion	$CaHPO_4 \cdot 2H_2O$; $CaHPO_4$	183	197

*MAL = Missouri Analytical Labs, data from various sources.
†OHRI = Oral Health Research Institute, Indianapolis, Indiana; data courtesy Dr George Stookey.

compared with a reference standard ($Ca_2P_2O_7$). Clearly, there will be some variation (about 10%) in actual numbers due to differences between teeth, as well as slight batch variation in the standard. For this reason, some prefer to classify dentifrices as low, moderate, or high in abrasivity. None of the currently marketed dentifrices in the United States are highly abrasive (Table 9-3). Clinically, the actual abrasion experienced will depend on the dentifrice and the patient's brushing habits (type of brush and force used), the presence of saliva, calculus or pellicle, and the effect of restorations and appliances. All of these characteristics make it impossible to be confident about the meaning of laboratory abrasiveness ratings in human experience.

A serious problem encountered in the development of a therapeutic dentifrice was an interaction between the fluoride ion and the abrasive salt, especially calcium, so that the fluoride ion was no longer available to react with the tooth enamel. Most modern fluoride dentifrices no longer use calcium carbonate (chalk). Usually the proportion of available fluoride gradually decreases during storage. An interesting development in Sweden has been the use of spherical acrylic particles (0.5 μm diameter), which take up very little of the fluoride.[29]

Synthetic silicas (SiO_2), in the form of silica gel or hydrated silica have also been prepared. The particle size is controlled by controlling the conditions under which the silica is precipitated. Silica is now widely used as the abrasive ingredient in many dentifrices. As well as being compatible with fluoride, it has the advantage that it allows the manufacture of clear gel dentifrices by careful matching of the refractive indices of the abrasive humectant systems.[55]

Humectants

Humectants are used in dentifrices to prevent loss of water and subsequent hardening of the paste when it is exposed to air. The most commonly employed humectants are glycerol, sorbitol, and propylene glycol. Sorbitol ($C_6H_{14}O_6$) is a white odorless powder that is freely soluble in alcohol. Glycerol, a liquid, is an extremely effective humectant. It gives a sheen to the prepared paste and is stable even at high temperatures. Propylene glycol ($C_3H_3O_2$) is an odorless, viscous, colorless liquid that is totally miscible in water and in alcohol. It is used as a substitute for glycerol. Glycerol and sorbitol have a sweet taste, whereas propylene glycol has a slightly acrid taste.

Binders

Binders are hydrophilic colloids that stabilize the formulation and prevent separation of the solid and liquid phases during storage. The binders disperse or swell to form a viscous material.

Gum arabic, gum karaya, and gum tragacanth are natural tree exudations that are being used as binders. Seaweed colloids such as the alginates, Irish moss extract, and gum carrageenan have gained popularity and are among the most widely used binders in the United States. Xanthan gum is a cross-linked polysaccharide consisting of glucose, mannose, and glucuronic acid. Water-dispersible derivatives of cellulose, as represented by methyl cellulose and carboxymethyl cellulose, have also been utilized in commercial toothpastes. The latter have become increasingly popular in recent years for economic reasons. Another synthetic water-soluble binder is carbomer-940, which is a cross-linked polymer of acrylic acid and has numerous free carboxylic groups. It also serves as an emulsifying agent.

Surface-active detergents

These are agents that lower the surface tension, penetrate and loosen surface deposits, and emulsify or suspend the debris that the dentifrice removes from the tooth surface. The newer synthetic compounds have largely replaced the natural soaps used in the past. These detergents are soluble in water, will function in acid or alkaline solution, and will not form precipitates in hard water or saliva. There is no evidence to indicate that the detergents alone clinically can remove plaque; an abrasive is required for this purpose. Detergents contribute to the foaming property of the mixture. The foaming action gives a pleasant sensation. Some detergents are listed in Table 9-4. Sodium lauryl sulfate is the most commonly used surface active agent in dentifrices. In addition to its ability to lower surface tension, or possibly because of this effect and perturbation of membrane structure of taste-receptor cells, sodium lauryl sulfate is a taste modifier and can reduce the perceived taste of certain substances.[14] Sodium coconut monoglyceride sulfonate is a mixture of fatty acid esters of monoglyceride sulfonate. The source of the fatty acids is coconut oil.

Sodium *N*-lauroyl sarcosinate is formed through the condensation of a fatty acid (lauric acid) and an amino acid (sarcosine or *N*-methyl glycine):

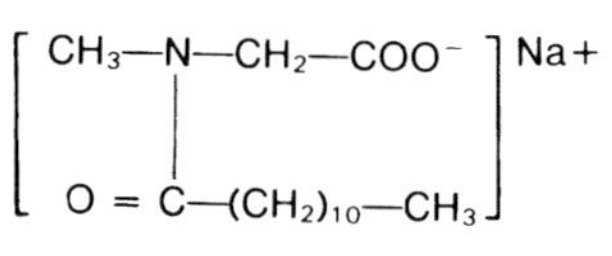

The surface activity resides in the anionic carboxyl group of the amino acid.

Sarcosinate has been claimed to have a therapeutic effect by virtue of its "antibacterial" and "antienzyme" action. Although the anticaries effectiveness of sarcosinate dentifrices has been reported, subsequent investigations have not found any protective effect against dental caries.

Table 9-4 Detergents used in dentifrices

Name	Properties	Formula
Dioctyl sodium sulfosuccinate	White solid, slightly soluble in water	$C_{20}H_{37}NaO_7S$
Sodium alkyl sulfoacetate (sodium lauryl sulfoacetate)	Faint coconut odor	$ROCOCH_2SO_3Na$
Sodium lauryl sulfate	Water-soluble, characteristic slight odor	$CH_3(CH_2)_{10}CH_2OSO_3Na$
Sodium *N*-lauroyl sarcosinate (Colgate Gardol)	White powder, water-soluble	$CH_3(CH_2)_{10}CON(CH_3)$-CH_2COONa
Sodium cocomonoglyceride sulfonate	White, neutral, mild flavor	$RCOOCH_2CH(OH)CH_2SO_3Na$

Brushing with a sarcosinate solution decreases plaque formation[53]; however, for a variety of reasons, including untoward soft tissue responses, sarcosinate is no longer used in dentifrices in the United States. Poloxalene (Pluronic), which consists of chains of hydrophobic polyoxypropylene condensed with hydrophobic polyoxyethylene, has been used in a dentifrice as a nonionic surfactant polymer. Nasadent (Scherer Laboratories), a dentifrice without any detergents in it, was developed by Shannon[48] for use in space flights and does not require expectoration. As an ingestable paste it may find broader application and is currently being tested in the Veterans Administration Hospitals on patients with handicaps such as paraplegia, quadriplegia, oral facial paralysis, and emphysema.

Flavors

Quantitatively, flavoring ingredients constitute only a minor part (1% to 2%) of a dentifrice. Nevertheless the taste of a dentifrice, both the initial impact and the aftertaste, is one of the most important properties as far as public acceptance is concerned. Advertisements suggest that this will give the user a "seductive breath"—but this will last only about as long as it takes to get out of the bathroom. Preparing a dentifrice with a satisfying flavor is more of an art than a science; however, the selected flavor ingredients must be compatible with the other ingredients and must remain unchanged during manufacture, aging, and storage of the paste.

The flavor in a toothpaste usually blends several components. The most common principal flavors used are in the mint spectrum (spearmint, peppermint, spice mint, wintergreen) and may be modified with other essential oils of anise, clove, caraway, pimento, eucalyptus, citrus, menthol, nutmeg, thyme, or cinnamon. Children prefer a tutti-frutti-flavored dentifrice, which uses a combination of fruit flavors.

In addition, most dentifrices contain a synthetic sweetener such as saccharin (0.1% to 0.3%) and formerly contained cyclamate. Chloroform, after a long history of use in dentifrices in countries overseas, was introduced in dentifrices in the United States (eg, Close-Up, ~1%, Macleans, ~3%, Ultrabrite, ~3%). It imparts a type of flavor impact and freshness that is not possible to duplicate with other materials. Excessive ingestion of chloroform can cause hepatotoxicity. However, studies of liver function following long-term daily use of a dentifrice containing 3.4% chloroform and a mouthrinse containing 0.43% chloroform indicate the safety of these concentrations.[46] In 1976 the Food and Drug Administration (FDA) banned the use of chloroform in foods, drugs, and cosmetics because of evidence indicating chloroform might cause cancer. Dentifrice manufacturers have voluntarily discontinued the use of this ingredient. Chloroform and certain aromatic oils (eg, eugenol) have the capacity to dissolve polymethyl methacrylate and/or release internal stresses, thereby causing crazing or increased abrasion.

Preservatives

Most dentifrice humectants and certain of the organic binders are susceptible to attack by microorganisms or molds. Therefore preservatives such as dichlorophene, benzoates, *p*-hydroxybenzoates, formaldehyde, or paraben (methyl, ethyl, propyl, butyl) are included at a level of 0.05% to 0.5%.

Other ingredients

Many dentifrices include a coloring agent to make the product more attractive to the consumer. Coloring agents used include FD&C blue #1, FD&C green #3, FD&C red #3 (erythrosine), FD&C yellow #5 (tartrazine), FD&C yellow #20, FD&C red #33, and FD&C red #37. Titanium dioxide, an insoluble white powder, is also widely used to give dentifrices a white color. A small amount of titanium dioxide is frequently used to convert gels to pastes.

Packaging

Shelf life

Problems of drying can be overcome by using a humectant. Separation of ingredients during storage is prevented by including various stabilizers and binders. Spoilage by bacterial contamination can be avoided by using preservatives.

Toothpaste tubes

The pH of dentifrices may range from mildly acidic to alkaline. Pastes with neutral pH are packaged in aluminum tubes. However, acidic pastes (eg, containing stannous fluoride) or pastes containing insoluble sodium metaphosphate, an aluminum sequestrant, must be packaged in tubes lined with a chemically inert compound to prevent interaction with the aluminum tube. Use of plastic containers avoids the problem of lead contamination from tubes.[6]

Toothpaste pumps

Pumps have become popular toothpaste containers. Two types of design are employed. One uses the "pole-climber" principle with an internal piston climbing a central rod after each use. The other type uses vacuum pressure to pump out paste. It has been suggested that pumps can add to domestic tranquility by avoiding family fights over the proper way to squeeze and roll up the toothpaste tube.[9]

Ingestion

Ingestion of dentifrice during toothbrushing may be measured either by the use of a marker that is recovered from urine and feces and subsequently analyzed,[3] or by measuring the amount of toothpaste that enters the mouth and subtracting the amount subsequently recovered.[21] Either method has disadvantages and is subject to error. The average amount of dentifrice used by adults and most children in a single brushing is about 1 g and does not vary appreciably with age, though mothers of infants under 3 years of age tend to dispense less toothpaste on their children's brushes, about 0.5 g.[15] However, the amount *ingested* varies considerably with age: children swallow more dentifrice than adults. In one study, children 2 to 4 years of age swallowed about one third of the dentifrice (0.3 g), and children 11 to 13 years of age swallowed only 0.07 g.[3] In another study the youngest children, 5 to 6 years of age, also ingested the highest amount of dentifrice (0.27 g), whereas older children 7 to 16 years of age usually ingested about 0.19 g or about 20% of the dentifrice.[4] Preschool children vary in their ability to expectorate toothpaste; however, those who can expectorate tend to do so consistently. Rinsing with water after brushing reduces the amount of dentifrice that is swallowed.[4] Adults swallow very little dentifrice.

Calcium phosphate and carbonate polishing agents prevent a considerable fraction of the fluoride content of dentifrices from being absorbed.[11]

Contact sensitivity and irritation due to dentifrice ingredients

Hypersensitivity to toothpaste is uncommon. Occasionally, the flavoring and coloring agents employed in dentifrices may give rise to allergic reactions in some patients. These may include desquamation and edema of lips and tongue, perioral dermatitis, angular cheilitis, gingivitis, and intraoral ulceration.[28] Cinnamon oil (approximately 80% cinnamic aldehyde) in a commercial toothpaste can cause acute allergic gingivostomatitis.[16,30,37] Perioral leukoderma manifesting as porcelain white depigmentation of the skin just lateral to the oral commissures and adjacent to the vermillion borders of the lips has also been associated with the use of toothpaste containing cinnamic aldehyde.[35] Such patients may experience mild irritation while using the toothpaste, which usually disappears a few minutes after ceasing to brush. Other dentifrice flavoring agents that have been reported to be allergenic include menthol, eugenol, and oil of peppermint. Flavoring agents in cosmetics and chewing gums may cause similar stomatitis.[26,27] A thorough history of the patient may suggest the causative agent, which must then be confirmed by patch testing.

In addition to individual hypersensitivity, which is relatively rare, certain dentifrice ingredients are capable of irritating the oral mucosa in the general population. Clinically these dentifrices cause erythema at the test site. Histologically, epithelial changes ranging from a parakeratinlike surface layer to necrosis and intraepithelial abscess formation have been observed.[2] Local irritation may result from chloroform, sodium *N*-lauroyl sarcosinate, sodium lauryl sulfate,[44] or from the essential oil ingredients.

Persons with lesions of the mucous membranes induced by therapeutic irradiation or vesiculoerosive disease often find commercial dentifrices irritating to the tissues. A bland dentifrice containing half the customary flavoring agents is more acceptable to such patients.[20] Conversely, people with healthy oral mucous membranes generally prefer the more flavored dentifrices and find that a bland dentifrice lacks the tingling sensation and does not make the mouth feel fresh and clean.

Therapeutic dentifrices

Dentifrices for which therapeutic effects are claimed are subject to the drug testing provisions of the 1962 Kefauver-Harris amendment to the Federal Food, Drug and Cosmetic Act. Evidence of both safety and effectiveness must be demonstrated. Manufacturers of therapeutic dentifrices are also required to submit preliminary animal safety data and test protocols for FDA approval prior to extensive testing in humans. After marketing, manufacturers are required by law to forward all adverse reaction reports to the FDA.

Ammonia and urea

Acid formation by cariogenic microorganisms has long been recognized. It was hypothesized that dentifrices containing ammonia and/or urea might neutralize such acids. Many commercial dentifrices containing dibasic ammonium phosphate and urea were made available to the public as a result of initial promising reports regarding the anticaries effectiveness of these additives. The dentifrices were marketed as "ammoniated" dentifrices. The Council on Dental Therapeutics[10] classified such dentifrices in group C because the evidence for the usefulness of these products in the hands of the general public was either so limited or inconclusive or so contradictory that the dentifrices could not be accurately evaluated.[54]

At one time Block Drug Company marketed a product called "Super Amm-i-dent," which contained fluoride, urea, and detergent:

Concentration (%)	*Ingredient*	*Claimed mode of action*
0.2	NaF	Improving crystal surface
13.0	Urea	Antacid
1.7	Sodium *N*-lauroyl sarcosinate	Antienzyme

The manufacture of this product has been discontinued.

Chlorophyll

Chlorophyll, the major chromogen of green plants, contains modified pyrrole nuclei and is classified as a porphyrin. By chemical modification of the chlorophyll molecule, it can be made water-soluble and the central magnesium atom can be replaced by other metallic ions. Dentifrices containing chemically modified chlorophylls have been marketed. There is no evidence based on clinical trials that such dentifrices are effective in reducing tooth decay. In only one of four different clinical trials did the chlorophyll dentifrices reduce gingivitis. Chlorophyll dentifrices are no longer listed in *Accepted Dental Therapeutics*.[1] Chloresium, "the therapeutic chlorophyll toothpaste" (Ryston) is still sold.

Antibiotic and chemotherapeutic agents

Penicillin was included in dentifrices on a trial basis. Results in caries reduction have been conflicting. Furthermore, there are some inherent problems in its use:

1. Sensitization—the tendency to induce allergic reactions following prolonged topical use
2. Development of penicillin-resistant strains
3. Overgrowth of unwanted microorganisms (eg, *Candida albicans*)

Because of these concerns penicillin dentifrices have not been further tested.[40]

A reduction in caries with a tyrothricin dentifrice has been reported. Certain other antibiotics (bacitracin, erythromycin, lincomycin, spiramycin, virgimycin, streptomycin, tetracycline, and vancomycin) can reduce the bacterial population associated with caries activity in experimental animals.

Chlorhexidine has been incorporated into test dentifrices and applied to the teeth by splints to avoid the effect of toothbrushing.[19] It has been shown that these test dentifrices reduced plaque formation.[22]

The antibacterial activity of oxygenating agents is well known, and several of them are currently used in commercial mouthwashes. A toothpaste containing 3.5% hydrogen peroxide has been reported to reduce plaque formation and selectively repress the plaque flora, particularly the anaerobic fusobacteria.[45]

However, the efficacy of dentifrices containing chemotherapeutic agents in caries reduction in humans has not been adequately tested.

Fluorides

Certain fluoride-containing dentifrices have been classified by the Council on Dental Therapeutics of the ADA as therapeutic agents that provide limited protection against the development of dental caries. Commercially available fluoride dentifrices contain either sodium fluoride, stannous fluoride, sodium monofluorophosphate (MFP), or organic amine hydrofluoride. Fluoride dentifrices are discussed in Chapter 11 and reviewed in detail elsewhere.[25]

Other claims

In addition to claims of anticaries activity, dentifrices are being promoted to the public and the profession for relieving hypersensitivity of teeth, for removing calculus or retarding its formation, for removing stains, for controlling mouth odors, and even for improving sex appeal. Apparently dentifrice manufacturers have been quite successful in their advertising, because annual sales in the United States approximate $1 billion. Fluoride-containing dentifrices account for about 95% of this market. Some dentifrices are bought for reasons other than protection against decay, such as cosmetic appeal, enhanced whitening, preferred flavor, package, reduced tartar formation, and relief of sensitive dentin.

Desensitizing dentifrices

Many agents have been used to treat dentinal sensitivity, including formaldehyde, potassium nitrate, silver nitrate, zinc chloride, sodium citrate, sodium fluoride, sodium silicofluoride, strontium chloride, liquefied phenol, benzyl alcohol, hot mineral oil, and glycerin. Although a plethora of active ingredients and treatment procedures have been suggested as effective means to treat this persistent problem, which affects about 15% of patients visiting private dental offices, no treatment appears to eliminate the problem completely for all patients.[8]

Sensodyne (Block Drug Company), a dentifrice containing 10% strontium chloride as the active ingredient, is claimed to relieve hypersensitivity by "biocolloidal binding and blocking actions believed to interrupt transmission of stimuli." Sensodyne contains no carbonate, phosphate, calcium, or magnesium so that the strontium ions remain available. Other ingredients include glycerin (12%), sorbitol (12%), diatomaceous earth (15%), water (43.3%), and miscellaneous agents (8%). Based on studies using quantitatively controlled stimuli, the Council on Dental Therapeutics has recognized the usefulness and safety of this dentifrice for the relief of pain and discomfort from dentinal sensitivity.[12] Thermodent (Mentholatum Co, Inc) also contains 10% strontium chloride hexahydrate as the active ingredient. Protect (International Pharmaceutical Corporation) is a dentifrice advertised as protecting sensitive teeth against stimuli such as cold and touch. It contains sodium citrate in a surfactant gel of poloxalene. This formulation has been reported to be highly effective in controlling dental sensitivity when compared with other dentifrices containing strontium chloride or stannous fluoride.[59] Denquel (Vicks Toiletry Products) is marketed for the protection of sensitive teeth and has been found acceptable as a desensitizing dentifrice by the Council on Dental Therapeutics.[11] The active ingredient is 5% potassium nitrate. Promise (Block Drug Company) also contains 5% potassium nitrate and has been accepted by the Council on Dental Therapeutics. Potassium ions may act to relieve pain by depolarizing nerve fiber membranes to reduce pulpal sensory nerve activity.

To assess the efficacy of any agent or procedure, an objective clinical means of measuring altered dentinal sensitivity is desirable. Many of the earlier investigations relied on subjective evaluation by patients, but unfortunately such studies had little scientific basis and belong to the realm of testimonials. More recently, clinical studies have been using devices whereby the stimulus (electrical or thermal) can be closely controlled and measured.[51,52] Nevertheless, the individual patient's pain threshold is still used as the endpoint and is therefore variable depending on cultural, psychological, and other factors. A further complication in attempting to evaluate desensitizing agents is that placebo treatments produce almost half as much improvement in desensitization as the active ingredients. Changes of such magnitude in the baseline response to placebo agents create statistical problems in evaluating the active agent. The most widely accepted mechanism to explain dentinal sensitivity is based on the hydrodynamic theory, which states that movement of tubule contents or tubule fluid, in either direction, causes the sensitivity. A corollary of that theory is that anything that can decrease dentinal fluid movement or dentinal permeability should decrease dentinal sensitivity. A variety of physicochemical mechanisms can reduce permeability and sensitivity of exposed dentin. These include the growth of intratubular crystals derived from minerals in salivary or dentinal fluid, adsorption of plasma proteins to the inner surface of dentinal tubules, or formation of a smear layer on the exposed dentin surface.[39] All of these procedures result in partial occlusion of the tubule.

Anticalculus dentifrices

Several toothpastes that have been shown to reduce the formation of supragingival calculus are commercially available. The active ingredient in two such products (Colgate Tartar Control, Colgate-Palmolive Co; Crest Tartar Control, Procter & Gamble Co) is 3.3% pyrophosphate. One formulation uses a combination of tetrasodium pyrophosphate and disodium pyrophosphate, while the other one uses a combination of tetrasodium and tetrapotassium pyrophosphate; the reason for such formulations is to maintain the solubility of the pyrophosphate salt. Other products (Prevent Antitartar, Johnson & Johnson Dental Products; Aim Antitartar and Close-Up Tartar Control, Chesebrough-Pond's Inc) use zinc chloride or zinc citrate as the active agent. Both pyrophosphate and zinc ion interfere with calcium binding, thereby inhibiting crystal growth and mineralization. Using such dentifrices once or twice a day reduces accumulation of supragingival calculus on the lingual surfaces of mandibular incisor teeth by 30% to 50%.[31-33,47,58] These products have not been shown to prevent the accumulation of subgingival calculus, and thus their benefits are primarily cosmetic. Since several of these dentifrices contain fluoride, they have been accepted by the Council on Dental Therapeutics as effective in reducing caries, but not periodontal disease.

Antiplaque claims

Several manufacturers of dentifrices have made specific claims that their products fight or reduce plaque formation. There is no doubt that any dentifrice containing some abrasive ingredient, when used on a toothbrush, will reduce plaque, more effectively than the toothbrush and water alone. Accordingly, such a claim for reducing plaque could be made for every dentifrice; however, the effectiveness and extent of plaque removal depend more on the time taken and techniques used in brushing and on the devices used (eg, dental floss, interproximal brushes, toothpicks) than on the particular brand of dentifrice that is employed (see discussion on mechanical removal of plaque, chapter 6).

Organic and cosmetic dentifrices

For those who prefer products with "natural" or "organic" ingredients there is Barth's Natural Toothpaste (Barth Vitamin Corporation), Weleda Pink Toothpaste, and New Concept Organic Dentifrice (Shaklee Marketing Corporation). Barth's contains papain, calcium carbonate, "natural" oil of peppermint, and a binder that is extracted from pure

Table 9-5 Dentifrice claims

Prevents caries	Retards calculus	Desensitizes dentin	Whitens teeth	Treats gum disease	Fights plaque
Aim*	Aim AT	Denquel*	Caroid	Chloresium	Aim
Aqua-Fresh*	Colgate TC	Promise*	Close-Up	Dentagard	Aqua-Fresh
Close-Up	Close-Up TC	Protect*	Kolynos	Dental Care	Check Up
Colgate MFP*	Crest TC	Sensodyne*	Listerine	Shane	Colgate
Colgate TC*	Prevent AT	Thermodent	Peak		Crest
Crest*	Pycopay		Pearl Drops		Dentagard
Crest TC			Pepsodent		Peak
Dentagard*			Topol		Viadent
Elmex			Ultra Brite		
Gleem					
Macleans*					
Promise*					
Sensodyne F*					
Ultra Brite					
Zact*					

*Accepted by ADA Council on Dental Therapeutics for this therapeutic effect.

"natural" seaweed. Weleda uses no detergent but is claimed to have a gentle astringent action due to its content of plant extracts: myrrh, rhatany root, clove, and sage.

Leading the sales of "cosmetic" dentifrices is Pepsodent (Chesebrough-Pond's, Inc), followed by Pearl Drops Tooth Polish (Carter). The exact composition of many dentifrices is not disclosed by the manufacturers. The various claims made for some of the major-brand products are summarized in Table 9-5.

Cost of dentifrices

A great variety of dentifrices are marketed, including both American and foreign-made brands. Some generalizations concerning costs are as follows:

1. Supermarket and chain drugstore brands are cheapest.
2. Fluoride-containing dentifrices are no more expensive than those without fluoride and often may be cheaper.
3. Imported brands and special products (eg, desensitizing and "smokers" pastes) are the most expensive.
4. The larger the tube, the cheaper the dentifrice, on a cost per unit weight basis.

Table 9-6 Comparison of cost of dentifrices*

Brand	Cost (cents/oz)			
	Supermarket		Pharmacy	
	Tube	Pump	Tube	Pump
Aim	30	40	49	—
Aim Antitartar	29	—	47	62
Aim Extra Strength	30	—	—	—
Aqua-Fresh	27	34	—	—
Aqua-Fresh Triple	—	—	45	62
Aqua-Fresh Kids	—	—	52	57
Binaca	—	—	113	—
Check Up	—	53	—	67
Close-Up	23	—	49	—
Close-Up Tartar Control	—	—	47	62
Colgate MFP	40	—	44	64
Colgate Tartar Control	27	42	—	67
Craig Martin	—	—	29	—
Crest	27	34	46	58
Crest Kids	23	—	—	—
Crest Tartar Control	27	34	46	—
Denquel	77	—	102	—
Dentagard	28	42	—	65
Gleem	26	—	44	—
Macleans	—	—	46	—
Oral B Muppets	—	51	—	—
Pearl Drops	—	96	—	132
Pepsodent	23	40	49	—
Promise	—	—	102	—
Protect	—	—	99	—
Pyco-Pay (powder)	—	—	52	—
Sensodyne	82	—	107	—
Thermodent	—	—	84	—
Tom's Natural	60	—	—	—
Topol Smokers	120	—	85	—
Ultrabrite	25	30	47	—
Vademecum	—	—	57	—
Viadent	—	—	85	—
Zact Smokers (paste)	96	—	115	—
Zact Smokers (gel)	107	—	133	—

*Survey conducted in San Francisco Bay Area, November 1987. Cost per ounce based on purchase of largest available tube in store.

5. Cooperatives and supermarkets are slightly cheaper than pharmacies.
6. Dentifrices sold in tubes are cheaper than in pumps.

Because of the recognized caries-reducing effect of fluoride dentifrices and the fact that they are no more expensive than other dentifrices (Table 9-6), patients in a caries-susceptible age group would be well advised to use dentifrices containing fluoride.

Chapter review

- List the components of a dentifrice and indicate the functions of each component.
- List the factors that influence how much abrasion occurs during toothbrushing.
- State how the abrasiveness of a dentifrice can be measured.
- Group dentifrices according to their commercial claims.
- Specify what problems arise in formulating fluoride dentifrices and how they can be overcome.
- List ingredients in dentifrices that are potentially allergenic and state how this can be confirmed.
- State how one can measure the amount of a dentifrice ingested during toothbrushing.
- Indicate how habitual dentifrice ingestion could be of clinical significance.

Selected readings

Accepted Dental Therapeutics. 1984. Dentifrices. 40th ed. Chicago: American Dental Association, pp. 421–428.

Baker, K.A., and Helling, D.K. 1986. Oral Health Products. In *Handbook of Non-Prescription Drugs,* 8th ed, Washington, D.C.: American Pharmaceutical Association, pp. 477–505.

Gershon, S.D., and Pader, M. 1972. Dentifrices. In *Cosmetics: Science and Technology,* vol. 1, M.S. Balsam and E. Sagarin (eds), New York: Wylie-Interscience Publishers, Inc, pp. 243–531.

Heifetz, S.B., and Horowitz, H.S. 1986. Fluoride dentifrices. In *Fluorides and Dental Caries,* 3rd ed, E. Newbrun (ed), Springfield, Ill.: Charles C Thomas, pp. 50–70.

Pader, M. 1971. Dentifrices. Problems of growth. *Drug Cosmet Ind* 109:36–103.

Pader, M. 1988. Oral Hygiene Products and Practice. *Cosmetic Science and Technology Series,* vol. 6, New York: Marcel Dekker.

United States Department of Health and Human Services. 1982. Over-the-Counter Oral Health Care and Discomfort Drugs. *Federal Register* 47:22710–22930.

Volpe, A.R. 1982. Dentifrices and mouthwashes. In *A Textbook of Preventive Dentistry,* 2nd ed, R.E. Stallard (ed), Philadelphia: W.B. Saunders, pp. 170–216.

References

1. American Dental Association. *Accepted Dental Therapeutics.* 1984. Dentifrices. 40th ed. Chicago: American Dental Association, pp. 421–428.
2. Allen, A.L., Hawley, C.E., Cutright, D.E., and Seibert, J.S. 1975. An investigation of the clinical and histologic effects of selected dentifrices on human palatal mucosa. *J Periodontol* 46:102–112.
3. Barnhart, W.E., Hiller, L.K., Leonard, J.G., and Michaels, S.D. 1974. Dentifrice usage and ingestion among four age groups. *J Dent Res* 53:1317–1322.

4. Baxter, P.M. 1980. Toothpaste ingestion during toothbrushing by schoolchildren. *Br Dent J* 148:125–128.
5. Baxter, P.M., Davis, W.B., and Jackson, J. 1981. Toothpaste abrasive requirements to control naturally stained pellicle. *J Oral Rehabil* 8:19–26.
6. Berman, E., and McKiel, K. 1972. Is that toothpaste safe? *Arch Environ Health* 25:64–65.
7. Bull, W.H., Callender, R.M., Pugh, B.R., and Wood, G.D. 1968. The abrasion and cleaning properties of dentifrices. *Br Dent J* 125:331–337.
8. Clark, D.C., Al-Joburi, W., and Chan, E.C.S. 1987. The efficacy of a new dentifrice in treating dentin sensitivity: effects of sodium citrate and sodium fluoride as active ingredients. *J Periodont Res* 22:89–93.
9. Consumers Union. 1986. Toothpastes. *Consumer Reports* 51:144–149.
10. Council on Dental Therapeutics. 1970. Abrasivity of current dentifrices. *J Am Dent Assoc* 81:1177–1178.
11. Council on Dental Therapeutics. 1981. List of accepted products. *J Am Dent Assoc* 103:827.
12. Council on Dental Therapeutics. 1985. Acceptance of Sensodyne toothpaste for sensitive teeth. *J Am Dent Assoc* 110:394–395.
13. Davis, W.B., and Winter, P.J. 1976. Measurement in vitro of enamel abrasion by dentifrice. *J Dent Res* 55:970–975.
14. DeSimone, J.A., and Heck, G.L. 1980. Surface active taste modifiers: a comparison of the physical and psycophysical properties of gymnemic acid and sodium lauryl sulfate. *Chem Senses* 5:317–330.
15. Dowel, T.B. 1981. The use of toothpaste in infancy. *Br Dent J* 150:247–249.
16. Drake, T.E., and Maibach, H.I. 1976. Allergic contact dermatitis and stomatitis caused by cinnamic aldehyde-flavored toothpaste. *Arch Dermatol* 112:202–203.
17. Forsman, B., and Ericsson, Y. 1973. Fluoride absorption from swallowed fluoride toothpaste. *Community Dent Oral Epidemiol* 1:115–120.
18. Gershon, S.D., and Pader, M. 1972. Dentifrices. In *Cosmetics: Science and Technology*, vol. 1, M.S. Balsam and E. Sagarin (eds), New York: Wylie-Interscience Publishers, Inc, pp. 243–531.
19. Gjermo, P., and Rolla, G. 1970. Plaque inhibition by antibacterial dentifrices. *Scand J Dent Res* 78:464–470.
20. Greenspan, D., and Silverman, S. 1979. Study of a bland dentifrice for persons with radiation-induced mucositis and vesiculo-erosive disease. *J Am Dent Assoc* 99:203–204.
21. Hargreaves, J.A., Ingram, G.S., and Wagg, B.J. 1972. A gravimetric study of the ingestion of toothpaste by children. *Caries Res* 6:237–243.
22. Harrap, G.J. 1974. Assessment of the effect of dentifrices on the growth of dental plaque. *J Clin Periodontol* 1:166–174.
23. Hefferren, J.J. 1976. A laboratory method for assessment of dentifrice abrasivity. *J Dent Res* 55:563–573.
24. Hefferren, J.J., Kingman, A., Stookey, G.K., Lehnhoff, R., and Muller, T. 1984. An international collaborative study of laboratory methods for assessing abrasivity of dentin. *J Dent Res* 63:1176–1179.
25. Heifetz, S.B., and Horowitz, H.S. 1986. Fluoride dentifrices. In *Fluorides and Dental Caries*, 3rd ed, E. Newbrun (ed), Springfield, Ill.: Charles C Thomas, pp. 50–70.
26. Kerr, D.A., McClatchey, K.D., and Regezi, J.A. 1971. Allergic gingivostomatitis (due to gum-chewing). *J Periodontol* 42:709–712.
27. Kerr, D.A., McClatchey, K.D., and Regezi, J.A. 1971. Idiopathic gingivostomatitis. *Oral Surg* 32:402–423.
28. Kowitz, G., Lucatorto, M.S., and Bennett, W. 1973. Effects of dentifrices on soft tissues of the oral cavity. *J Oral Med* 28:105–109.
29. Koch, G. 1967. Effect of sodium fluoride in dentifrice and mouthwash on incidence of dental caries in school children. *Odontol Revy* 18:Suppl. 12.
30. Laubach, J.L., Malkinson, F.D., and Ringrose, E.J. 1953. Cheilitis caused by cinnamon (Cassia) oil in toothpaste. *J Am Med Assoc* 152:404–405.
31. Lobene, R.R. 1982. Clinical studies on the cleaning functions of a dentifrice. *J Am Dent Assoc* 105:798–802.
32. Lobene, R.R. 1986. A clinical study of the anticalculus effect of a dentifrice containing soluble pyrophosphate and sodium fluoride. *Clin Prev Dent* 8:5–7.
33. Lobene, R.R., Soparkar, P.M., Newman, M.B., and Kohut, B.E. 1987. Reduced formation of supragingival calculus with the use of fluoride-zinc chloride dentifrice. *J Am Dent Assoc* 114:350–352.
34. Mallatt, M.E., Beiswanger, B.B., Stookey, G.K., Swancar, J.R., and Hennon, D.K. 1985.

Influence of soluble pyrophosphate on calculus formation in adults. *J Dent Res* 64:1159–1162.

35. Mathias, C.G.T., Maibach, H.I., and Conant, M.A. 1980. Perioral leukoderma simulating reitiligo from use of a toothpaste containing cinnamic aldehyde. *Arch Dermatol* 116:1172–1173.
36. Meister, F., Braun, R.J., and Gerstein, H. 1980. Endodontic involvement resulting from dental abrasion or erosion. *J Am Dent Assoc* 101:651–653.
37. Millard, L. 1973. Acute contact sensitivity to a new toothpaste. *J Dent* 1:168–170.
38. Pader, M. 1971. Dentifrices. Problems of growth. *Drug Cosmet Ind* 109:36–103.
39. Pashley, D.H. 1986. Dentin permeability, dentin sensitivity, and treatment through tubule occlusion. *J Endo* 12:465–474.
40. Peterson, J.K. 1968. The current status of therapeutic dentifrices. *Ann NY Acad Sci* 153:334–349.
41. Redmalin, G., and Rydén, H. 1979. Dentifrice abrasivity. The use of laser beams for comparative studies in vitro of surface changes. *Swed Dent J* 3:91–100.
42. Redmalin, G., and Rydén, H. 1984. Dentifrice abrasivity. The use of laser light and supplemental techniques for characterizing toothpastes containing different abrasives. An in vitro study. *Swed Dent J* 8:57–66.
43. Robinson, H.B.G. 1969. Individualizing dentifrices. The dentist's responsibility. *J Am Dent Assoc* 79:633–636.
44. Rubright, W.C., Walker, J.A., Karlsson, U.L., and Diehl, D.L. 1978. Oral slough caused by dentifrice detergents and aggravated by drugs with antisialic activity. *J Am Dent Assoc* 97:215–220.
45. Rundergren, J., Fornell, J., and Ericson, T. 1973. In vivo and in vitro studies on a new peroxide-containing toothpaste. *Scand J Dent Res* 81:543–547.
46. Salva, S. de, Volpe, A., Leigh, G., and Regan, T. 1975. Long-term safety of a chloroform-containing dentifrice and mouth rise in man. *Food Cosmet Toxicol* 13:529–532.
47. Schiff, T.G. 1986. The effect on calculus deposits of a dentifrice containing soluble pyrophosphate and sodium fluoride. *Clin Prev Dent* 8:8–10.
48. Shannon, I.L. 1972. Personal communication.
49. Stookey, G.K., Hudson, J.R., and Muhler, J.C. 1966. Studies concerning the polishing properties of zirconium silicate on enamel. *J Periodontol* 37:200–207.
50. Stookey, G.K., and Muhler, J.C. 1968. Laboratory studies concerning the enamel and dentin abrasion properties of common dentifrice polishing agents. *J Dent Res* 47:524–532.
51. Tarbet, W.J., Silverman, G., Stolman, J., and Fratarcangelo, P.A. 1979. An evaluation of two methods for quantitation of dentinal hypersensitivity. *J Am Dent Assoc* 98:914–918.
52. Trash, W.J., Dorman, H.L., and Smith, F.D. 1983. A method to measure pain associated with hypersensitive dentin. *J Periodontol* 54:160–162.
53. van Betterav, W., and Riethe, P. 1973. The plaque inhibiting activity of surface-active substances—Sodium *N*-laurylsarcosinate and sodium sulphoricinoleate. *Caries Res* 7:85–88.
54. Volker, J.F., and Thomas, J.P. 1973. Prophylactic and operative techniques in dental caries prevention. In *Clinical Pedodontics*, 4th ed, S.B. Finn (ed), Philadelphia: W.B. Saunders, pp. 544–548.
55. Wason, S.K. 1978. Cosmetic properties and structure of fine-particle synthetic precipitated silicas. *J Soc Cosmet Chem* 29:497–521.
56. Wictorin, I. 1972. Effect of toothbrushing on acrylic resin veneering material. II. Abrasive effect of selected dentifrices and toothbrushes. *Acta Odontol Scand* 30:383–395.
57. Wright, K.H.R., and Stevenson, J.I. 1967. The measurement and interpretation of dentifrice abrasiveness. *J Soc Cosmet Chem* 18:387–411.
58. Zacherl, W.A., Pfeiffer, H.J., and Swancar, J.R. 1985. The effect of soluble pyrophosphates on dental calculus in adults. *J Am Dent Assoc* 110:737–738.
59. Zinner, D.D., Duany, L.F., and Lutz, H.J. 1975. Effects of five dentifrices on hypersensitive tooth surfaces. *J Dent Res* 54: Sp. Issue A, Abstr. L340, p. L85.

Chapter 10

Occlusal Sealants

Bikinis for Bicuspids

Now a stunning thing to wear
For a groovy tooth that's bare
Is a plastic coat to fit;
It is better than knit.
It protects against pollution
Even more than evolution
And it also must be stated
That the coat comes out X-rated,
For it has a see-through quality
That shows complete morphology.

A. Rizzo, June 22, 1973.

Susceptibility of occlusal surfaces

The occlusal surfaces of posterior teeth have repeatedly been noted to be the most vulnerable locations for dental caries. The high caries susceptibility of this area is directly related to the morphology of the pits and fissures. Occlusal pits and fissures vary in shape but are generally narrow (~0.1 mm wide) and tortuous, with invaginations or irregularities where bacteria and food are mechanically retained. Saliva does not readily reach to the base of fissures, nor can those areas be mechanically cleaned. An explorer tip or toothbrush bristle, for example, is too large (0.2 mm diameter) to penetrate most fissures. The thickness of enamel at the base of deep fissures is minimal. In many cases, fissures extend practically to the dentinal surface. Whereas enamel thickness in most tooth locations is approximately 1.5 to 2.0 mm, it is only 0.2 mm or less under deep fissures.

Differences in caries susceptibility between occlusal surfaces and other tooth areas are further emphasized in individuals who have had access to fluorides, because the protective effect of fluoride is much greater on smooth tooth surfaces than in pits and fissures. The reasons for this variation are not well understood but are attributed to the differences in enamel thickness and to the inaccessibility of the base of pits and fissures to topical fluoride sources.

Historical efforts at prevention of occlusal caries

Since the high incidence of pit and fissure caries has long been recognized by clinicians and research dentists, it is not surprising that numerous and varied procedures for decreasing the vulnerability of these surfaces have been proposed.

Extension for prevention

M. H. Webb introduced the concept that cavity preparations on teeth under treatment for occlusal caries be extended to eliminate noncarious fissures. This principle was subsequently popularized by G. V. Black. Although developed a century ago, this procedure is still widely accepted and practiced.

Prophylactic odontotomy

Hyatt[26] advocated the placement of small amalgam restorations in pits and fissures of newly erupted teeth *before* the appearance of clinical signs of decay.

Fissure eradication

Bodecker[4] recommended shaping noncarious pits and fissures into wide, nonretentive grooves rather than placing restorations. He contended that any dentin exposed by the grinding procedures would undergo secondary changes and become resistant to caries. Hyatt's and Bodecker's procedures did not become commonly employed, because there was a reluctance to perform operative procedures on teeth with no apparent lesions. Furthermore, considering the professional time and costs involved in such procedures, their public health applications were very limited.

Application of impregnating solutions

Howe[25] proposed that ammoniacal silver nitrate solutions be applied to sterilize tooth surfaces. The material has been reported to diffuse into enamel and dentin and increase the resistance of the area by forming complexes with protein components and by depositing reduced silver. Younger[56] reported dramatic caries reductions after applications of silver nitrate precipitated with saturated calcium chloride. Another solution, consisting of zinc chloride and potassium ferrocyanide, was also reported to be effective in reducing caries. The use of impregnating solutions was based largely on the theory that the primary route for the initiation of caries was by proteolytic action of organisms on organic structures in enamel. This concept was not supported by later evidence, and controlled clinical studies showed no significant cariostatic effects of these procedures.[3,29]

Application of nonadhesive dental materials

Numerous dental materials, including zinc phosphate and copper cement, were used in an attempt to physically block pits and fissures. These substances, however, had limited value due to their high solubility and poor retention to tooth structure.

Development of occlusal sealants

In recent years, interest in nonoperative methods for increasing the resistance of pits and fissures has focused on developing polymeric materials capable of adhering to tooth structure. A material of this type could then be applied to occlusal surfaces to "seal" caries-susceptible areas from external sources of substrate.

Requirements of a sealant material

The sealant is not necessarily required to fill the entire depth of the fissure, but it must extend along its entire length, bonding firmly at the fissure orifice. There should be an absence of microleakage at the enamel/sealant interface to prevent nutrients from diffusing to organisms remaining in the fissure and to prevent new organisms from entering. Although some bacteria sealed within fissures may remain viable for extended periods of time, they do not produce sufficient acid to initiate caries if deprived of a continuous external source of fermentable carbohydrate. The requirements of a sealant material are listed in Table 10-1.

Table 10-1 Requirements for occlusal sealants

Adhesion to enamel for extended periods
Simple clinical application
Noninjurious to oral tissues
Free flowing and capable of entering narrow fissures by capillary
Rapidly polymerized
Low solubility in oral fluids

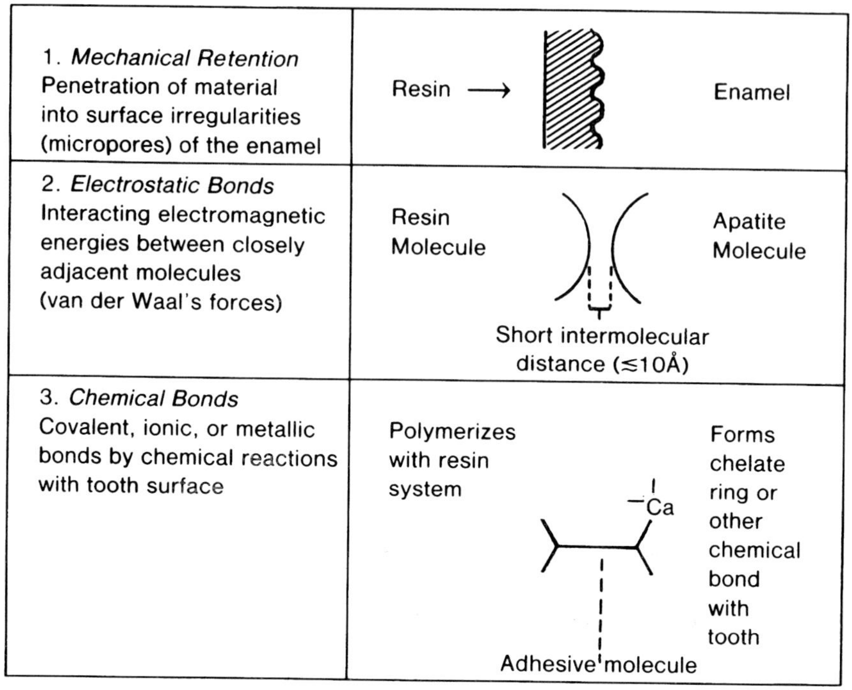

Fig 10-1 Adhesion of dental materials.

Principles of adhesion

Adhesion is the molecular attraction existing between the surfaces of contacting bodies.[14] Retention can result from multiple points of mechanical interlocking in natural or artificially created surface irregularities.[8] Electrostatic bonds result from interacting electromagnetic energies within closely adjacent molecules (dipoles, induced dipoles, and nonpolar effects). Hydrogen bonding may be considered to be a special type of electrostatic interaction. An adhesive can also form covalent or ionic bonds if it reacts chemically with the surface of the substrate. Primary chemical bonds (covalent) are generally stronger than either mechanical or electrostatic bonds (Fig 10-1). Under clinical circumstances it has not been possible to effectively use primary chemical bonds for retention of restorative materials. The carboxyl groups in the long chain polyacrylic acid (eg, carboxylate cements) may chelate calcium in the mineral phase of the tooth. Direct evidence of this type of interaction is based on infrared spectroscopy. At the present time the available occlusal sealants depend upon mechanical retention for their adhesion. The sealing ability of the occlusal sealants is good when assessed for microleakage.[38,49]

Table 10-2 Effects of enamel conditioning on retention

Increases surface wettability and approximation between sealant and substrate by removing contaminants and superficial enamel
Produces a modified outer surface, more suitable for retention
Increases the surface area for bonding
Produces surface irregularities for sealant penetration

Pretreatment of enamel surfaces

Close approximation at the molecular level between sealant and substrate is an absolute requirement for retention. Close approximation can only be achieved if the surface of the substrate is clean and thoroughly wetted by the sealant liquid. Wetting, or molecular dispersion of the sealant liquid on the substrate, will not occur effectively on inert or contaminated surfaces.

Unmodified enamel is a poor substrate for occlusal sealants because its hygroscopic nature favors the displacement of the sealant molecules by water.[31] Furthermore, plaque, pellicle, and other contaminants inhibit the dispersion of the sealant and prevent close approximation with tooth structure. A major breakthrough in the efforts to produce an effective sealant occurred when Buonocore[7] reported greatly enhanced retention of an acrylic filling material to an enamel surface that had been etched with a 50% phosphoric acid solution. The etchant (referred to clinically as a "conditioning agent") removes surface contaminants and part of the enamel surface to a depth of 5 to 10 μm and creates an outer surface more representative of the underlying tooth structure. There is also a marked increase in surface area and topographical irregularity, that is, roughness, due to the selective removal of enamel rods or interprismatic substance by the acid (Table 10-2). A multitude of micropores and protrusions are created. Tags of resin, between 20 and 50 μm in length, have been noted projecting from the resin bulk after the enamel has been demineralized.[12,52] It is apparent that the resin material can penetrate and polymerize in the enamel micropores created by the etchant and form mechanical bonds with the tooth (Fig 10-2).

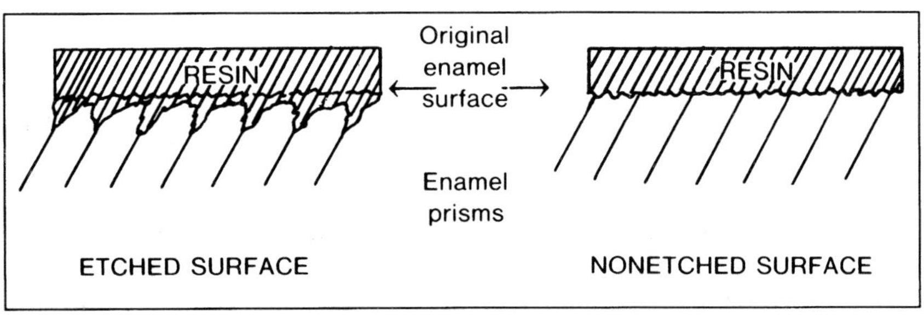

Fig 10-2 Diagram of enamel/resin interface in etched and nonetched enamel indicating penetration of resin into etched surface (adapted from Buonocore[11]).

Phosphoric acid is the conditioning agent of choice, although other acids such as citric and formic acid have been tried.[33] In most cases, a solution of 50% phosphoric acid containing 7% dissolved zinc oxide by weight has been used. A 25% phosphoric acid solution without zinc oxide also appears to be effective. Paradoxically, more dilute phosphoric acid (at least 25% to 30%) is more effective than 50% phosphoric acid, presumably because at the higher concentration the common ion phosphate would decrease the dissolution of the enamel. Strong acids such as hydrochloric are too destructive to be used effectively, while chelating agents such as ethylenediaminetetraacetic acid work too slowly to be of clinical value. The characteristics of an etched surface are also related to chemical and structural conditions in the enamel. In primary teeth, the outer enamel usually consists of tightly packed prisms with crystallites oriented parallel to the long axis of the prism. This so-called prismless enamel remains generally smooth and uniform after etching and provides a less favorable surface for retention of sealants. Accordingly, a 2-minute rather than 1-minute etching time is indicated for primary teeth. Teeth with a high fluoride content in the outer enamel resist normal acid etching procedures and require longer conditioning times.[20]

Once an enamel surface has been conditioned, it is important that it not be contaminated by saliva, compressor oil, or other substances prior to placement of the sealant material. The use of topical fluorides at this time is also contraindicated because the resultant reaction products decrease surface wettability and interfere with the penetration of the sealant.

The phosphoric acid etching solution is considered safe for use because an etched surface that remains uncovered appears clinically to return to normal within a few days, although remineralization continues for weeks and months. Furthermore, similar concentrations of acid are in general use in zinc phosphate cements. Clinical studies indicate that etched uncovered surfaces or surfaces from which the sealant has been lost are not more susceptible to caries than untreated surfaces.[23,39]

Materials assessed for use as sealants

Cyanoacrylate

The first material with adhesive potential to be clinically tested as a sealant was methyl 2-cyanoacrylate (Eastman 910 adhesive) in combination with a powdered filler.[13] Although early tests with this product were encouraging, later clinical studies showed mixed or negative results.[44] The material is relatively unstable (short shelf life) and was never marketed commercially. Alkyl-cyanoacrylate and isobutyl-cyanoacrylate were also tested as sealants but not produced for commercial sale. A fluorocyanoacrylate material prepared by the 3M Company was developed as a long-term topical fluoride treatment rather than as a true sealant. The material is generally lost within weeks but reportedly greatly enhances surface fluoride absorption. Although this class of materials is potentially useful, its anticaries effects must be tested clinically and compared to the effects of conventional topical fluoride applications.

Polyurethane

A polyurethane product, Epoxylite #9070, containing 10% disodium monofluorophosphate, was marketed (1970 to 1972) originally as a sealant and later as a prolonged topical fluoride application.[32] Following several reports[15,16,43,46] of poor retention, solubility, and ineffectiveness, this material was withdrawn from the market. Elmex Protector (Gaba A.G.), a polyurethane resin containing amine fluoride, is currently available in Europe. In a clinical study with this material, however, Rock[46] found almost no sealant retention after 6 months and no caries reduction over a 2-year period.

Two urethane dimethacrylate sealants are commercially available, both manufactured by Vivadent. They are Contact-Seal, a chemically cured material with a shelf life of 24 months when refrigerated, and Helioseal, which is polymerized by visible light. Helioseal contains 2% titanium oxide as an opaquer and has a shelf life of 36 months unrefrigerated.

BIS-GMA

In an effort to improve the physical properties of existing resin filling materials, Bowen[5] developed a new cross-linking thermo-setting dimethacrylate monomer. The monomer is formed as the reduction product of bis-(4 hydroxyphenol)-dimethylmethane, a dihydroxyphenol, and glycidyl methacrylate, an epoxy acrylic monomer (Fig 10-3). This product, BIS-GMA, is currently the resin component of most composite resin materials.[6] BIS-GMA was diluted with methyl methacrylate or other comonomers, to improve flow characteristics, and was adapted for use as a sealant. The monomer mixture undergoes less polymerization shrinkage and has a lower coefficient of thermal expansion than methyl methacrylate alone and is, therefore, more likely to form and maintain bonds with enamel. Polymerization of BIS-GMA is initiated by the conventional chemical method (benzoyl peroxide catalyst) or by long-wave ultraviolet (UV) radiation (3,600 Å) applied after the composition is made sensitive to UV radiation by the addition of 2% benzoin methyl ether (catalyst).

In the first reported clinical study using BIS-GMA sealant,[48] 29% fewer new carious surfaces were observed in sealed compared to unsealed teeth. In later studies, caries was reduced from 65% to 100% (Table 10-3).

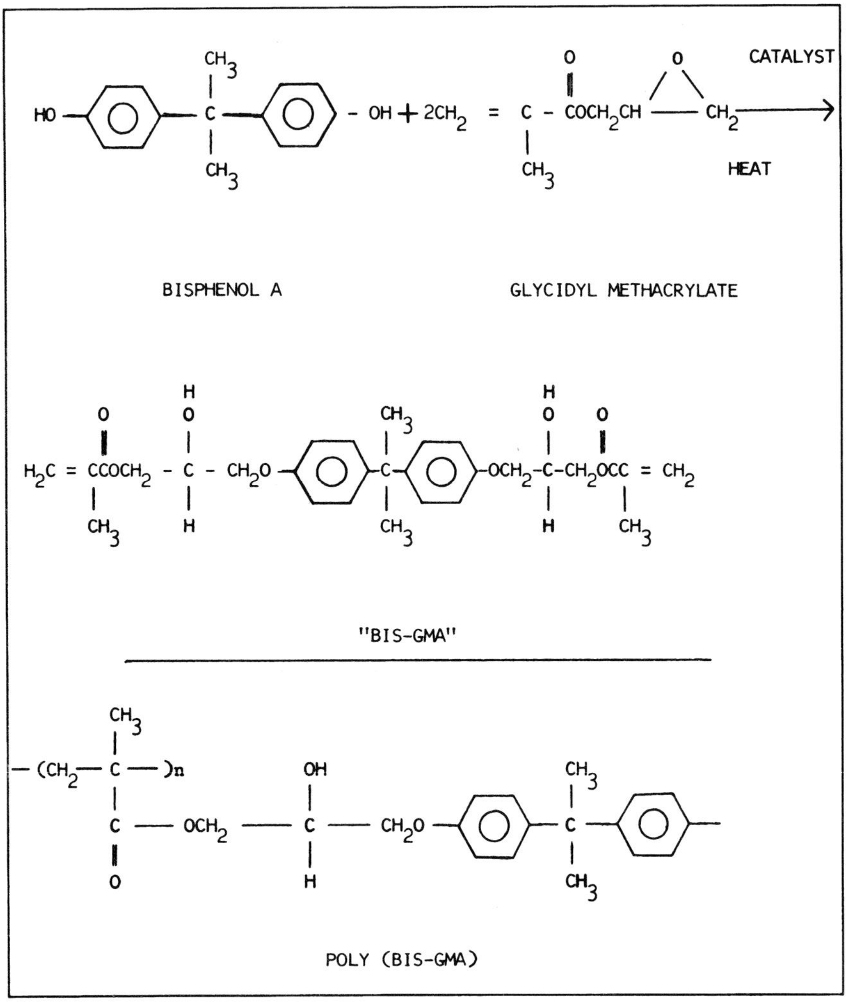

Fig 10-3 BIS-GMA is the resin component of most composite resin materials.

Currently, there are several sealants commercially available in the United States that have been evaluated and found acceptable by the ADA Council on Dental Materials, Instruments, and Equipment, based on submission of information from laboratory test results on mechanical and physiological properties and biological acceptability as well as on clinical data on biocompatibility and effectiveness as a caries-preventive material.[2] The following pit and fissure sealants have been rated as acceptable:

Concise Brand White Sealant (3M Dental Products)
Delton (Johnson & Johnson Dental Products)
Delton (tinted) (Johnson & Johnson Dental Products)
Nuva-Seal P.A. (L.D. Caulk Co, Div. Dentsply International, Inc)

Table 10-3 Clinical studies of BIS-GMA sealants

Study	Time (mo)	Sealant retained* (%)	Caries reduction (%)
Roydhouse[48]	36		29
Buonocore[9]	24	87	99
Rock[46]	24	80	99
Horowitz et al[24]	60	42	39
Gourley[19]	24	78	57
Merrill et al[38]	15	55	
Going et al[18]	24	69	55
Meurman and Helminem[40]	36	80	88
Messer and Cline[39]	36	42	44
Richardson et al[45]	36	75	64
McCune et al[35]	36	88	85

*Completely present, data for permanent teeth.

Oralin Pit and Fissure Sealant (S.S. White Dental Products, Inc)
Prisma-Shield (L.D. Caulk Co, Div. Dentsply International, Inc)
Prisma-Shield (tinted) (L.D. Caulk Co, Div. Dentsply International, Inc)
Visio-Seal (E.S.P.)

In addition, Helioseal (Vivadent U.S.A.) and Delton Light Cure (Johnson & Johnson Dental Products) have been rated provisionally acceptable. The Council stresses that the technique of application is critical.[1,2]

Other sealants

Duraphat (Woelm Pharma), a varnish preparation containing sodium fluoride, has been released in Europe. The material sets on moist tooth surfaces as a thin film.[50] Duraphat appears to function as an extended fluoride application rather than as a true sealant.

Aspa II is a glass ionomer cement formed by the hardening reaction between aluminosilicate glass powders and polyacrylic acid. This ionic polymer cement is hydrophilic, unlike the hydrophobic organic resins. It has been tested in England,[36,59] and its cariostatic effect is impressive. This may be due in part to the cement's high fluoride content (16%), which is probably released slowly.

Technique for the use of sealants

Tooth preparation

Proper tooth preparation is absolutely essential for bonding the sealant to enamel. Teeth to be sealed are first mechanically cleaned using motor-driven polishing brushes or cups, with or without a dentifrice. Fine-grained abrasives have a tendency to be retained in fissures and are not recommended. The teeth are then isolated with a rubber dam or cotton rolls and are etched for 1 minute with conditioning solution (50% H_3PO_4 containing 7% wt/vol ZnO). The etchant is moved gently over the enamel surface with a cotton pellet or brush and then washed away using an air-water spray and a high velocity aspirator. The teeth are dried using a clean air spray for 20 seconds.

Sealant application

The sealant is mixed thoroughly with catalyst and painted into the pits and fissures with a fine camel's hair brush or cotton pellet. Polymerization is induced either by UV radiation transferred through a clear quartz rod or by visible light depending on the product used. The tip of the rod is held 2 mm from the tooth surface for approximately 30 seconds. Epoxylite 9075 (Lee Pharmaceuticals) is applied in a three-step procedure. A priming agent is first applied to the tooth surface and allowed to dry. The base monomer is painted into the pits and fissures, and then the catalyst solution is applied. Initial polymerization occurs in 30 to 60 seconds. The Delton system uses an applicator with a disposable tube. Sealant is drawn up into the tube by depressing and releasing the lever. The applicator tip is applied to the occlusal surface and sealant is discharged by depressing the level of the applicator. After sealant application, occlusion is checked and, if necessary, adjusted. Excess material outside the fissures is usually removed quickly by normal attrition.[10]

Factors affecting clinical use of available sealants

Effectiveness

Although clinical studies using BIS-GMA sealant show varied results,[57] the material has a definite protective effect extending over several years. Second-year results of a study conducted in Kalispell, Montana, by the Public Health Service Division of Dental Health show that 73% of treated teeth still had sealant completely present and that the sealant was 67% effective in preventing occlusal caries.[20] In a study conducted in Rochester, New York, Buonocore[10] reported 87% sealant retention and 99% caries reduction after 2 years on teeth treated with the BIS-GMA material (see Table 10-3). The variation in results between those two studies may be attributed in part to differences in tooth selection, facilities and equipment used, and evaluation criteria. Buonocore utilized only teeth with well-defined fissures, where the sealant is more likely to be retained; occlusal anatomy was not a consideration in the Montana study. Montana study subjects were treated under mass application conditions using portable equipment, while operatory facilities were used for the Rochester project. Also, in the Montana study, sealed teeth that subsequently received mesial-occlusal or distal-occlusal restorations for proximal decay were counted as sealant treatment failures. It is not stated whether such teeth were assessed by Buonocore. Naturally, the longer the sealant is in the mouth, the greater the chance it will be lost. In the Montana study, complete retention of sealant after 5 years was 42%, and prevention of occlusal caries was 39%.[24] The retention of Delton, a cold-cured autopolymerized BIS-GMA system, is superior to that of Nuva-Seal polymerized by ultraviolet light.[34,40] Ten years after a single office application of Concise White Sealant, 57% of first permanent molars retained the sealant and only 16% of the occlusal surfaces were restored or carious.[53]

Another cause of differences in caries reduction can be the posteruptive time of sealing. Teeth that have been present in the mouth for several years at time of sealing will be from the more caries-resistant part of the population. Clinical trials on children of varying ages constitute a disparate sample leading to heterogeneous results.[47]

Retention of sealant is better on premolars than on molars, the poorest retention being the distal pits of the maxillary second molars.[18] Presumably this is related to the difficulty of isolating and keeping dry those teeth that may not be fully erupted. The importance of preventing contamination by saliva must be stressed. Inadequate exposure of Nuva-Seal to UV radiation is another possible cause for sealant losses in some clinical trials with this resin.[55] Small quantities of cured resin on the tip of the quartz rod drastically reduce the output intensity of the UV light. Accordingly, the tip should be cleaned with chloroform following the treatment of each patient. BIS-GMA containing filler particles (Concise Enamel Bond, 3M Dental Products) provides better retention and caries prevention than unfilled BIS-GMA (Nuva-Seal).[58] However, the improved performance may be due not to the presence or absence of filler, but to the use of a double-film technique in which unfilled BIS-GMA is first applied as a thin film, then covered by a filled composite resin. Leakage and permeability of a fissure sealant are less when a double-film method is employed.

Rock[46] and other investigators consider that much sealant loss results shortly after the material is placed and is due to improper application. In practice, therefore, it is recommended that sealant be applied before the patient's last visit so that a short-term evaluation of the treated teeth can be made.

Sealing carious lesions

In vitro and in vivo evidence suggest that small lesions sealed within the tooth structure do not advance. In an in vitro study utilizing tooth sections,[42] carious lesions in enamel became arrested after the application of sealant. The etchant and sealing procedure produces an immediate bactericidal effect.[54] Gross reductions occur in the number of viable bacteria in carious dentin of sealed teeth.[21,27,28,37] Clinical and radiographic findings indicate that incipient lesions inadvertently sealed will not progress. Until further long-term data are available, however, teeth with detectable caries should be treated according to conventional operative techniques.

Indications for use

Some general guidelines can be established for the clinical use of the currently available sealants, based on the physical properties of the material and reports from clinical studies. Sealants are especially indicated for newly erupted teeth with pronounced pits and fissures and for patients with considerable previous occlusal caries experience. On the other hand, caries-free teeth that have been present in the mouth for over 4 or 5 years or those with shallow wide grooves need not be sealed. Patients with high proximal caries activity may not be good candidates for a sealant, because compound restorations are generally extended into the occlusal fissures. Sealants applied in these cases must be accompanied by other preventive procedures, especially fluoride applications.

Available sealants are not retained by amalgam, gold, or silicate and cannot be used on the margins of restorations made of those materials. Sealants do, however, adhere chemically to composite resins and can be used to improve the adhesion and marginal seal of composite resin restorations.

Public health and private practice application

Utilization of currently available sealant materials on a public health basis is very limited due to the professional time and costs involved. Teeth must be examined, diagnosed for caries, and carefully prepared prior to sealing. Equipment to dry and isolate teeth must be available. Following application of the sealant, regular careful checks should be made for retention of sealant and for carious lesions. If the sealant is lost and there are no carious lesions, the conditioning and sealant application should be repeated.

In one school program, after 4 years, the cost of implementating sealing was almost 4 times the cost of the saving in treatment.[30] The low occlusal caries reduction (22%) and poor retention results are probably due to the difficulty of maintaining a dry field using portable equipment. Sealing all susceptible fissures takes more time than restoring only those teeth that become decayed. Use of sealants would be more efficient in fluoridated communities where there is less proximal caries. For example, in fluoridated Bloomington, Minnesota, a matched pair analysis comparing sealed and unsealed surfaces found that the necessary restorations cost 1.64 times the cost of sealing the surfaces.[53] In young adults (17 to 23 years old), sealant therapy is not cost effective because of the relatively low caries attack rate.[15] Greater utilization of auxiliary personnel, who must be adequately trained and sufficiently motivated to apply sealants, will help to lower unit cost.[22] New, less demanding sealant materials and procedures are probably needed before the technique has effective mass application potential.

Although the retention of sealants and the resultant caries reduction have been quite good (see Table 10-3), the acceptance by dentists of this technique has generally been low.[17] Most dentists are not yet convinced of the effectiveness of the procedure and are also concerned about the longevity of the material in the mouth. Increased use will depend on improved communication regarding the function and value of sealants.

Chapter review

- Indicate why occlusal fissures are so vulnerable to caries.
- Define prophylactic odontotomy.
- List the principles of adhesion.
- State the requirements of an ideal occlusal sealant.
- State the objective of occlusal sealing.
- List the types of materials that have been tested as sealants.
- Explain the purpose of the etching (conditioning) step in the application of a sealant.
- List the possible causes of failure of sealant retention.
- State what happens if initial caries has been covered by the sealant.
- State the nature of the enamel/sealant bond.
- Explain why dryness is critical to successful retention.
- State the effectiveness of sealants in reducing caries.

Selected readings

Buonocore, M.G. 1975. Pit and fissure sealing. *Dent Clin North Am* 19:367–383.

Buonocore, M.G. 1975. *The Use of Adhesives in Dentistry*. Springfield, Ill.: Charles C Thomas.

Horowitz, A.M. (Chair). 1984. Dental sealants in the prevention of tooth decay. National Institutes of Health Concensus Development Conference: *J Dent Educ* (Suppl.) pp. 1–131.

Murray, J.J., and Williams, B. 1975. Fissure sealants and dental caries. A review. *J Dent* 3:145–152.
Ripa, L.W. 1980. Occlusal sealants. Rationale and review of clinical trials. *Int Dent J* 30:127–139.
Ripa, L.W. (ed) 1986. *Preventing pit and fissure caries: a guide to sealant use.* Massachusetts Department of Health. Boston, Massachusetts.
Silverstone, L.M., and Dogon, I.L. (eds) 1975. *The Acid Etch Technique.* Proceedings of the International Symposium. St. Paul, Minn.: North Central Publishing Co.
Simonsen, R.J. 1980. *Clinical Applications of the Acid Etch Technique.* Chicago: Quintessence Publ Co.
Simonsen, R.J. 1981. Preventive aspects of clinical resin technology. *Dent Clin North Am* 25:291–305.

References

1. American Dental Association, Council on Dental Materials and Devices. 1976. Pit and fissure sealants. *J Am Dent Assoc* 93:134–135.
2. American Dental Association, Council on Dental Materials, Instruments and Equipment. 1987. Pit and Fissure Sealants. *J Am Dent Assoc* 114:671–672.
3. Ast, D.B., Bushel, A., and Chase, H.C. 1950. A clinical study of caries prophylaxis with zinc chloride and potassium ferrocyanide. *J Am Dent Assoc* 41:442.
4. Bodecker, C.F. 1929. The eradication of enamel fissures. *Dent Items* 51:859.
5. Bowen, R.L. 1963. Properties of a silica-reinforced polymer for dental restorations. *J Am Dent Assoc* 66:57–64.
6. Bowen, R.L. 1970. Crystalline dimethacrylate monomers. *J Dent Res* 49:810–815.
7. Buonocore, M.G. 1955. Simple method of increasing the adhesion of acrylic filling materials to enamel surfaces. *J Dent Res* 34:849–853.
8. Buonocore, M.G. 1963. Principles of adhesive retention and adhesive restorative materials. *J Am Dent Assoc* 67:382–391.
9. Buonocore, M.G. 1971. Caries prevention in pits and fissures sealed with an adhesive resin polymerized by ultraviolet light. A two year study of a single adhesive application. *J Am Dent Assoc* 82:1090–1093.
10. Buonocore, M.G. 1972. Adhesives for pit and fissure caries control. *Dent Clin North Am* 16:693–708.
11. Buonocore, M.G. 1973. Sealing of pits and fissures with an adhesive for caries prevention. *J Can Dent Assoc* 39:841–850.
12. Buonocore, M.G., Matsui, A., and Gwinett, A.J. 1968. Penetration of resin materials into enamel surfaces with reference to bonding. *Arch Oral Biol* 13:61–70.
13. Cueto, E.I., and Buonocore, M.G. 1967. Sealing of pits and fissures with an adhesive resin. Its use in caries prevention. *J Am Dent Assoc* 75:121–127.
14. de Bruyne, N.A. 1962. Action of adhesives. *Sci Am* 206:114–122.
15. Eden, G.T. 1976. Clinical evaluation of a pit and fissure sealant for young adults. *J Prosthet Dent* 36:51–57.
16. Frank, R.M., Sommermater, J., and Locoste, J.L. 1971. Essai clinique de prévention de la carie dentaire par scellement des fissures. *Schweiz Monatsschr Zahnheilkd* 81: 543–547.
17. Gift, H.C., Frew, R., and Hefferren, J.J. 1975. Attitudes toward use of pit and fissure sealants. *J Dent Child* 42:460–466.
18. Going, R.E., Haugh, L.D., Grainger, D.A., and Conti, A.J. 1976. Two-year clinical evaluation of a pit and fissure sealant. *J Am Dent Assoc* 92:388–397, 578–585.
19. Gourley, J.M. 1975. A two year study of fissure sealant in two Nova Scotia communities. *J Public Health Dent* 35:132–137.
20. Gwinett, A.J., and Matsui, A. 1967. A study of enamel adhesives. The physical relationship between enamel and adhesive. *Arch Oral Biol* 12:1615–1620.
21. Handleman, S.L., Washburn, F., and Wepperer, P. 1976. Two-year report of sealant effect on bacteria in dental caries. *J Am Dent Assoc* 93:967–970.
22. Horowitz, H.S. 1980. Pit and fissure sealants in private practice and public health programmes. Analysis of cost-effectiveness. *Int Dent J* 30:117–126.

23. Horowitz, H.S., Heifetz, S.B., and McCune, R.J. 1974. The effectiveness of an adhesive sealant in preventing occlusal caries. Findings after two years in Kalispell, Montana. *J Am Dent Assoc* 89:885–890.
24. Horowitz, H.S., Heifetz, S.B., and Poulsen, S. 1977. Retention and effectiveness of a single application of an adhesive sealant in preventing occlusal caries. Final report after five years of study in Kalispell, Montana. *J Am Dent Assoc* 95:1133–1139.
25. Howe, R.R. 1917. A method of sterilizing and at the same time impregnating dentinal tissues. *Dent Cosmos* 59:89.
26. Hyatt, T.P. 1923. The cutting into the tooth for the prevention of the disease. *Dent Cosmos* 65:234–241.
27. Jensen, Ø.E., and Handelman, S.L. 1980. Effect of an autopolymerizing sealant on viability of microflora in occlusal dental caries. *Scand J Dent Res* 88:382–388.
28. Jeronimus, D.J., Till, M.J., and Sveen, O.B. 1975. Reduced viability of microorganisms under dental sealants. *J Dent Child* 42:275–280.
29. Klein, J., and Knutson, J.W. 1942. Studies on dental caries. XIII. Effect of ammoniacal silver nitrate on caries in first permanent molars. *J Am Dent Assoc* 29:1420–1426.
30. Leake, J.L., and Martinello, B.P. 1976. A four year evaluation of a fissure sealant in a public health setting. *J Can Dent Assoc* 8:409–415.
31. Lee, H.L. 1969. Adhesion between living tissue and plastics. I. Adhesion of epoxy and polyurethane resins to dentin and enamel. *J Biomed Mater Res* 3:349–367.
32. Lee, H.L., Cupples, A.L., Schubert, R.J., and Swartz, M.L. 1971. An adhesive dental restorative material. *J Dent Res* 50:125–132.
33. Lee, H.L., and Swartz, M.L. 1971. Sealing of developmental pits and fissures: I. In vitro study. *J Dent Res* 50:133–140.
34. Li, S.H., Swango, P.A., Gladsden, A.N., and Heifetz, S.B. 1981. Evaluation of the retention of two types of pit and fissure sealants. *Community Dent Oral Epidemiol* 9: 151–158.
35. McCune, R.J., Bojanini, J., and Abodeely, R.A. 1979. Effectiveness of a pit and fissure sealant in the prevention of caries. Three-year clinical results. *J Am Dent Assoc* 99:619–623.
36. McLean, J.W., and Wilson, A.D. 1976. Fissure sealings and filling with an adhesive glass-ionomer cement. *Br Dent J* 136:269–276.
37. Mednick, G.A., Corpron, R.E., and Loesche, W.J. 1974. A bacterial evaluation of an occlusal sealant as a barrier system in humans. *J Dent Child* 41:356–360.
38. Merrill, S.A., Leinfelder, K.F., Oldenburg, T.R., and Taylor, D.F. 1975. Methods of evaluating pit and fissure sealants. *J Dent Child* 42:43–47.
39. Messer, L.B., and Cline, J.T. 1980. Relative caries experience of sealed versus unsealed permanent posterior teeth. A three year study. *J Dent Child* 47:175–182.
40. Metz-Fairhurst, E.J., Fairhurst, C.W., Williams, J.E., Della-Giustina, V.E., and Brooks, J.D. 1984. A comparative clinical study of two pit and fissure sealants: 7-year results in Augusta, GA. *J Am Dent Assoc* 109:252–255.
41. Meurman, J.H., and Helminen, S.K.I. 1976. Effectiveness of fissure sealant 3 years after application. *Scand J Dent Res* 84:218–223.
42. Micik, R.E. 1972. Fate of in vitro caries-like lesions sealed within tooth structure. Proceedings, International Association for Dental Research, 50th General Session, Abstr. 710, p. 225.
43. Newbrun, E., Plasschaert, A.J.M., and König, K.G. 1974. Progress of caries in fissures of rat molars treated with occlusal sealant. *J Am Dent Assoc* 89:121–126.
44. Parkhouse, R.C., and Winter, G.B. 1971. A fissure sealant containing methyl-2-cyanoacrylate as a caries preventive agent. A clinical evaluation. *Br Dent J* 130:16–19.
45. Richardson, A.S., Gibson, G.B., and Waldman, R. 1980. Chemically polymerized sealant in preventing occlusal caries. *J Am Dent Assoc* 46:259–260.
46. Rock, W.P. 1974. Fissure sealants, further results of clinical trials. *Br Dent J* 136: 317–321.
47. Rock, W.P. 1977. Fissure sealants, results of a 3-year clinical trial using an ultraviolet sensitive resin. *Br Dent J* 142:16–18.
48. Roydhouse, R.H. 1968. Prevention of occlusal fissure caries by use of a sealant. A pilot study. *J Dent Child* 35:253–262.
49. Rudolph, J.J., Phillips, R.W., and Swartz, M.L. 1974. In vitro assessment of microleakage of pit and fissure sealants. *J Prosthet Dent* 32:62–65.
50. Schmidt, H.F.M. 1971. Duraphat in dental caries prophylaxis. *Odont Prat* 6:261–263.
51. Silverstone, L.M. 1974. Fissure sealants. Laboratory studies. *Caries Res* 8:2–26.
52. Silverstone, L.M. 1975. The acid etch technique. In vitro studies with special reference to the enamel surface and the enamel resin interface. In *Proc Int Symp Acid Etch*

Technique, L.M. Silverstone and I.L. Dogon (eds), St. Paul, Minn.: North Central Publishing Co, pp. 13–39.

53. Simonsen, R.J. 1987. Retention and effectiveness of a single application of white sealant after 10 years. *J Am Dent Assoc* 115:31–36.
54. Theilade, E., Fejerskov, O., Migasena, K., and Prachyabrued, W. 1977. Effect of fissure sealing on the microflora in occlusal fissures of human teeth. *Arch Oral Biol* 22:251–259.
55. Young, K.C., Hussey, M., Gillespie, F.C., and Stephen, K.W. 1977. The performance of ultraviolet lights used to polymerize fissure sealants. *J Oral Rehabil* 4:181–191.
56. Younger, H.B. 1949. Clinical results of caries prophylaxis by impregnation. *Texas Dent J* 67:96.
57. Williams, B., Casson, M.H., and Winter, G.B. 1974. A clinical study using a new ultraviolet light polymerized fissure sealant. *J Dent* 2:101–105.
58. Williams, B., Price, R., and Winter, G.B. 1978. Fissure sealants. A 2-year clinical trial. *Br Dent J* 145:359–364.
59. Williams, B., and Winter, G.B. 1976. Fissure sealants, a 2-year clinical trial. *Br Dent J* 141:15–18.

Chapter 11

The Uses of Fluorides in Preventive Dentistry

For thou must know, Sancho, that a mouth without teeth is like a mill without a stone; and that a diamond is not so precious as a tooth.

Miguel de Cervantes Saavedra, from *The Adventures of Don Quixote de la Mancha*

Fluorides

Fluorine is a member of the halogen family. It is the most electronegative of all the elements, which makes it extremely reactive. It combines with almost every element and also reacts with organic radicals. It is rarely found in the free state in nature but is widely distributed in the earth's crust, ranking 17th in abundance (0.06% to 0.09%). Fluorine usually occurs in minerals, such as fluorspar (CaF_2), cryolite (Na_3AlF_6), or fluorosilicates (Na_2SiF_6), and in rocks in the forms of mica, hornblende, and pegmatites. In biological mineralized tissue, such as bones and teeth, it occurs as the apatite salt—not as fluorapatite ($Ca_{10}(PO_4)_6F_2$), but rather as fluoridated hydroxyapatite ($Ca_{10}(PO_4)_6(OH)_{2-x}F_x$, where x is much smaller than 2). In other words, only some of the hydroxyls of the apatite lattice are replaced by fluoride ions, yet this change profoundly alters the resistance of enamel to demineralization.

There is no doubt of the anticaries effectiveness of fluoride, yet there is no unanimity as to the exact mechanism of how fluoride reduces decay. Table 11-1 lists several hypotheses that have been prepared to explain its action.

That fluoride acts on the hydroxyapatite of the enamel per se and on the bacteria of dental plaque is generally accepted, having been supported in part by laboratory tests and in part by clinical findings. The hypotheses that fluoride acts on the enamel surface or alters tooth morphology are more speculative and less widely accepted. The mechanism by which fluoride works also depends on the conditions of its use. For example, at the high fluoride concentrations (12,000 to 22,600 ppm F) used for office topical therapy, there is at least a temporary effect on bacterial metabolism, inhibiting glycolysis and suppressing *Streptococcus mutans*. At lower fluoride concentrations, such as systemic fluoride provided by water fluoridation or supplements or topical fluoride from

Table 11-1 Hypotheses regarding fluoride's anticaries mechanism of action

Fluoride acts on the hydroxyapatite of the enamel per se:
Decreasing its solubility
Improving its crystallinity
Remineralizing calcium-depleted mineral
Action on the bacteria of dental plaque:
Inhibiting enzymes
Suppressing cariogenic flora
Action on the enamel surface:
Desorbing proteins and/or bacteria
Lowering the free surface energy
Alteration of tooth morphology

dentifrices and mouthrinses, there is an uptake of fluoride by hydroxyapatite, rendering it less soluble and improving its crystallinity. More recently, much emphasis has been placed on the ability of fluoride to promote and accelerate remineralization of calcium-depleted tooth structure. Remineralization is the process whereby partially demineralized enamel is repaired through recrystallization of tooth enamel by mineral salts. Even small amounts of fluoride accelerate this process, as documented by increases in microhardness and radiopacity observed by microradiographic techniques.[1]

In most dental textbooks it is convenient and customary to discuss fluoride therapy for the prevention of dental caries under two main headings: systemic fluoride acting preeruptively, and topical fluoride acting posteruptively. *Systemic fluoride* refers to that intended for ingestion, whereas *topical fluoride* is not meant to be swallowed. Although such division is convenient for didactic purposes and serves to distinguish between the very low dosages used systemically and the somewhat higher concentrations of fluoride used topically, it has become increasingly clear that such a distinction is not absolute. Fluorides being ingested for their systemic effect can also have a topical posteruptive benefit on teeth that are already erupted. Conversely, topical fluoride agents may be swallowed, particularly by young children, and thereby exert a systemic preeruptive effect on teeth that are still undergoing mineralization. With this proviso we will consider fluoride therapy on the basis of systemic and topical treatment.

Systemic fluoride

Fluoridation of communal water supplies

Classic epidemiological surveys of the prevalence of dental caries carried

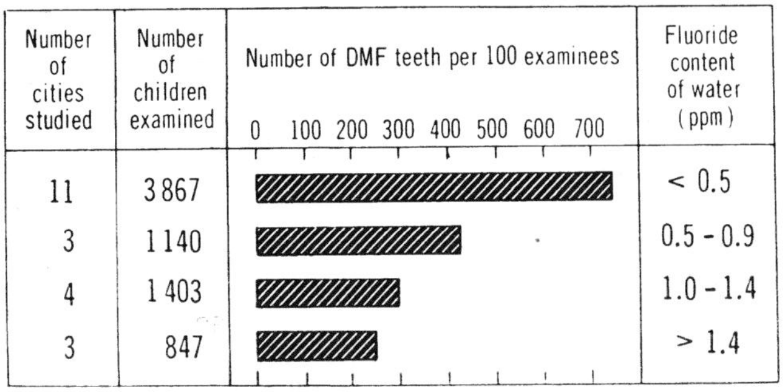

Fig 11-1 Data from 21 US cities grouped according to fluoride content of drinking water, showing inverse relationship between caries prevalence and fluoride content of water. (Courtesy of Newbrun.[46])

out by Dean [14,15] and others, working for the United States Public Health Service during the late 1930s and early 1940s, demonstrated an inverse relationship between caries prevalence and fluoride concentration in the drinking water. Initially these surveys were limited to school-age children residing in different cities with naturally high or low levels of fluoride in the public water supplies (Fig 11-1). It was later shown that adults, as well as children, who have continually consumed fluoridated water lose fewer teeth and have lower scores of decayed, missing, and filled teeth (DMFT).[44,53] Root caries is a soft, progressive lesion of the root surface that mainly affects adults. Lifelong residence in communities with naturally occurring fluorides in the water is associated with a significant reduction in the prevalence of root caries and root fillings.[2,8]

Endemic dental fluorosis (mottling) is a condition that can range from mild (a few opaque white flecks) to severe (extensive yellow to brown staining and multiple pitting). The extent of dental fluorosis has also been directly related to the concentration of fluoride in the drinking water. An *optimal* level of fluoride in the water supply, however, provides significant protection against caries yet entails *low* risk of fluorosis (Fig 11-2). The optimal concentration depends on the annual average maximum daily air temperature in the community (temperature influences the amount of water ingested). In temperate zones of North America, where the annual average maximum daily air temperature ranges between 14.7° and 17.7°C (58.4° to 63.8°F), the optimal level of fluoride is 1 ppm. In Africa and Asia the optimal level is not known and may differ because of different dietary practices and/or greater physical activity, requiring increased water consumption. Between 1950 and 1979, carefully controlled independent studies from 20 countries showed that if fluoride is added to the domestic water supply to bring it up to optimal levels (controlled water fluoridation), the modal caries reduction for permanent teeth was 50% to 60% (Fig 11-3). These clinical trials have been conducted throughout the world, not only in the United States and Canada, which were the first countries to initiate such programs, but in

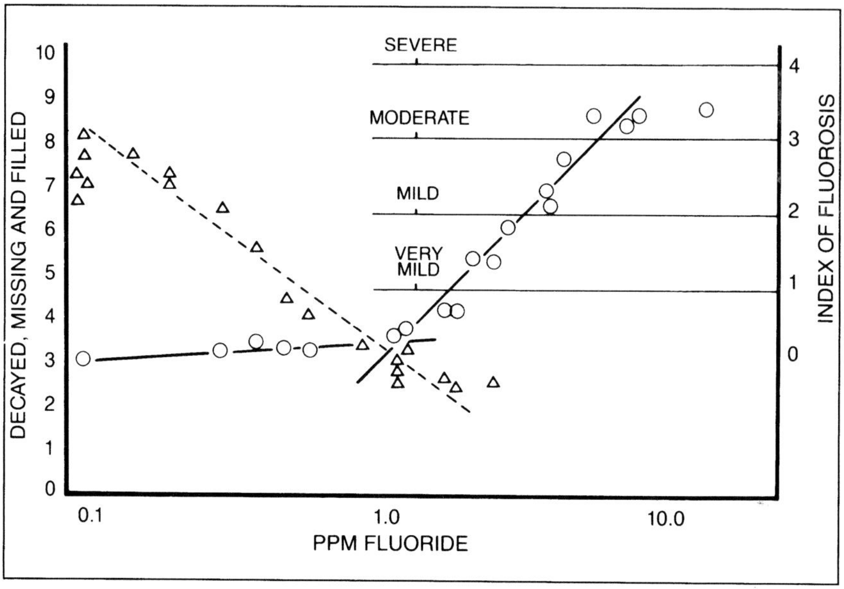

Fig 11-2 Relationship between the logarithm of the fluoride content of the drinking water, caries prevalence, and dental fluorosis. DMF (- - - - - - - -), DFI (———). Data points represent mean caries prevalence (△) and mean fluorosis index (○) for children in each community. (Courtesy of Hodge.[33])

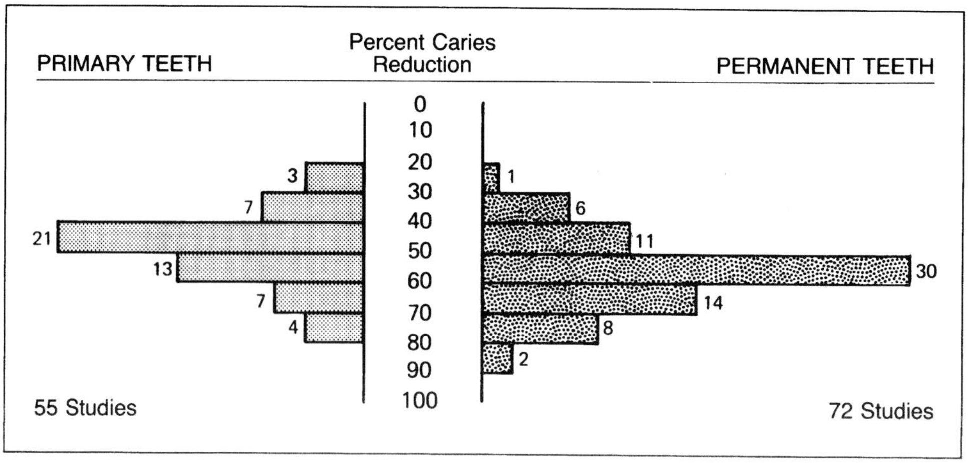

Fig 11-3 Percentage caries reductions observed in 95 studies on the effectiveness of controlled fluoridation in 20 countries. Fifty-five studies gave results for the primary dentition (dmft) and 72 for the permanent dentition (DMFT). (Courtesy of Murray and Rugg-Gunn.[15])

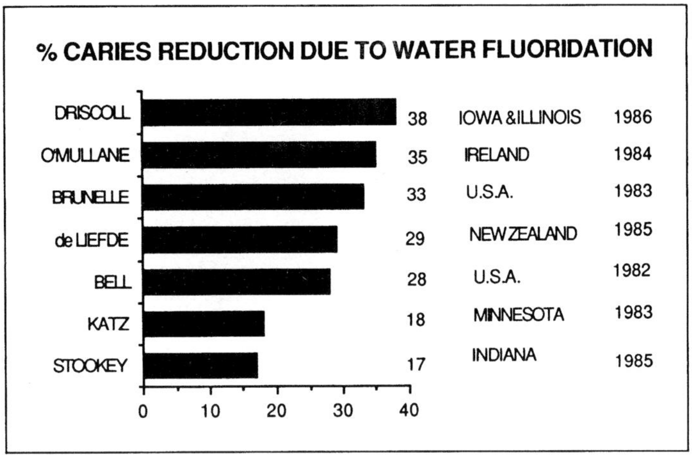

Fig 11-4 Percentage caries reductions, ranging from 17% to 38%, observed since the 1980s in seven studies comparing the prevalence of caries in optimally fluoridated communities with that in nearby nonfluoridated communities. Dates shown indicate year of publication; actual surveys were done 1 or more years earlier.

diverse populations in Australia, Hong Kong, Ireland, Germany, The Netherlands, New Zealand, and the United Kingdom. Worldwide, more than 300 million persons are now consuming water that either is adjusted to or naturally contains an optimal concentration of fluoride.

During the past 20 years, a steady decline in the prevalence of caries in children and young adults has been observed in most Western industrialized countries. This has occurred in communities with suboptimal fluoride levels and in communities with optimal fluoride levels. Undoubtedly the decrease in communities lacking optimal fluoride in the water supply can be attributed to the introduction of caries-preventive methods. These methods include the adoption of many other forms of fluoride, particularly the widespread daily use of fluoride dentifrices, the introduction of extensive fluoride rinse programs in schools and at home, topical fluoride therapy in dental offices, and the ingestion of fluoride tablets or drops by some children. Indeed, because of the ready availability of these additional forms of fluoride, some dentists in Australia, Canada, and Denmark have questioned the continuing need for communal water fluoridation, suggesting that it "may have outlived its usefulness."[11,29,57,64] Before dismissing such proposals as totally heretical, it is worth looking at currently available data on the prevalence of caries in communities with and without optimal water fluoridation. State and national surveys and one demonstration project in the United States and studies of communities in Ireland and New Zealand show caries reductions in the range of about 20% to 40% due to water fluoridation, rather than the 50% to 70% observed 30 to 40 years ago (Fig 11-4).

Since the caries-preventive benefits of topical fluorides and systemic fluorides are additive,[35] and since topical use of fluoride was much more limited 30 to 40 years ago, it is not surprising that recent epidemiological surveys of caries prevalence are finding less difference between optimally fluoridated and nonfluoridated communities. Furthermore, in states

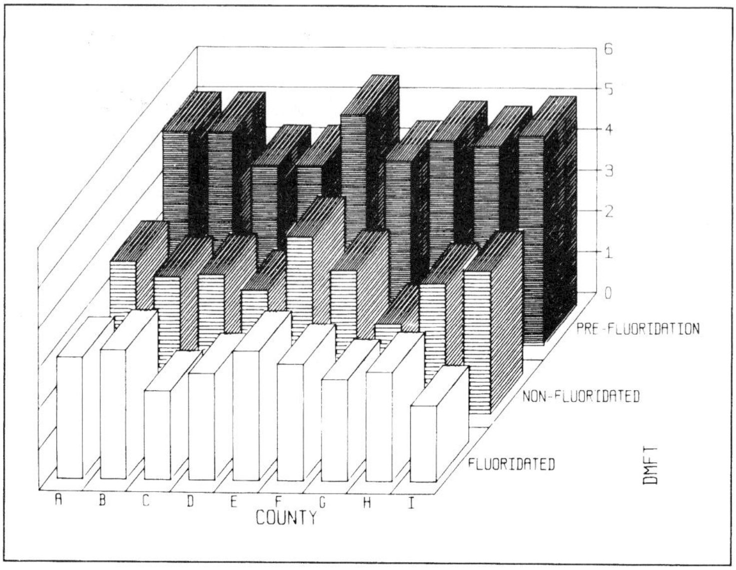

Fig 11-5 Caries prevalence in 12-year-old children in Ireland surveyed pre-fluoridation (1961 to 1963) and again in 1984. The 1984 data for each county (A to I) cover children exposed only to topical fluorides (marked "nonfluoridated") and children exposed to both communal water fluoridation and topical fluorides (marked "fluoridated"). This latter group consistently shows the greatest caries reductions. *(A)* Clare; *(B)* Cork; *(C)* Donegal; *(D)* Galway; *(E)* Kerry; *(F)* Limerick; *(G)* Louth; *(H)* Offaly; *(I)* Waterford. (Adapted from O'Mullane et al.[47])

such as Indiana, Illinois, Iowa, and Minnesota, where 65% to 88% of the population are already served by optimally fluoridated water supplies, it is probable that the small proportion of the population residing in nonfluoridated areas is in fact receiving foods and beverages manufactured in fluoridated areas of those states. Accordingly, these "nonfluoridated" populations are in fact getting not only topical but some systemic fluoride, albeit not optimal, which would account for the decrease in caries.

However, such findings of a secular decline in the prevalence of caries in nonfluoridated communities should not be interpreted as meaning that water fluoridation is no longer necessary. Caries reductions are greatest where water fluoridation *and* topical fluorides are used, as illustrated in Ireland (Fig 11-5). In every county surveyed, caries had decreased between 1964 and 1984,[47] but the decrease was consistently greatest in those communities in the same county where the schoolchildren were exposed to both communally fluoridated water and topical fluoride. An unfortunate lesson of stopping water fluoridation should not be forgotten; in Antigo, Wisconsin, where water fluoridation was begun in 1949 but discontinued in November 1960 and not reinstated until October 1965, the caries prevalence increased remarkably (about

100%) between 1960 and 1966.[40] Similarly, in Wick, Scotland, which had fluoridated water in 1969 but stopped fluoridation in 1979, the caries prevalence in 5- to 6-year-old children increased by 27% between 1979 and 1984, despite a national decline in caries and the universal availability of fluoridated dentifrices.[59] Clearly, abandoning water fluoridation and relying only on topical forms of fluoride therapy is a mistake and is not borne out by the available evidence.

Opponents of water fluoridation have questioned its safety, yet careful comparison of communities with optimal versus those with suboptimal levels of fluoride in the water supplies reveals no significant differences in the frequency of birth defects or in mortality statistics (including heart disease, cancer, and stroke).[30] Very thorough medical examinations of children in fluoridated and nonfluoridated communities were undertaken in some of the initial studies of controlled water fluoridation; no significant differences in health or in growth and development were found. One study was very detailed and included tonsillectomy rates, height and weight, onset of menstruation, bone density by radiographic examination of hands and knees, skeletal maturation, hemoglobin level, erythrocyte count, leukocyte count, urinalysis, and skin moisture, texture, color, and eruptions. The conclusion of this long-term pediatric study was that, aside from reduced caries, there was no indication of any systemic effects, adverse or otherwise, from the use of fluoridated water.[54] Subsequent studies on the effects of water-borne fluoride on general health have focused on cancer, heart disease, allergies, mental and neurological abnormalities, endocrine function, eyes, liver, kidney, skin, bones, joints, and the digestive, circulatory, and respiratory systems. These investigations have failed to show any significant differences in mortality and morbidity attributable to fluoridation at the recommended levels.[52]

Communal water fluoridation continues to be the cornerstone of an ideal caries prevention program. Its efficacy in reducing caries prevalence has been amply demonstrated. Its safety has also been well established. The cost-benefit ratio is impressive, but even more important are the value of teeth saved from extraction and the avoidance of pain and discomfort and of time lost from school and work.

Fluoridation of school water supplies

Because central water supplies are not available to large segments of the world's population, other methods of delivering the benefits of water-borne fluorides have been sought. In rural areas remote from any community water fluoridation, research has shown that adjusting the fluoride content of a school's water supply will produce a reduction in dental caries with no objectionable dental fluorosis. Children spend annually from 20% to 25% of their total waking hours in school. To compensate for this part-time exposure to fluoride, the currently recommended level for school water fluoridation is 4.5 times the optimum amount recommended for community water fluoridation in the same geographic area. The main disadvantage of school fluoridation is that children are 5 to 6 years old before they begin attending school and drinking the water. Maximum caries prevention accrues when fluoridated water is consumed from birth.

Fluoride supplements

Communal water fluoridation is the method of choice in providing systemic fluoride: the benefits accrue automatically with no conscious effort required. Where communal water fluoridation is not feasible because people have individual wells (about 20% of the US population) or where apathy and political opposition prevent its implementation, fluoride supplements offer an alternative source of systemic fluoride. Fluoride tablets, drops, or lozenges have been proven unequivocally to be effective cariostatic agents, provided such supplements are taken continuously on a daily basis from birth to about 14 years of age. The cariostatic effects of fluoride supplements have ranged from less than 10% to more than 80%, depending on how soon after birth supplementation starts, on the degree of compliance, and the dosage.[20] The highest caries reductions have been reported in private pediatric practices, where there has been a high degree of motivation on the part of the professionals who prescribe the supplements, parents who give the supplements to their young children, and the children themselves, as they get older and assume responsibility for taking them. Furthermore, the dosage used (0.5 mg fluoride from birth) exceeded what is currently recommended (0.25 mg fluoride from birth to 2 years of age). When fluoride supplements have been distributed on a large scale, such as by community health centers, well-baby clinics, and county health departments, caries reductions were generally lower because long-term compliance was not as good. The failure to comply has been due, in a large part, to inadequate patient education and an insufficiently informed health provider.

The correct dosage in prescribing fluoride supplements depends on two factors: the age of the child, and the existing fluoride concentration in the water supply (Table 11-2). The latter information can be obtained from the local water supply authority or, in the case of private wells, will require individual analysis. Failure to determine the fluoride concentration in the water source can result in overdosage and consequent dental fluorosis. For young infants, drops are more convenient because they can be dispensed directly into the child's mouth with a medicine dropper or added to foods (such as cereals) or beverages (such as milk, formula, or juices). For older children whose primary teeth have erupted, fluoride tablets or lozenges are indicated, as these provide both systemic benefits when swallowed and topical benefits as they are swished around the mouth. Fluoride tablets or lozenges are available in 0.25, 0.50, and 1 mg dosages. Not more than 120 mg of fluoride (264 mg sodium fluoride) should be dispensed in any one container, and the container should be

Table 11-2 Supplemental fluoride dosage schedule (mg/d*) according to fluoride concentration of drinking water

	Concentration of fluoride in drinking water (ppm)		
Age (yr)	Less than 0.3	0.3 to 0.7	Greater than 0.7
Birth to 2	0.25	0	0
2 to 3	0.50	0.25	0
3 to 16	1.00	0.50	0

*2.2 mg sodium fluoride contains 1 mg fluoride.

Table 11-3 Sample fluoride prescription for a 4-year-old child residing in a community where the water contains 0.1 ppm fluoride

Name:	Jane Doe
Address:	23 Eighth Avenue, Santa Rosa, CA
Age:	4 years
R_x:	Tabs sodium fluoride 2.2 mg
Disp:	120 tablets
Directions:	One tablet daily to be chewed and swished in mouth for 1 minute before swallowing.
Warning:	Keep out of reach of children.
Refill:	3 times
	E. Oldspring, DMD

provided with a child-proof top and labeled: "Caution—store out of reach of children." A sample prescription of a fluoride supplement for a 4-year-old child residing in a community with 0.1 ppm fluoride in the water supply is shown in Table 11-3.

Not enough data exist to establish the efficacy of prenatal supplements, given to pregnant mothers, in reducing caries in the offspring.[21] Accordingly, the Food and Drug Administration does not permit any fluoride preparation to be labeled, represented, or advertised "for prenatal use." Only a portion of the enamel of the primary teeth (mostly of the incisors) is formed at birth, and no permanent teeth are mineralized except the tips of the first molars. It is therefore more important to ensure that, when indicated, adequate fluoride supplements are taken regularly after birth. The concentration of total fluoride in human milk is about 0.05 ppm, and of cow's milk about 0.1 ppm. Hence, both types of milk are a negligible source of fluoride. Nevertheless, in most cases there is no need to supplement breast-fed children who reside in optimally fluoridated communities. Because the median duration of nursing in the United States is only 4 months and exclusive breast-feeding is uncommon, the amount of fluoride obtained from the optimally fluoridated water, used in preparing formula and baby food, will suffice. However, if the infant resides in a suboptimally fluoridated community, the dosage schedule shown in Table 11-2 should be followed. Vitamins do not enhance or potentiate the caries-preventive effects of fluoride supplements, but they do increase the cost to the patient. If the child needs vitamins, a fluoride-vitamin combination may be more convenient, but children are unlikely to require vitamins from birth to their teens, as they do fluoride. Unfortunately, some fluoride-vitamin preparations contain as much as 60% total sugar as a sweetener to mask the taste of some of the B vitamins. Such products are contraindicated for caries prevention.

Topical fluoride

Professional application

The topical application of concentrated fluoride preparations (2% sodium fluoride, 8% stannous fluoride, or acidulated phosphate fluoride containing 1.23% fluoride) by a dentist or dental hygienist is an established caries-preventive procedure. Neutral sodium fluoride solutions (2%) were first tested in the early 1940s and were shown to reduce caries by about 30%. Teeth were first cleaned with pumice paste and the solution was applied to the teeth for 3 minutes. The application, but not the pumicing, was repeated at weekly intervals for a total of four applications each at ages 3, 7, 11, and 13.[38] This sequence of application was used more widely in public health programs than in private practice. In the 1950s stannous fluoride (8%) solutions were introduced. The procedure again involved coronal polishing, and the stannous fluoride was applied for 4 minutes semiannually.[23] Aqueous stannous fluoride solutions, however, have several disadvantages: they undergo rapid hydrolysis and oxidation (and thus must be prepared freshly for each treatment), and they are astringent and have an unpleasant taste.

By far the most popular form of office fluoride therapy is the application of acidulated phosphate fluoride (APF) in the form of a solution or a gel. Use of these agents provides a 25% to 40% reduction in caries. APF agents should have a pH of approximately 3 and contain 1.23% fluoride and 0.1 M orthophosphoric acid.[65] The low pH favors more rapid fluoride uptake by enamel, and the presence of the orthophosphate prevents enamel dissolution by the common ion effect. Application of these solutions or gels is often preceded by a coronal polishing. This removes exogenous stains and temporarily removes plaque but does not affect the cariostatic potential of the topical fluoride agent. Recent clinical trials indicate the efficacy of the gels was similar whether there was a coronal polishing or not.[49] The agent itself should be applied for 4 minutes, usually in a disposable tray applicator. Some commercial products have been promoted based on claims that they need be applied for only 1 minute instead of 4 minutes. Such claims have not been supported by clinical trials demonstrating caries reductions. Until such time, a 4-minute application of the agent is the method of choice, and the procedure should be repeated semiannually.

APF preparations contain hydrogen and fluoride ions that react with glass components in restorative materials. Single applications may not cause a problem, but repeated applications (particularly if used daily in a self-applied prevention program) may result in loss of material, surface roughening, and changes in the esthetic appearance of porcelain or composite resin restorations. Accordingly, for patients with extensive restorations of this type who require frequent fluoride therapy, nonacidic fluoride preparations are recommended.[12]

To allow topical fluoride more time to react with the enamel and thereby increase its uptake, fluoride varnishes have been developed. Two such products are currently available in Canada, Europe, and some other countries, but they are not marketed in the United States. Duraphat (Woelm Pharma) contains 2.26% fluoride (as sodium fluoride) in an alcoholic suspension of rosin. Fluor Protector (Vivadent) contains 0.7% fluoride (as difluorosilane) in a polyurethane varnish. Application of the fluoride varnishes is quick and easy, as they set rapidly and stick to the teeth. Clinical studies of caries prevention show a range of efficacy, depending on study design and frequency of application.[10,54] Generally, Duraphat has provided caries reductions equivalent to those of APF solutions and gels, whereas Fluor Protector has not resulted in equivalent reductions.

Safety considerations

Because topical agents used in the dental office contain relatively high concentrations of fluoride (12,000 to 22,600 ppm), the operator should take certain precautions to prevent the patient from inadvertently ingesting these agents.[31] If solutions are used, the teeth should be carefully isolated with cotton rolls or gauze swabs and only enough solution applied to wet the surfaces of the teeth and keep them wet. If gels in trays are to be used, only a minimum amount of gel should be dispensed in the tray, sufficient to cover the teeth but not to exude from the tray. A saliva ejector, or better still, high-vacuum suction, should be maintained during the 4-minute application of the agent. On removal of the tray, any excess gel should be wiped away from the teeth and gingiva with gauze; the patient should be instructed to expectorate thoroughly. The recommended procedures to reduce fluoride ingestion from professional gel tray applications are summarized in Table 11-4.

Table 11-4 Recommended procedures to reduce fluoride ingestion from professional gel-tray applications

- Place patient in upright position
- Warn patient not to swallow the gel
- Use small amounts (no more than 2.5 ml per tray)
- Use custom-fitted or stock trays with absorptive liners
- Use suction
- Remove excessive gel from teeth and gingiva with gauze
- Have patient expectorate thoroughly after treatment

Self-applied topical fluoride in the home

One of the most effective means of caries reduction involves the daily self-application of 0.5% fluoride gel (5,000 ppm F, about 40% of the concentration used for professional office applications) in custom-fitted trays for 5 minutes daily. The custom-fitted maxillary and mandibular trays (Toplicators) are fashioned by vacuum drawing heat-treated sheets of polyvinyl over plaster models of the teeth. This procedure, first tested in supervised school programs, reduced decay in a nonfluoridated community by about 75% and in a fluoridated community by about 30% after 2 years.[25,26] This form of self-therapy is best suited for high-caries-risk patients who are sufficiently motivated to conform with the daily regimen. It is not intended for very young children, but it is appropriate for those of school age and also benefits adults with xerostomia secondary to therapeutic irradiation of the head and neck region.[19] The advantage of the technique is that fluoride preparations are held in intimate contact with the teeth daily for 5 minutes. Saliva is excluded from the field of application, thereby maintaining the effective concentration of the active agent in the gel. Intermittent biting pressure on the plastic trays tends to pump the gel into pits, fissures, and interproximal spaces. Because the trays are custom-made, a minimum amount of gel (usually 0.5 ml) is required in each tray. The main disadvantages are the relatively high cost of fabricating individual trays for each patient and the dependence on the patient's cooperation.

Self-application by brushing with 0.4% stannous fluoride gel (1,000 ppm F) has been used as an alternative to the custom-fitted tray method and has been actively promoted by several commercial manufacturers of these products. Many of these stannous fluoride gels have been accepted by the ADA Council on Dental Therapeutics; however, they vary considerably in the amount of available tin ion,[62] which also exerts some antibacterial effect. The original formulation, developed at the Veterans' Administration Hospitals, had an unpleasant taste, so that many of the high-caries-risk patients either refused to use the gel or used it only sporadically. The commercial products have more acceptable flavors, which encourage better compliance. Because fluoride uptake is time-dependent,[36] applying a gel containing 1,000 ppm fluoride for approximately 1 minute by brushing will not provide as much fluoride uptake as from a gel in a custom-fitted tray containing 5,000 ppm fluoride applied for 5 minutes. No direct comparisons of the clinical efficacy of these two techniques are available.

Fluoride mouthrinses

In the mid 1960s, Scandinavian researchers studying a population with very high caries activity that included many smooth surface lesions, showed that a biweekly rinse for 1 minute with a solution of 0.2% sodium fluoride (900 ppm F) was as effective in reducing decay as were professionally applied topical fluoride treatments, and about as effective as the daily use of the fluoride dentifrices then available.[63] Furthermore, daily rinsing for 1 minute with an even more dilute solution containing 0.05% sodium fluoride (230 ppm F) gave even greater caries protection. The benefits from fluoride mouthrinsing range from 20% to 50% less decay. The original Scandinavian findings have since been reproduced in many different countries in the world, so that now a weekly fluoride rinse has become widely adopted in many school-based preventive dentistry programs. The popularity of the weekly rinse is based on the fact that it is safe, effective, relatively inexpensive, easy to learn, requires little time (about 5 minutes of class time weekly), and can be supervised by non-dental personnel. Compliance may vary and is generally better in elementary schools than in junior and senior high schools. Compliance will also depend on whether the classroom teachers and the administration of the school are successfully motivated and interested in the preventive dentistry program. Fluoride mouthrinses, when originally introduced, were prescription items, and the 0.2% sodium fluoride rinse still is. But in 1983 the Food and Drug Administration approved the sale of 0.05% sodium fluoride mouthrinses, 0.1% stannous fluoride mouthrinse, and 0.4% stannous fluoride gels for sale as over-the-counter products.[27] In the case of the 0.05% sodium fluoride rinse, 10 ml of the solution, the recommended dosage, contains only 2.3 mg of fluoride. The products are packaged with child-proof caps, and their labels state that use is restricted to persons 6 years of age and older.[32] The rinse should be swished between the teeth for 1 minute and then expectorated. The patient, parent, or teacher needs to be advised of these instructions, both to ensure that the agent is present for sufficient time and to avoid unnecessary ingestion of the rinse.

Fluoride dentifrices

In the 1940s the first clinical evaluations of dentifrices containing fluoride were undertaken. These were products in which fluoride was simply incorporated into existing dentifrice formulations. Because the abrasive systems used in these early dentifrices ($CaHPO_4$, $CaCO_3$) contained calcium ions, which interfered with the availability of the fluoride ion, these products were ineffective in reducing decay. The first fluoride-containing dentifrice reported to decrease the incidence of caries, as compared with the similar use of a nonfluoride dentifrice, contained stannous fluoride (0.4%) together with calcium pyrophosphate that had been heat-treated to increase its compatibility with fluoride.[43] In 1960 this dentifrice was given provisional acceptance, and in 1964 full acceptance, by the ADA Council on Dental Therapeutics. This acceptance stimulated other manufacturers to develop and test various fluoride formulations and abrasive systems. The sale of these products in 1987 was about $1.2 billion annually in the United States, where over 95% of all toothpastes sold contain some form of fluoride. With few exceptions, similar changes have occurred in the dentifrice market in most Western industrialized countries. The original stannous fluoride market has been superseded by more compatible and more effective formulations. Clinically effective fluoride-abrasive systems that are more-or-less compatible are summarized in Table 11-5.

Sodium monofluorosphosphate (MFP) (Fig 11-6) was first tested as a therapeutic agent in dentifrices in the early 1960s. Numerous clinical trials of dentifrices containing 0.76% or 0.8% MFP have since been conducted by different groups in various countries. In almost all these trials some degree of effectiveness, about 25% less caries, has been demonstrated.[17] In the United States, MFP at 0.76%, or 1,000 ppm fluoride, is the most commonly used therapeutic ingredient in commercial toothpastes.

Sodium fluoride was the first form of fluoride to be tested in a toothpaste and was originally found ineffective because of incompatibility with the earlier abrasive systems used.[5] Later, when tested with acrylic particles or hydrated silica as the abrasive, sodium fluoride was found to give significant cariostatic benefits. Several commercial products now use sodium fluoride as the active therapeutic ingredient.

A dose-response effect has been documented both with sodium fluoride and with MFP dentifrices (Table 11-6). A sodium fluoride toothpaste tested at 0, 250, 500, and 1,000 ppm fluoride gave the greatest caries reduction at the highest fluoride concentration.[48] A sodium fluoride formulation (1,100 ppm F) with silica abrasive was found more effective than the earlier stannous fluoride–calcium pyrophosphate dentifrice, undoubtedly because of the greater availability of the fluoride ion in this newer system.[3,66] A sodium fluoride–silica abrasive dentifrice showed significantly more caries reduction at 2,800 ppm fluoride than at 1,100 ppm fluoride.[41] Similarly, dentifrices with less MFP are less effective,[42] and dentifrices with more MFP (1,500 ppm F) are more effective.[7,34,59] Dentifrices with these higher concentrations of fluoride should bear a clear warning label that children under 6 years of age should apply only a pea-sized amount of dentifrice on the brush, and that the dentifrice should be expectorated after use to avoid unintentional ingestion and the potential risk of enamel fluorosis.

In Europe, an amine fluoride dentifrice containing two compounds, diethanol aminopropyl-N-ethanol octadecylamine-dihydrofluoride and

Table 11-5 Clinically effective fluoride-abrasive systems in dentifrices

Fluoride compound	Abrasive system	Formula
Stannous fluoride (SnF_2)	Calcium pyrophosphate	$Ca_2P_2O_7$
	Insoluble sodium metaphosphate	$(NaPO_3)_x$
	Silica	SiO_2
Sodium fluoride (NaF)	Calcium pyrophosphate	$Ca_2P_2O_7$
	Insoluble sodium metaphosphate	$(NaPO_3)_x$
	Polymethylmethacrylate	$H\text{-}(OR\text{-}CO)_nOH$
	Silica	SiO_2
Sodium monofluorophosphate (Na_2PO_3F)	Calcium carbonate	$CaCO_3$
	Aluminum oxide	Al_2O_3
	Insoluble sodium metaphosphate	$(NaPO_3)_x$
	Silica	SiO_2
	Dicalcium phosphate	$CaHPO_4$
	Calcium pyrophosphate	$Ca_2P_2O_7$
Amine fluoride	Insoluble sodium metaphosphate	$(NaPO_3)_x$

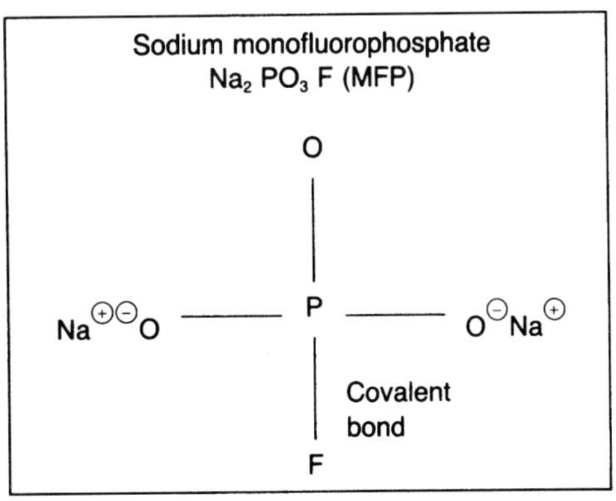

Fig 11-6 Chemical structure of sodium monofluorophosphate (MFP).

cetylamine hydrofluoride (Fig 11-7), at a concentration providing 1,250 ppm fluoride, has been used for many years. Both substances have a long aliphatic chain, containing 16 or 18 carbon atoms, which is responsible for the dentifrice's property of lowering surface tension. This dentifrice is effective in reducing dental decay,[55] but is not superior to the inorganic fluoride dentifrices available in North America.

There is no doubt that widespread use, most commonly twice a day,

Table 11-6 Dose/response efficacy of fluoride dentifrices in reducing caries

Study	Fluoride, ppm (agents)	Duration, (yr)	Supervised use	Diagnostic radiographs	Fluoride dose/response	Comment
Reed (1973)[48]	0/250/500/1000 (NaF)	2	—	√	√	Used $Ca_2P_2O_7$ abrasive, F only partly available
Forsman (1974)[28]	0/250/1000 (MFP & NaF)	2	—	√	√/—	Supervised use of 0.2% NaF rinse biweekly, relatively low caries increments
Hodge et al (1980)[34]	0/1000/1450 (MFP & NaF)	3	√	√	√	Girls demonstrated efficacy more dramatically than boys and had better oral hygiene
Koch et al (1982)[39]	250/1000 (MFP & NaF)	3	—	√	—	Insufficient sample size, chance of not detecting differences
Buhe et al (1984)[7]	0/1000/1500 (MFP)	3	—	√	√	Increasing F level resulted in increased efficacy
Mitropoulos et al (1984)[43]	250/1000 (MFP)	2.7	√	√	√	Reducing F level resulted in lower efficacy
Diodati et al (1986)[18]	1000/1450/2000 (MFP & NaF)	3	—	—	√	Increased efficacy at higher F levels, no significant difference between the higher levels
Stephen et al (1987)[59]	1000/1500/2500 (MFP)	3	—	√	√	Increased efficacy at higher F levels
Lu et al (1987)[41]	1100/2800 (NaF)	3	—	√	√	Increased efficacy at higher NaF levels
Ripa et al (1988)[1]	1000/2500 (MFP & NaF)	3	—	—	—	Poor compliance, dentifrice distasteful, high withdrawal rate

√ Supervised use, diagnostic radiographs available, and positive dose/response observed.
— No supervised use, no diagnostic radiographs available, and no dose/response observed.

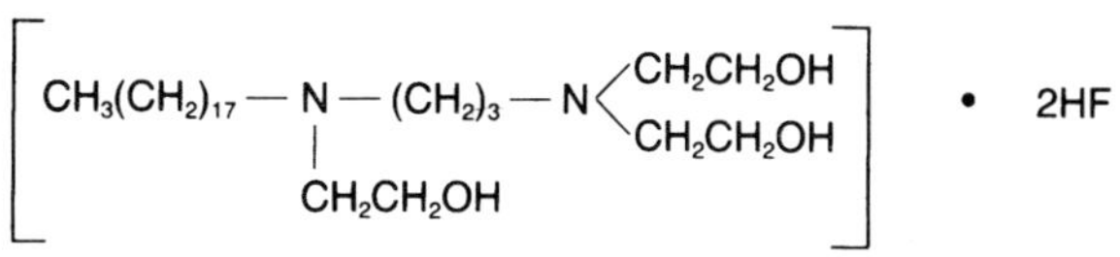

Diethanol aminopropyl-N-ethanol octadecylamine-dihydrofluoride

$CH_3(CH_2)_{15}NH_3^+F^-$

Cetylamine hydrofluoride

Fig 11-7 Chemical structure of the active ingredients in amine fluoride dentifrices: diethanol aminopropyl-N-ethanol octadecylamine-dihydrofluoride and cetylamine hydrofluoride.

of fluoride-containing dentifrices has had a profound effect in reducing caries in many developed countries and accounts for some of the secular decline in caries observed in communities lacking optimal fluoride levels in the water supply. The degree of effectiveness varies with different dentifrice formulations. Dentifrices containing sodium fluoride have been reported as the most effective,[41,60] although the differences are small and not precise enough to draw firm conclusions. Those products that have received acceptance by the ADA Council on Dental Therapeutics, based on clinical trials and/or laboratory testing, are to be recommended in preference to products lacking such evidence of efficacy.[13]

Agents and systems used for topical fluoride therapy

In the previous sections several fluoride compounds have been mentioned that are presently in use (Table 11-7). Those used for professional topical application in the office include sodium fluoride, stannous fluoride, acidulated phosphate fluoride, and fluoride varnishes. Fluoride mouthrinses usually contain either sodium fluoride or stannous fluoride. Currently marketed fluoride dentifrices contain sodium fluoride, sodium monofluorophosphate, or amine fluoride.

In addition, ammonium fluoride and titanium tetrafluoride have been tested in vitro and found to deposit fluoride into enamel. However, when tested clinically, neither of these compounds was superior to sodium fluoride or acidulated phosphate fluoride for preventing caries. Taste considerations make ammonium fluoride a poorer choice than conventional fluoride compounds.

Considerable research has been directed toward increasing the uptake of fluoride by enamel, especially in incipient lesions. One approach has been to increase the time in which fluoride can react with hydroxyapatite

Table 11-7 Topical fluoride agents and systems

Agent
Sodium fluoride (NaF)
Stannous fluoride (SnF_2)
Sodium monofluorophosphate (Na_2PO_3F)
Acidulated phosphate fluoride
Amine fluoride
Titanium fluoride (TiF_4)
System
F + varnish (rosin; polyurethane)
F + complexing agent (aluminum)
F + pretreatment (dicalcium phosphate dihydrate)
F + cationic surfactant (Lodyne; Zonyl FSC)
F + soluble calcium (calcium chloride; calcium glycerophosphate)
F + cationic polyelectrolyte (polyacrylic acid)

by using a varnish film that remains on the teeth for up to 12 hours; however, clinical tests of such varnishes have not found them to be better than APF solutions or gels or biweekly NaF rinses. Pretreatment of the tooth with a complexing agent, such as aluminum, increases fluoride uptake and decreases caries in rats more than does topical NaF alone. Pretreating enamel with dicalcium phosphate dihydrate also enhances fluoride uptake. Fluoride in combination with cationic surfactants gives increased deposition in the enamel and less caries in rodents than the fluoride alone. In vitro artificial carious lesions of enamel show enhanced fluoride uptake from MFP in combination with soluble calcium (calcium chloride) than from MFP alone, but in clinical trials dentifrices containing MFP with soluble calcium (calcium glycerophosphate) were only slightly better in reducing caries than MFP alone.

Cationic polyelectrolytes exhibit a tremendous capacity for increasing fluoride reactivity, resulting in a several times greater uptake of fluoride in sound and carious enamel. Adsorption of these polymers on a solid surface is accomplished by the attachment of numerous functional groups along the macromolecular backbone. Based on this technology, a delivery system, consisting of sodium fluoride and polyacrylic acid with a strontium bridge to form a "polyampholyte" (containing both positive and negative charges), has been developed that can enhance fluoride uptake in vitro and provides significant caries reduction in rats. The sodium fluoride–strontium polyacrylate system has recently been introduced in a commercial fluoride dentifrice and mouthrinse.

Fluoride toxicology

Paracelsus said, "All substances are poison; there is none which is not a poison. The right dose differentiates a poison and a remedy." Fluoride falls into the category of Class 4 "very toxic" drugs, together with aspirin, phenobarbital, quinidine, and chlorpromazine. When ingested in amounts of 1 to 3 mg per day, as would be the case in optimally fluoridated communities, it is perfectly safe. However, 5 to 10 grams of sodium fluoride (2.5 to 5 g fluoride) are certainly a lethal dosage for an adult, and lesser amounts are toxic for children. Incidents of acute fluoride poisoning have been recorded, either as a result of accidents from the use of household insecticides containing fluoride, or from deliberate attempts at suicide. Persons with severe fluoride poisonings characteristically exhibit:

1. Nausea; vomiting; diarrhea
2. Progressive hypotension; intense hypocalcemia and hypomagnesemia; acidosis
3. Cardiac irregularities; ventricular tachycardia and fibrillation; sometimes asystole

Successful treatment is based on early initiation of the following procedures:

1. Cardiac monitoring; preparation for endotracheal intubation and for direct-current cardioversion
2. Prompt and frequent blood analyses, especially for calcium, magnesium, potassium, pH
3. IV infusion as needed of fluids to restore blood volume of calcium gluconate or chloride, and of magnesium, potassium, and bicarbonate to restore calcium and magnesium levels to normal ranges and to correct other imbalances observed in serum analyses or inferred from electrocardiographic signs
4. Alkaline diuresis to speed fluoride excretion
5. Appropriate treatment of severe cardiac arrhythmias

Only two dentally related fluoride fatalities have been recorded. One case followed office topical therapy in which inappropriate agents and procedures were used and no adequate treatment was provided for management of this overdose.[9] The other case resulted from a child's ingesting 200 fluoride tablets from a container that did not have a childproof cap.[24] When normal procedures are followed, as outlined in the preceding sections, the topical application of fluoride agents in the office or the self-application of fluoride agents in the home does not pose a risk of acute toxicity.

Guide to the use of fluoride agents

Several studies have documented that the cariostatic benefits of fluoride therapy can be increased by combining the use of one vehicle with that of another. In other words, the caries-preventive effects are additive. The forms of fluoride treatment that are best indicated for the individual patient depend on his or her caries risk, which is best assessed as discussed in chapter 8.

Systemic fluoride supplements are indicated for all children under 16 years of age who reside in communities with suboptimal fluoride concentrations in the water supplies. Fluoride dentifrices, in preference to fluoride-free dentifrices, are recommended for all patients, children and adults, irrespective of whether they live in fluoridated or nonfluoridated communities. Since fluoride dentifrices cost no more than other dentifrices and their regular use inhibits caries by 20% to 30%, they should be used throughout life.

For patients with active caries who continue to develop new or recurrent lesions in spite of using fluoride dentifrices, additional forms of fluoride therapy are required. Such patients should receive semiannual topical fluoride applications of APF gel in the dental office and should also use a daily fluoride mouthrinse concurrently with a fluoride dentifrice. Such combined therapy is appropriate for anyone over 6 years of age.

If these combined measures fail to control caries in patients at extreme caries risk, such as those with xerostomia, or in patients with rampant caries involving tooth surfaces that do not commonly develop caries, more intensive fluoride therapy is required. More frequent (four times per year) professionally applied topical fluoride (1.23%) with APF gel has been proposed.[50] In addition, the daily self-application of 0.5% fluoride gel in a custom-fitted tray is recommended. Of course, other preventive measures, such as sealing occlusal fissures, suppressing *S mutans* levels with antibacterial agents, and restricting sugar intake, should all be included as part of a comprehensive caries prevention program. Furthermore, the need to continue such intensive and demanding preventive intervention should be reevaluated at regular intervals. If no caries has occurred for two recall visits or 1 year, the daily gel application can be discontinued and a low-concentration fluoride rinse used instead. Similarly, semiannual rather than quarterly office applications of APF gels can be resumed.

Chapter review

- List the various hypotheses that have been proposed to explain the caries-preventive mechanism of fluoride action. Indicate which ones are considered to be the most important. Explain how the mechanism of action is dependent on the fluoride concentration.
- Graph the relationships between caries prevalence, endemic dental fluorosis, and the fluoride content of the water supplies.

- Define optimal fluoridation. State how the level of optimal fluoridation varies with air temperature.
- State the modal percent caries reduction observed as a result of water fluoridation in studies conducted between the 1950s and 1970s, and the range of percent caries reductions reported in the 1980s. Explain the difference.
- State the concentration of fluoride used in school water fluoridation and explain why this is in excess of the optimal level set for community water fluoridation.
- State the maximum amount of *(1)* sodium fluoride and *(2)* fluoride ion that may be dispensed at any one time for home use.
- State the amounts of fluoride recommended at *(1)* birth to 2 years old, *(2)* 2 to 3 years old, *(3)* 3 years and older, for children living in a community with known amounts of fluoride in the communal water supplies (from 0.1 to 1 ppm).
- Write a prescription for a fluoride supplement *(1)* in drop form and *(2)* in tablet form for a child, given the child's age and the fluoride concentration in the communal water supply.
- State the policy of the Food and Drug Administration concerning claims of efficacy for prenatal fluoride products.
- List the advantages and disadvantages of using fluoride-vitamin combination supplements.
- List *(1)* the compounds used for professional topical application of fluoride, *(2)* the concentration of each agent used for such application, and *(3)* the recommended frequency for each of these topical applications.
- List the disadvantages of stannous fluoride for topical application.
- List the various techniques for self-administration of topical fluorides. Identify which has given maximum caries reduction.
- List the recommended clinical procedures for reducing unintentional fluoride ingestion by children during the professional application of a topical fluoride gel.
- Tabulate the fluoride concentrations (in ppm) of self-applied fluoride rinses, stannous fluoride gels and fluoride dentifrices, and professionally applied stannous fluoride solutions and APF gels.
- Identify the fluoride compounds currently used in commercial dentifrices.
- State the problems encountered in formulating a therapeutic dentifrice.
- Graph the relationship between the available fluoride content of a dentifrice and caries increments during use of the dentifrice.

- List the signs and symptoms that follow an acute lethal dose of fluoride. State the steps necessary to treat such an overdose.
- Outline a sequence of self-applied and/or professional treatments with available fluoride agents for patients at *(1)* low, *(2)* moderate, and *(3)* high caries risk.

Selected readings

Ekstrand, J., Fejerskov, O., and Silverstone, L.M. (eds) 1988. *Fluoride in Dentistry*. Copenhagen: Munksgaard.

Johansen, E., Taves, D.R., and Olsen, T.O. (eds) 1979. Continuing evaluation of the use of fluorides. AAAS Selected Symposium 11. Boulder: Westview Press.

McClure, F.J. 1962. Fluoride drinking waters. Washington, D.C.: U.S. Government Printing Office, Public Health Service Publication No. 825.

Mellberg, J.R., and Ripa, L.W. 1983. *Fluoride in Preventive Dentistry*. Chicago: Quintessence Publ Co.

Murray, J.J. (ed) 1986. *Appropriate Use of Fluorides for Human Health*. Geneva: World Health Organization.

Newbrun, E. (ed) 1986. *Fluorides and Dental Caries*. 3rd ed. Springfield, Ill.: Charles C Thomas.

Ripa, L. (ed) 1986. *A Guide to the Use of Fluorides for the Prevention of Dental Caries*. 2nd ed. Denver: National Foundation of Dentistry for the Handicapped.

Wei, S.H.Y. (ed) 1985. *Clinical Uses of Fluorides*. Philadelphia: Lea & Febiger.

References

1. Arends, J., and Gelhard, T.B.F.M. 1983. In vivo remineralisation of human enamel. In *Demineralisation and Remineralisation of the Teeth*, S.J. Leach and W.M. Egar (eds), Oxford: IRL Press, pp. 1–6.
2. Banting, D.W. 1984. Dental caries in the elderly. *Gerodontology* 3:55–61.
3. Beiswanger, B.D., Gish, C.W., and Mallatt, M.E. 1981. A three-year study of the effect of a sodium fluoride-silica abrasive dentifrice on dental caries. *Pharmacol Ther Dent* 6:9–16.
4. Bell, R.M., Klein, S.P., Bohannan, H.M., Graves, R.C., and Disney, J.A. 1982. Results of baseline dental exams in the national preventive dentistry demonstration program. R2862-RWJ, Rand Corporation, Santa Monica, CA 90406, p. 31.
5. Bibby, B.G. 1945. Test of the effect of fluoride-containing dentifrices on dental caries. *J Dent Res* 24:297–303.
6. Brunelle, J.A., Miller, A.J., and Smith, J.I. 1983. DMFS in U.S. children with and without lifelong exposure to water fluoridation. *J Dent Res* 62:(Sp. Issue, Abstr. 302): 203.
7. Buhe, H., Buttner, W., and Barlage, B. 1984. Uber einen dreijahrigen klinischen Zahncremetest mit Zahnpasten unterschiedlicher Fluoridkonzentration 0.8% und 1.2% Natriummonofluorphosphat. *Quintessenz* 1:103–111.
8. Burt, B.A., Ismail, A.I., and Eklund, S.A. 1986. Root caries in an optimally fluoridated and a high-fluoride community. *J Dent Res* 65:1154–1158.
9. Church, L.E. 1976. Fluorides—use with caution. *J Md State Dent Assoc* 19:106.
10. Clark, D.C. 1982. A review on fluoride varnishes: an alternative topical fluoride treatment. *Community Dent Oral Epidemiol* 10:117–123.
11. Consensus Report. 1985. *Prevention and Treatment of Caries*. Copenhagen: Danish Medical Research Council.
12. Council on Dental Materials, Instruments, and Equipment. 1988. Status report: effect of acidulated phosphate fluoride on procelain and composite restorations. *J Am Dent Assoc* 116:115.

13. Council on Dental Therapeutics. 1986. Guidelines for the acceptance of fluoride-containing dentifrices. *J Am Dent Assoc* 110:545–547.
14. Dean, H.T. 1942. The investigation of physiological effects by the epidemiological method. In *Fluorine and Dental Health,* F.R. Moulton (ed), Washington, D.C.: American Association for the Advancement of Science, Pub. no. 19, pp. 23–31.
15. Dean, H.T. 1946. Epidemiological studies in the United States. In *Dental Caries and Fluorine,* F.R. Moulton (ed), Washington, D.C.: American Association for the Advancement of Science, pp. 5–31.
16. de Leifde, B., and Herbison, G.P. 1985. Prevalence of developmental defects of enamel and dental caries in New Zealand children receiving differing fluoride supplementation. *Community Dent Oral Epidemiol* 13:164–167.
17. DePaola, P.F. 1983. Clinical studies of monofluorophosphate dentifrices. *Caries Res* 17(Suppl. 1):119–135.
18. Diodati, R.R., Triol, C.W., Kranz, S.M., Korn, L.R., and Volpe, A.R. 1986. Clinical anticaries effect of various fluoride dentifrices. *J Dent Res* 65(Sp. Issue, Abstr. 258): 198.
19. Dreizen, S., Brown, L.R., Daly, T.E., and Drane, J.B. 1977. Prevention of xerostomia-related dental caries in irradiated cancer patients. *J Dent Res* 56:99–104.
20. Driscoll, W. 1974. The use of fluoride tablets for the prevention of dental caries. In *International Workshop on Fluorides and Dental Caries Reductions,* D. Forrester and E. Schulz (eds), Baltimore: University of Maryland, pp. 25–96.
21. Driscoll, W. 1981. A review of clinical research on the use of prenatal fluoride administration for prevention of dental caries. *J Dent Child* 48:109–177.
22. Driscoll, W.S., Heifetz, S.B., Horowitz, H.S., Kingman, A., Meyers, R.J., and Zimmerman, E.R. 1986. Prevalance of dental caries and dental fluorosis in areas with negligible, optimal, and above-optimal fluoride concentrations in drinking water. *J Am Dent Assoc* 113:29–33.
23. Dudding, N.J., and Muhler, J.C. 1962. Technique of application of stannous fluoride in a compatible prophylactic paste and as a topical agent. *J Dent Child* 29:219–224.
24. Eichler, H.G., Lenz, K., Fuhrmann, M., and Hruby, K. 1982. Accidental ingestion of NaF tablets by children—report of a poison control center and one case. *Int J Clin Pharmacol Ther Toxicol* 20:334–338.
25. Englander, H.R., Keyes, P.H., Gestwicki, M., and Sultz, H.A. 1967. Clinical anticaries effect of repeated topical sodium fluoride applications by mouthpieces. *J Am Dent Assoc* 75:638–644.
26. Englander, H.R., Sherrill, L.T., Miller, B.G., Carlos, J.P., Mellberg, J.R., and Senning, R.S. 1971. Incremental rates of dental caries after repeated topical sodium fluoride applications in children with lifelong consumption of fluoridated water. *J Am Dent Assoc* 82:354–358.
27. Food and Drug Administration. 1983. Prescription drugs switched to OTC. FDA *Drug Bulletin* 13:29.
28. Forsman, B. 1974. Studies on the effect of dentifrices with low fluoride content. *Community Dent Oral Epidemiol* 2:166–175.
29. Gray, A.S. 1987. Fluoridation, time for a new base line? *J Can Dent Assoc* 53:763–765.
30. Hagan, T.L., Pasternack, M., and Scholz, G.C. 1954. Water-borne fluorides and mortality. *Public Health Rep* 69:450–454.
31. Heifetz, S.B., and Horowitz, H.S. 1984. The amounts of fluoride in current fluoride therapies: safety considerations for children. *J Dent Child* 51:257–269.
32. Heifetz, S.B., and Horowitz, H.S. 1986. Amounts of fluoride in self-administered dental products: safety considerations for children. *Pediatrics* 77:876–882.
33. Hodge, H.C. 1950. The concentration of fluorides in drinking water to give the point of minimum caries with maximum safety. *J Am Dent Assoc* 40:436–439.
34. Hodge, H.C., Holloway, P.J., Davies, T.G.H., and Worthington, H.V. 1980. Caries prevention by dentifrices containing a combination of sodium monofluorophosphate and sodium fluoride. *Br Dent J* 149:201–204.
35. Horowitz, H. 1980. Combinations of caries-preventive agents and procedures. *J Dent Res* 59:2183–2189.
36. Joyston-Bechal, S., Duckworth, R., and Braden, M. 1973. The mechanism of uptake of ^{18}F by enamel from sodium fluoride and acidulated phosphate fluoride solution labeled with ^{18}F. *Arch Oral Biol* 18:1077–1089.
37. Katz, R.V., Jensen, M.E., and Meskin, L.H. 1983. Dental caries prevalence in a community of schoolchildren: fluoridated vs. non-fluoridated. *J Dent Res* 62(Sp. Issue, Abstr. 296): 202.
38. Knutson, J.W. 1948. Sodium fluoride solutions: technic for application to the teeth.

J Am Dent Assoc 36:37–39.
39. Koch, G., Petersson, L.-G., Kling, E., and Kling, L. 1982. Effect of 250 and 1000 ppm fluoride dentifrice in caries. *Scand Dent J* 6:233–238.
40. Lemke, C.W., Doherty, J.M., and Arra, M.C. 1970. Controlled fluoridation: the dental effects of discontinuation in Antigo, Wisconsin. *J Am Dent Assoc* 80:782–786.
41. Lu, K.H., Ruhlman, C.D., Chung, K.L., Sturzenberger, O.P., and Lehnhoff, R.W. 1987. A three-year clinical comparison of a sodium monofluorophosphate dentifrice with sodium fluoride dentifrices on dental caries in children. *J Dent Child* 54: 241–244.
42. Mitropoulos, C.M., Holloway, P.J., Davies, T.G.H., and Worthington, H.V. 1984. Relative efficacy of dentifrices containing 250 or 1000 ppm F in preventing dental caries—report of a 32-month clinical trial. *Community Dent Health* 1:198–200.
43. Muhler, J.C., Radike, A.W., Nebergall, W.H., and Day, H.G. 1954. The effect of stannous fluoride-containing dentifrice on caries reduction in children. *J Dent Res* 33:606–612.
44. Murray, J.J. 1971. Adult dental health in fluoride and non-fluoride areas. *Br Dent J* 131:391–395, 437–442.
45. Murray, J.J., and Rugg-Gunn, A.J. 1982. *Fluorides and Dental Caries.* 2nd ed. Bristol: John Wright & Sons, Ltd.
46. Newbrun, E. (ed) 1986. *Fluorides and Dental Caries.* 3rd ed. Springfield, Ill.: Charles C Thomas, p. 9.
47. O'Mullane, D., Clarkson, J., Holland, T., O'Hickey, S., and Whelton, H. 1986. Children's dental health in Ireland. 1984. Stationery Office, Dublin: Government Publications, p. 39.
48. Reed, M.W. 1973. Clinical evaluation of three concentrations of sodium fluoride in dentifrices. *J Am Dent Assoc* 80:1401–1403.
49. Ripa, L.W. 1984. Need for prior toothcleaning when performing a professional topical fluoride application: review and recommendations for change. *J Am Dent Assoc* 109:281–285.
50. Ripa, L. (ed). 1986. *A Guide to the Use of Fluorides for the Prevention of Dental Caries.* 2nd ed. Denver: National Foundation of Dentistry for the Handicapped.
51. Ripa, L., Leske, G., Forte, F., and Varma, A. 1988. Caries inhibition of mixed NaF-Na_2PO_3F dentifrices containing 1,000 and 2,000 ppm F: 3-year results. *J Am Dent Assoc* 116:69–73.
52. Royal College of Physicians. 1976. *Fluoride, Teeth and Health.* London: Pitman Publishing Ltd.
53. Russell, A.L., and Elvove, E. 1951. Domestic water and dental caries, VII. A study of fluoride-dental caries relationship in adult population. *Public Health Rep* 66: 1389–1401.
54. Schlesinger, E.R., Overton, D.E., and Chase, H.C. 1954. A long-term medical study of children in a community with a fluoridated water supply. In *Fluoridation as a Public Health Measure,* J.H. Shaw (ed), Washington, D.C.: American Association for the Advancement of Science, pp. 131–147.
55. Schmid, R., Barbakow, F., Mühlemann, H., and DeVecchi, P. 1984. Amine fluoride and monofluorophosphate: I. Historical review of fluoride dentifrices. *J Dent Child* 51:99–103.
56. Seppa, L. 1982. Fluoride varnishes in caries prevention. *Proc Finnish Dent Soc* 78: Suppl. 8.
57. Smith, G.E. 1987. Fluoridation: forty years on. *Endeavour* 11:16–20.
58. Stephen, K.W., Creanor, S.L., Russell, J.I., Burchell, C.K., and Huntington, E. 1987. Three-year oral health trial with zinc-containing monofluorophosphate dentifrices. *J Dent Res* 66(Sp. Issue, Abstr. 459): 65.
59. Stephen, K.W., McCall, D.R., and Tallis, J.I. 1987. Caries prevalence in northern Scotland before, and 5 years after, water defluoridation. *Br Dent J* 163:324–326.
60. Stookey, G.K. 1985. Are all fluoride dentifrices the same? In *Clinical Uses of Fluorides,* S.H.Y. Wei (ed), Philadelphia: Lea & Febiger, pp. 105–131.
61. Stookey, G.K., Sergent, J.W., Park, K.K., Jackson, R.D., and Drook, C.A. 1985. Prevalence of dental caries in Indiana schoolchildren: results of 1982 survey. *Pediatr Dent* 7:8–13.
62. Tinanoff, N. 1985. Stannous fluoride in clinical dentistry. In *Clinical Uses of Fluorides,* S.H.Y. Wei (ed), Philadelphia: Lea & Febiger, pp. 25–34.
63. Torell, P., and Ericsson, Y. 1965. Two-year clinical tests with different methods of local caries-preventive fluorine application in Swedish schoolchildren. *Acta Odontol Scand* 23:287–322.

64. Thylstrup, A., and Fejerskov, O. (eds) 1986. *Textbook of Cariology*. Copenhagen: Munksgaard, p. 324.
65. Wellock, W.D., and Brudevold, F. 1963. A study of acidulated fluoride solutions. II. The caries-inhibiting effect of a single annual topical application of an acidic fluoride and phosphate solution. A two-year experience. *Arch Oral Biol* 8:179–182.
66. Zacherl, W.A. 1981. A three-year clinical caries evaluation of the effect of a sodium fluoride-silica abrasive dentifrice. *Pharmacol Ther Dent* 6:1–7.

Chapter 12

Control and Prevention of Dental Caries

Regimen autem conſeruatiuum;dentiū decē cōpletur
canonibus. Primus vitet corruptionē cibi,& potus in ſto
macho,& per conſequens omnē cauſam corruptionis, vt
puta ea,quæ merito ſuæ ſubſtātiæ corrūpuntur, ſicut lac,
piſces ſaliti,& ſimilia,poſtpoſitionem cibi ſubtilis craſſo.
Motus fortes poſt cibi aſſumptionem,& ante deſcenſum
D eius è ſtomacho,nutriētia diuerſa,coitum, & balneū poſt
cibū,& ſimilia.Secundus,caueat à vomitu,& multo ma-
gis ſi vomeret rem acetoſam. Tertius,euitet cibaria craſ-
ſa,viſcoſa,& proprie dulcia,viſcoſa, ſicut ſunt confectio-
nes de melle,et ficus ſiccas.Quartus,vitet res duras ad frā
gendum.Quintus,congelantia dentes,ſiue ſtupefacientia
fugiat. Sextus, res vehementis frigoris non comedat , &
proprie poſt aſſumptionē calidi. Item omnia vehemēter
calida,& amplius poſt frigidi aſſumptionem. Septimus,
res dentib.nocentes ſua proprietate,ſunt porri.Octauus,
mundificet dentes ſibi immediate poſt cibum ab eo ſuper
fluo,quod ingreditur inter ipſos, & proprie cū ligno ſub-
tili non acuto,nec incidēti,ſed ſit obtuſum cum latitudine
quadam.ſicut eſſet ramuſculus cypreſſi, ligni aloes,pini,
roriſmarini , iuniperi , & ſimilium , & hoc faciat abſque
multa perſcrutatione ne noceat gingiuæ ipſam mouendo
aut dentes ipſos, & ſint hæc proprie participantia amari-

Io.Arculani k iiij tudinem

tudinem cum quadam ſtipticitate. Nonus,facta tali mun E
dificatione immediate poſt cibum , vt ſupra lauentur den
tes,& proprie cum aliquo ex infraſcriptis vinis mediæ vi
noſitatis & ſaporis medij inter dulce, & acre nobiliter ſti-
pticis. Et ex cōuenientibus ad hoc eſt,vt in quatuor libris
muſti cōditionati,vt ſupra,poſtq̄ bullierit ſub racemis cir
ca tres dies , & extractum ſit de ſub racemis , bulliat in eo
vna libra ſaluiæ recentis inciſæ in fruſtra mediocria,& nō
piſtatæ,nec lotæ vſq; ad ſufficientem clarificationē ipſius
vini:deinde extrahatur, & obſeruetur in vaſe bene obtu-
rato,vel accipiatur cinnamomi electi. ℥.1.maſtichis. ℥.s.
galliæ muſcatæ,cubebarū,ana.ʒ.2.ſem.iuniperi.ʒ.3.radi-
cis ciper.ʒ.1.s.fol.roriſma. ℥.6.cōtundātur omnia craſſo
modo exceptis ſol.roriſma.& bulliāt omnia ſimul in vna
brenta vini,vt ſupra conditionati,& fiat per omnia, vt ſu
pradictum eſt,& hoc multum valet in paſſionibus neruo
rum. Decimus canon. Fricentur dentes ſuauiter, & tē-
pore breui,nam fortis frictio.aut diuturna deſtruit dentiū
humiditates naturales,& ad eos trahit rheuma, & vapo- F
res à ſtomacho aſcendentes , aut ſaltem ipſos præparat ad
hoc recipiendum,ſed frictio cum æqualitate abſtergit dē-
tes,& carnem gingiuarum confortat,et prohibet lapides,
ſeu gypſum circa ipſos generari,& facit oris odorē bonū.

Johannes Arculanus, *Practica Particularium Morborum Omnium,* Venice Junta 1557. Chap. 47. *De passionibus dentium,* f. 76^{R} D-f. 76^{V} E-F.

The regimen for saving the teeth comprises ten rules. First rule: one should avoid the corruption of the mouth and stomach. Consequently avoid . . . milk, salt fish and such things, avoid taking light food after heavy food, avoid violent motion after taking food . . . , avoid diverse nutriments, . . . avoid sexual intercourse and bathing after food. Second rule: avoid vomiting, more so if one should vomit acidified matter. Third rule: avoid rich and sticky foods, especially those which are sweet and sticky as are confections of honey and dried figs. Fourth rule: avoid things which chill and numb the teeth. Sixth rule: one should not eat things which are cold after things which are hot and likewise from cold to hot. Seventh rule: avoid things which of themselves are harmful to the teeth such as leeks. Eighth rule: one should cleanse one's teeth immediately after eating, even after eating superfluous things. This rubbing of the teeth should be done especially with light and fine grained wood; not sharp or cutting but with wood that has been blunted and with a certain width such as a twig of cyprus, pine or juniper and such things. One should do this without much poking between the teeth lest one harm the gums and the teeth themselves. . . . Ninth rule: that when such rubbing has been done after eating the teeth should be, in addition, washed especially with some of the wines . . . tasting between sweet and dry with a styptic quality. . . . [T]here can be added . . . cinnamon, mastichis, galliae mustcatae, cubebarii ana, seed of juniper and leaves of rosemary. . . . Tenth rule: the teeth should be gently rubbed for a short time, for a hard rubbing or a long rubbing destroys the natural moistures of the teeth. . . . Even a moderate rubbing cleanses the teeth, strengthens the flesh of the gums, prevents formation of toothstones and makes the breath smell good.

Table 12-1 Reasons for tooth extractions

Author	Country	Population age (range)	Proportion of extractions (%) Caries	Periodontics	Prosthodontics	Orthodontics	Other
Agerholm & Sidi (1988)[1]	England & Wales	<10 to >80	48	27	4	13	9
Ainamo et al (1984)[2]	Finland	16 to >70	60	18	12	1	8
Cahen et al (1985)[16]	France	<5 to >70	48	32	3	8	7
Chauncey et al (1987)[17]	United States	45 to 90	33	19	31	NA	16
Kay & Blinkhorn (1986)[34]	Scotland	<10 to >70	50	21	12	7	10

Extent of the problem

Almost everyone in the United States experiences dental caries to some degree, mostly before reaching adulthood but continuing even then. The disease is the leading cause of loss of teeth in both children and adults[1,2,14,16,17,34] (Table 12-1).

During the past 20 years there have been tremendous strides in our understanding of the causation of this disease, of the specific flora associated with smooth surface, fissure, and root caries, the transmissibility of the flora, the mechanisms involved in the adherence of the oral flora, and the formation of dental plaque. We now have a better appreciation of the unique role dietary sucrose plays in determining the numbers of cariogenic organisms able to colonize on tooth surfaces.[24]

Despite these creditable scientific advances and the fact that caries is preventable, the disease continues to be a major public health problem. Untreated, caries can cause considerable pain and discomfort; the repair or replacement of carious teeth involves millions of hours per year, as well as loss of time from school and work. Americans spend about $20 billion a year to treat all their dental/oral woes.[62] A major portion of this amount is for the treatment of decayed teeth, or the sequelae of caries.

Caries is the most prevalent affliction of childhood. The average American child has at least one decayed, missing or filled surface by age 8, four by age 12, and eleven by age 17.[61] Therefore, the average schoolchild has approximately one new decayed surface a year. Data from the US Army give a representative picture of the problem for young adults 18 to 21 years of age. Army surveys reveal that every 100 inductees required 600 fillings, 112 extractions, 4 bridges, 21 crowns, 18 partial dentures, and 1 full denture. Thus, the prevalence of dental caries is exceedingly high and its cost is considerable.

Approaches to prevention of caries

Because dental caries is a complex disease involving the simultaneous interplay of three principal factors—the microflora, the host, and the substrate (diet)—it is unlikely that any one approach will lead to its prevention and control. Accordingly, the major strategies currently directed at reducing or eliminating caries are:

1. Combat the microbial agent (eg, programs of personal oral hygiene, plaque removal, or plaque control)
2. Increase the resistance of teeth (eg, systemic and topical fluoride, occlusal sealants)
3. Modify the diet (eg, diet control, restriction of sucrose-containing foods and beverages, use of noncariogenic sweeteners, phosphate additives)

In addition, there has been an increasing awareness of the need to improve the delivery and acceptance of proven caries-preventive methods and to evaluate the cost effectiveness of these methods.

These strategies will now be reviewed in terms of their applicability and efficacy when used at home by the individual patient, when practiced in the dental office, and when employed at the community level. Naturally, these strategies are interdependent; what happens regarding caries prevention at home is influenced by what goes on in the dental office and in the community. The reason for following this sequence is that the success of any program of caries prevention requires the concurrence and interest of the patient at home.

Preventive programs for the individual at home

Oral hygiene

Undoubtedly toothbrushing is the most widely used and socially accepted form of oral hygiene. Bibby[13] has facetiously written, "It now rates close to motherhood in respectability." Yet it is not clear to what extent toothbrushing of itself, exclusive of therapeutic dentifrices, alters the caries attack. Most children spend less than 1 minute toothbrushing (Table 12-2) and fail to brush 38% of the tooth surfaces, especially the lingual.* Adults do not spend any more time than children in brushing, generally about 45 to 90 seconds, with an average of about 60 seconds.[20,23,41,54] The extent to which plaque is removed is related to the duration of

*References 19, 29, 35, 40, 42, 56.

Table 12-2 Duration of toothbrushing(s) found in different studies

Author	n	Age	Duration (s)
Robinson (1946)[54]	405	22	67*
Dahl & Davis (1954)[19]	514	6–15	65
Dahl & Muhler (1955)[20]	340	17–34	60 (15–135)
Rugg-Gunn et al (1979)[56]	57	13	51 (20–85)
MacGregor et al (1979)[40]	85	11–13	60.3 (SD = ±23.8)
Kleber et al (1981)[35]	180	10–16	54.3 (SE = ±2.5)
Emling et al (1981)[23]	154	33.7	56.7 (SD = ±27.2)
Honkala (1984)[29]	110	13.5	80.9 (SE = ±3.5)
Macgregor & Rugg-Gunn (1985)[41]	60	18–22	33.0* (SD = ±12.0)
Macgregor et al (1986)[42]	57	13	51.1 (SD = ±15.4)

*Subjects aware that toothbrushing was being observed.

brushing.[30] For adults, a minimum time of 5 minutes daily has been recommended for brushing and flossing or using other interproximal cleansing aids.[30] The thoroughness of toothbrushing is usually measured by plaque or oral hygiene scores. But epidemiologists have failed to demonstrate a consistent relationship between dental plaque scores and dental caries prevalence, perhaps because the two indices measure items that occur over considerably different time intervals. Caries prevalence measures total caries experience accumulated since the teeth erupted (usually years), whereas plaque and oral hygiene indices measure a transient state. Even when plaque scores have been determined repeatedly and compared to caries increments (not prevalence), it has not been possible to demonstrate a relationship between the standard of oral cleanliness and dental caries.[58] The oral hygiene and plaque indices themselves have serious limitations because they tend to emphasize the buccal and lingual surfaces and are more subjective in measuring interproximal deposits. The occlusal and interproximal surfaces are most likely to become carious but are least likely to be cleaned by toothbrushing alone. Little wonder that we have not been able to prove in self-administered oral hygiene programs that "a clean tooth does not decay."

As an alternative to measuring the efficacy of plaque removal, some investigators have studied the diligence of toothbrushing, using questionnaires about brushing frequency. For example, it has been reported that children who brushed twice or more per day had significantly less caries than children who brushed only once a day or less.[38] However, because 90% of the children used a fluoride-containing dentifrice, these results may be due to increased contact with a topical fluoride agent rather than to mechanical cleansing of tooth surfaces. No significant differences have been found between the oral hygiene practices of caries-free, moderately caries-susceptible, and highly caries-susceptible children.[53]

The limitations of self-administered toothbrushing and flossing (mechanical plaque removal) in preventing decay will be considered further under "Preventive programs for the community." Although these limitations exist, we should not tell our patients to stop brushing their teeth. Considerable evidence indicates that toothbrushing and other oral hygiene procedures can prevent or control periodontal disease. We should, however, stop promising our patients that if they simply brush their teeth they can prevent decay, because brushing is not synonymous with removal of plaque.[21] Very few patients, be they children or adults, ever come close to doing an effective job.

Fluorides

Fluoride therapy continues to be the cornerstone of any caries-preventive program. Fluoride-containing dentifrices, 0.76% sodium monofluorophosphate, or 0.22% sodium fluoride, are extensively advertised and cost no more than most other toothpastes. Accordingly, they are the most commonly purchased type of dentifrice, accounting for over 90% of the market in the United States. Used regularly, such toothpastes can effect a 20% or better reduction in caries.

Other self-application procedures for the delivery of topical fluorides involve prescription items and include mouthrinsing with fluoride solutions and applying fluoride gels in mouthpieces. Daily mouthrinsing with a 0.05% sodium fluoride solution for 1 minute in the home is both practical and efficacious: it can reduce decay significantly, as much as 50%.[59] Fluoride mouthrinses are not cheap if obtained from a pharmacy. Fluoride (0.5%) gels applied in individual trays for 5 minutes daily at home can also be an important adjunct to caries prevention. Reusable applicator trays are available for children in a mixed dentition stage. For adults, whose dentition is stable, custom-made trays allow a closer fit but are expensive to make. This form of fluoride therapy is especially beneficial for patients with xerostomia, who have a high risk of caries.[22] Until recently fluoride rinses and gels have been restricted to prescription use. Such products are now recommended for over-the-counter human use provided that they contain no more than 120 mg total fluoride and that they are packaged in containers with child-resistant closures.[60]

Systemic administration of fluoride in the form of drops, tablets, or lozenges can reduce decay maximally if the supplements are taken on a regular basis from birth until about 14 years of age. Details concerning dosage of fluoride supplements are described in chapter 11.

Self-administered fluoride supplements can reduce decay appreciably in children whose parents are sufficiently interested in their dental health to continue therapy on a regular basis for years. Unfortunately, numerous reports record a considerable fall-off in daily use by many children. In order to achieve better patient compliance, the dentist or physician who is prescribing the fluoride supplement must convey enthusiasm and confidence in its effectiveness, should stress the economic rewards and dental benefits, and should explain that this is a unique opportunity available only during mineralization of the dentition. Furthermore, regular follow-up every 3 to 6 months to check on the patient's use of the supplement is important. An alternative is the supervised administration of fluoride tablets in schools (see "Preventive programs for the community").

Diet modification

The importance of diet—particularly sucrose-containing food and beverages—in cariogenesis has already been covered in chapters 4 and 5. Dietary control in caries prevention depends first and foremost on the will and tenacity of the individual patient (or parent, in the case of a child). The dentist, dental hygienist, and/or dietitian consultant can provide information concerning "safe" foods and drinks and can give support and encouragement. But the ultimate responsibility for diet modification and restriction of between-meal sugary snacks lies with the individual. Often this means going against the prevailing social mores and is extremely difficult. Other members of the family and, in the case of a child, the parents have to cooperate; otherwise the program will not succeed. Parents are generally aware of the cariogenicity of cookies, soft drinks, candies, and chewing gum, yet in one Swedish survey 66% of parents did not express any desire to change their children's consumption habits.[36] Conversely, one of three parents was interested in modifying his or her children's dietary behavior.

Voluntary dietary restriction of sucrose may suit some patients and certainly reduces caries, as evidenced by persons who have hereditary fructose intolerance. Children of dentists generally have low decay rates, which may in part be due to more careful selection of foods and snacks.[15,39] Some patients may be motivated to exert such dietary control, but it certainly is not characteristic of all patients, all of the time.

Preventive programs for the dental office

Before evaluating the specific procedures that can be employed in the office for prevention of caries, it is important that the whole field of preventive dentistry be placed in perspective. First, caries is potentially preventable. Second, it is patently evident that caries continues largely unchecked primarily because of the limited acceptance of known caries-preventive procedures. A survey by the National Opinion Research Center revealed that only 46% of the population in the United States had visited a dentist during the previous year. Of these, 67% went for symptomatic reasons and only 33% went for a check-up or prophylaxis (ie, preventive care).[48] More patients could become interested in prevention if the dental office personnel themselves were more effective in teaching preventive measures and transmitting the necessary skills. It is extremely difficult to identify those patients who are open to such changes in their personal dental health care. Some are not amenable, and one should not impose preventive programs on them. Selected patients can be instructed in oral hygiene, dietary control, and other proven preventive measures, but expectations of, and demands on, patients must be reasonable. Mosteller[43] has pointed out: "If people will not lose weight, stop smoking or drinking, will not obey the speed limits, when they know all these things can kill them, how can we expect them to be too inconvenienced in order just to keep their teeth?"

Several dentists have outlined the preventive programs used in their offices.[3,4,10-12] All include oral hygiene instruction, diet control, and fluoride therapy, though naturally the emphasis varies. Some stress plaque control, not only teaching the mechanical principles of cleaning teeth but also attempting to change behavior. Because it takes time to change habits, patients are recalled frequently until they have demonstrated the skills of plaque control. The patient assumes an active rather than a passive role in the preventive program. Other offices promote dietary control by having patients keep dietary records, evaluating these diet histories, conducting caries activity tests, and supplying dietary instructions. Such advice must not only focus on foods and drinks to be avoided but must also provide lists of safe alternative foods and drinks. Finally, some practices accentuate the fluoride therapy component of the preventive program. Multiple fluoride therapy is used, including fluoride-containing prophylaxis paste and topical fluoride application in the office. Patients are instructed to use only fluoride toothpaste, and, in addition, fluoride supplements are prescribed for children.

There are strict limitations on the inferences that can be drawn from an experimental clinical trial. The results may differ if the same procedures are used under the real-life conditions of the dental office. It would be of interest to determine the effectiveness of such procedures and directives to patients. Regrettably, few office programs provide data on the caries reductions achieved when these measures are actually employed by the patients and the private practicing dentist. Success is all too frequently based on subjective clinical impressions. Objective studies are difficult but not impossible. If different practices are to be compared, criteria for assessment of caries need to be standardized. Lower caries increments have been demonstrated in one preventive practice that was compared with 11 other practices employing no specific preventive program.[12] Fluoride therapy appeared primarily responsible for the observed reduction. In some preventive programs the patients are self-selected, because only those who accept the original sequence of appointments, meet the criteria for success, and continue in the semiannual recall system are included in the findings.[49]

Oral hygiene

The traditional annual or semiannual dental "prophylaxis," with nontherapeutic pastes, may well be a misnomer. Prophylaxis implies prevention of disease, but there is no convincing evidence that mechanical polishing and cleaning of the teeth once or twice a year reduces caries or periodontal disease.[13] These office procedures, which patients cannot perform by themselves, can remove calculus and extrinsic stains but have no preventive effect.

However, several clinical trials in Scandinavia have demonstrated that *more frequent* professional tooth cleaning can produce a dramatic reduction in dental disease.[6-8,52] Teeth were carefully cleaned every 2 weeks by specially trained and highly motivated chairside assistants (dental nurses) using mechanical instruments, polishing paste, small brushes driven by a dental engine, and dental floss. This frequent treatment substantially prevented caries and reduced gingivitis. Furthermore, children in the control groups, who received regular detailed instruction in proper oral hygiene but no mechanical tooth cleanings, continued to develop new carious lesions. The combination of oral hygiene instruction and professional toothcleaning with a fluoride-containing paste (either 5% sodium monofluorophosphate or 0.22% sodium fluoride) and a 2-minute fluoride mouthrinse repeated every 3 weeks reduced caries by 51%, compared with a group that only used a fluoride mouthrinse.[26] In addition, the treated group had lower plaque and gingivitis scores. Reducing the frequency of professional tooth cleaning to once a month reduces the efficacy of the treatment so that the benefits no longer justify the costs when applied to nonselected children.[9] If only children with high caries experience are considered, the efficacy of monthly preventive treatments becomes more striking. The use of a prophylaxis paste containing fluoride complicates the interpretation of the results of several of these studies, namely whether the effect is due to oral hygiene alone or to frequent application of topical fluoride. When a group of English girls received a professional prophylaxis with a fluoride-free polishing paste every 2 weeks, there was no influence on the caries increments in the treated group, although the gingival health improved.[5] Studies in Canada also suggest that interproximal flossing performed by a trained assistant on children each school day reduces the incidence of proximal caries.[63,64] No reduction in caries has been observed when subjects floss their own teeth.[25]

While these findings are encouraging, the feasibility of such programs, when applied to larger populations, is open to serious question. The cost efficacy of such oral hygiene treatment also needs to be tested in a private practice situation, and the long-term effect of such frequent polishing requires close surveillance.

Fluoride therapy and occlusal sealants

Topical fluorides (such as 2% sodium fluoride, 8% stannous fluoride, or acidulated phosphate fluoride containing 1.23% fluoride) in solution or gel form have been used extensively for professional application in the dental office following a mechanical cleaning and polishing. Solutions are applied directly to the teeth for 4 minutes; gels can be applied either directly or within plastic, wax, or polystyrene trays. Such procedures, when conducted semiannually, reduce dental decay by about 40%. On a cost efficacy basis, however, they rank much lower than other forms of fluoride therapy because each patient requires individual professional attention.

The occlusal surface of newly erupted posterior teeth is vulnerable to decay and is the most frequently affected surface. Resins are now available that are capable of adhering to suitably prepared fissures and grooves of teeth, thereby protecting them from carious attack. These adhesive resins must be meticulously applied in a dry field according to manufacturer's instructions, by trained dental personnel, in a dental office or with portable dental equipment. The failure rate or loss of sealant can be high if not inserted correctly. Because they do not require any drilling and are totally painless to insert, patient acceptance is high. Several clinical trials of the current fissure sealants have demonstrated major protection against decay in the treated occlusal surfaces when compared with untreated teeth. Sealants only protect the occlusal surface and should be used in conjunction with fluoride therapy to protect the other surfaces.

Diet modification

Diet is very much a matter of individual choice, influenced of course by age, ethnic and religious customs, family and peer group, advertisements, and economics. The function of the dental office personnel in diet modification is one of counseling, providing information, motivation, and encouragement. To do this competently, the counselor should be properly trained in the science and practice of nutrition; in other words, he or she should be a dentist, dental hygienist, or dietitian. This responsibility should not be relegated to a dental auxiliary or plaque control nurse.

How to interview a patient, arrive at a nutritional diagnosis, and provide dietary guidance has been described by Nizel.[46,47] At the first visit the counselor should obtain a searching diet history, preferably starting with a 24-hour recall that includes when and how much of each food was eaten. Using this as a sample, the patient then keeps a detailed food diary for the next 4 days. At a subsequent visit the patient and counselor together evaluate the diet history, the patient being asked to identify all sugar-containing confections, foods, and drinks by circling them in red on the diet history form (Fig 12-1). An additional check-form can be used for totaling the frequency of mealtime versus between-meal ingestion of such foods and beverages (Fig 12-2). This emphasizes to the patient the importance of snacking habits in causing decay. Once the patient is familiar with these causative factors, the counselor can proceed to the individualized diet prescription, which consists of four parts[47]:

Name: Jane Doe
Sex: M (F) Birth Date: 10-1-69
Weight (lbs): 60 Height (ins): 51
Pregnant: Yes (No) Lactating: Yes (No)
Activity Factor 0-1: 0.2 Menu # of days: 1

Instructions

1. Please record everything you eat or drink in the order in which it is eaten.
2. Be sure to list all between-meal snacks, cream and sugar in coffee, etc.
3. Estimate the amount eaten using household measures, e.g., 1 cup, 2 slices, 4 oz., 1 stick.

Date:

	Item	Unit	Quantity
Breakfast	(Cap'n Crunch)	¾	cup
	Milk, whole	½	cup
Snack	(Mars Chocolate Almond)	1	bar
Lunch	Sandwich,	2	slices
	(peanut butter and jelly)	1	tablespoon
Snack	(Jelly beans)	5	each
Dinner	Hamburger	1	5 oz
	French fried potatoes	10	each
	Milk, whole	1	cup
Snack	(Fig Newton)	1	each
	(Kool-Aid)	¾	glass

Fig12-1 Sample food intake diary of patient with high caries activity.

SUGAR-CONTAINING FOODS AND DRINKS

Instructions: Place a chit mark (/) for each sugary item eaten or drunk.

Form of sugar	When eaten	1st day	2nd day	3rd day	4th day	5th day
Liquid	With meals	/				
	Between meals	/				
Solid	With meals	/ / / /				
	Between meals	/ / / /				

Fig 12-2 Diet evaluation chart of food as recorded in Fig 12-1. (Adapted from Nizel.[33])

1. The overall quality and balance of the diet
2. Avoidance of caries-producing foods and snacks
3. A personalized meal plan
4. A suggested list of snacks and foods to include or avoid

The diet used in caries prevention is essentially a healthy, adequate, balanced diet and resembles a normal diet except for the exclusion of a few foods and eating practices. The recommended daily pattern includes the right number of servings from each of four basic food groups: milk, meat, fruit-vegetable, and grain. Since a great number of foods can be used in reaching this goal, the diet is relatively unrestricted and nondirective. Patients should become involved in deciding which foods to include and which to omit from their diet. Because the dietary customs of patients vary greatly, there is no single regimen or pat diet suitable for each one, nor is everyone amenable to altering his or her eating habits. Patients are most likely to comply with advice about foods that fit in with their already established life-style. Positive recommendations of foods that are noncariogenic, tasty, and attractive are better than only telling patients what they should not eat.

Microbiological examination provides an objective method for the assessment of the patient's cooperation. Changes in dietary habits are reflected within a couple of weeks in corresponding reductions in the numbers of oral lactobacilli and *Streptococcus mutans*.[37] For simplicity, an *S mutans* screening test or dip slide technique can be used to obtain an approximation of the numbers of *S mutans* or lactobacilli (see chapter 8). These tests stimulate patients' interest in their oral health and monitor their sucrose consumption and oral hygiene. Current knowledge of the oral microbiota can be used to advantage in caries control programs. Regrettably, in general dental practice it is practically not used at all.

Follow-up visits are advised so that the patient's diet can be rechecked and further modifications adopted if necessary. Continuous reinforcement, with clarification and encouragement, is an important component of a nutritional counseling program in the dental office.

The cost of noncariogenic foods is no more and often less than that of cariogenic foods. Because dietary counseling requires special knowledge and time, like other clinical services it deserves a fee. Accordingly, the cost of caries prevention by dietary means is relatively high when performed in the office.

Preventive programs for the community

Oral hygiene

Children and adolescents are more susceptible to enamel caries than the rest of the population. Personal preventive activities have had limited or variable success. Schools provide ready access to large numbers of children who are highly susceptible to oral disease and who can be supervised in their conduct of a preventive program.

Many dental health education programs in schools have focused on teaching and checking of plaque control. Some have been more comprehensive, including diet instruction and fluoride therapy as well. Often there is intensive oral hygiene instruction during the first week or two of the program, followed by periodic reinforcement. Such sporadic information and instruction, even if technically detailed and repeated several times per year, results in negligibly small effects on caries increments.[18,51]

On theoretical grounds, thorough removal of plaque daily should markedly reduce the increment of new carious lesions.[28] Accordingly, government-supported school-based programs have been conducted for mass control of plaque. The regimens have included scrupulous removal of all visible soft deposits by toothbrushing without a dentifrice, interproximal flossing, and supervised checking with disclosing agents. The participants spend about 15 minutes each day during the school year performing these procedures. Three years of this regimen produced a consistent reduction in plaque and gingivitis, but the effect on caries incidence was marginal or insignificant.[31,57] Considering the difficulty in obtaining and maintaining the cooperation of all students in the treatment groups and other obvious drawbacks, one must conclude that mass programs of plaque control for caries prevention are not worth the time, effort, and cost.

Fluorides

Fluoridation of water supplies to an optimal concentration ranging from 0.7 to 1.2 ppm, depending on mean daily temperatures, is the community caries prevention program par excellence. It benefits children of all socioeconomic groups, irrespective of their cooperation or interest. The cost of water fluoridation is remarkably low, usually between 15¢/and 20¢/person/year. In these days of rising health care costs, it is a rare bargain. Fluoridation of communal water supplies is based upon extensive and thorough epidemiological surveys that have shown about 60% less dental caries occurs when fluoridated water is consumed from birth. The safety of water fluoridation has been carefully documented.[44] There is no evidence that water containing optimal concentrations of fluoride impairs general health. Clearly, one of the most persuasive arguments for the safety of water fluoridation is based on the health of communities where for generations the inhabitants have been drinking water with natural fluoride at a concentration of about 1 ppm. Currently, over 108 million people in the United States drink fluoridated water, representing 61% of the population on public water supplies.[45] This still leaves about 115 million people who are not receiving the benefits of communal water fluoridation and for whom alternative means of fluoride therapy need to be provided. In rural communities that lack a central water supply, fluoridation of the school's water is a practical alternative that results in about 40% reduction in dental caries and major reduction in the need for extractions.[32]

Second to water fluoridation, school-based fluoride mouthrinsing programs have the greatest public health potential. Weekly supervised rinsing with 0.2% sodium fluoride for 1 minute is most effective, with 20% to 40% caries reduction. Fluoride rinsing takes very little time, is easy to learn, and requires few materials. The cost of a weekly school mouthrinsing program can be kept low, about 50¢/child/year, by purchasing supplies in bulk and by using volunteers to prepare and distribute the mouthrinse solution for each class.

Public health programs making fluoride supplements available to families for distribution to their children at home have mostly been unsuccessful. However, dental caries can be reduced when fluoride tablets are administered daily in schools (150 to 200 days/year). Based on several studies in the United States and Europe, the anticipated caries reduction is from 20% to 40%. Such programs do not provide fluoride to preschool children, from birth to 6 years, when the permanent incisors and first permanent molars are becoming mineralized. The advantages of distributing fluoride supplements at schools are that the program takes little time, is cheap (approximately 50¢/child/school year for sodium fluoride tablets bought in bulk), is easy to learn, and requires no materials other than the tablets.

These fluoride programs are not mutually exclusive and can be used in combination. For example, in a nonfluoridated community, school children can be provided with a fluoride dentifrice for home use and be given daily fluoride supplements and weekly fluoride mouthrinses in the classroom.[33] It is doubtful whether the benefits from each procedure, when used in combination, are cumulative. The mode of action of fluoride dentifrices and rinses are primarily topical, though some fluoride is also swallowed unintentionally. Fluoride supplements, however, do provide both topical and systemic exposure.

Diet modification

The composition and ingredients of many foods and beverages consumed nowadays are determined by the food manufacturer, not by the consumer. Accordingly, caries control by dietary modification on a public health scale requires the help and cooperation of the food industry if it is to have any serious impact. Industry is not unaware of its responsibility in improving dental health and of the need for noncariogenic products. Strict statutory definitions cover claims that products are "anticavity," "noncariogenic," or "less cariogenic." The FDA stringently enforces the 1958 Food Additives Amendment to the Food and Drug Act that requires proof of safety. This means there is considerable regulatory restraint upon the introduction of food additives. The cost of clinical trials to demonstrate safety and efficacy is very high, often beyond the capability of a single manufacturer. Clearly, research and development of safe, noncariogenic sweetening agents or other anticavity food additives should be done on an industry-wide, shared basis. Clinical testing of "noncariogenic" foods on humans is by no means simple, particularly because it is unethical to use a sucrose-consuming control group. Volunteers cannot be given additional sucrose-containing products as part of a trial because of the predictable cariogenesis.

In some schools, the sale of "junk" foods, such as sweets, sweet biscuits (cookies) and iced buns (pastries), doughnuts and soft drinks, has been banned in the cafeteria and from vending machines. Modest reductions in decay have followed such action.[50,55]

Total replacement of sucrose in foods is most unlikely. Undoubtedly there is a hierarchy of foods needing modification, with highest priority given to eliminating sucrose and other easily fermentable sugars from snack foods. Snack foods can be defined as those that are consumed other than at breakfast, lunch, or dinner and usually need little or no preparation. Several sugar substitutes may be required to provide a broad range for stability, taste onset, and sweetness intensity. Further development and testing are necessary to provide a sufficient array of noncariogenic snack foods to the consumer. Such changes could potentially have a major public health impact in reducing dental caries.

Concluding remarks

Prevention of caries, not just its treatment, should have high priority in every dental office and public health program. However, the number of professional people necessary to deliver this service as well as the cost are limiting factors. In Table 12-3 various types of procedures are compared as regards practicality/compliance, as well as cost and efficacy. In selecting a preventive program, these parameters must all be considered. Regrettably for some preventive methods, such as diet modification and fluoride supplements, the observed efficacy in practice does not reach its potential, mostly because of incomplete acceptance by the patient. Some procedures rank high in cost yet are justified if a high caries risk exists.

The importance of selecting patients carefully for a particular program cannot be overemphasized. There is no standard caries prevention program suitable for everyone; rather, the program should fit the patient. High-risk patients with active caries need more attention so that all available home and office procedures can be marshalled effectively. Persons who are fatalistic or disinterested in their dental health will not institute adequate home oral hygiene or modify their diets. However, for interested and cooperative patients we can provide a rewarding service. Caries can be prevented by a combination of procedures employed in the home,

Table 12-3 Comparison of caries prevention programs for the home, dental office, and community*

Preventive program	Type of procedure	Practicality/ compliance	Cost	Caries prevention: Observed efficacy	Caries prevention: Potential efficacy
Home	Oral hygiene	Good/variable	Medium	Insignificant	Unknown
	Fluoride				
	dentrifice	Good	Low	Fair	Fair
	rinse	Good	Medium	Good	Good
	gels	Poor/fair	High	Good	Excellent
	supplements	Fair/poor	High	Variable	Excellent
	Diet modification	Good/poor	Low	Insignificant	Excellent
Dental office	Oral hygiene ("prophylaxis")				
	semiannual or annual	Fair	High	Insignificant	Insignificant
	biweekly	Poor	High	Excellent	Excellent
	Fluoride				
	topical	Fair	High	Good	Good
	Occlusal sealant	Good	High	Good	Good
	Diet modification	Good/variable	High	Insignificant	Excellent
Community, school, or institution	Oral hygiene				
	occasional	Fair	Medium	None	Insignificant
	daily	Fair	High	Insignificant	Good
	Fluoride				
	water	Excellent	Low	High	High
	rinse	Good	Low	Good	Good
	supplements				
	school	Good/good	Low	Good	Good
	health center	Good/poor	Low	Poor	Excellent
	Occlusal sealants	Fair	Medium	Good	Good
	Diet modification	Good	Unknown	Unknown	Excellent

*These are very simplified and subjective evaluations of the procedures. The compliance, cost, and efficacy can vary depending on conditions of use (see text).

the office, and the community. Bringing about the adoption of these procedures by the public represents a challenge to, and an opportunity for, the dental profession.

Chapter review

- State the practicality and observed efficacy of home oral hygiene in caries prevention.
- State the forms of fluoride therapy that can be used at home. Identify which have the best observed efficacy.
- Explain why diet modification at home has had limited or no success.
- List the caries-preventive procedures that can be used in the dental office. Indicate which patients require such treatment and how they can be selected.
- Compare the cost and observed efficacy of biweekly professional oral hygiene with self-administered daily plaque control in schools.
- Specify which community fluoride programs are your first and second choice. Explain your choice on the basis of practicality, cost, and observed efficacy.
- Compare the practicality/compliance, cost, and observed efficacy of fluoride supplements when supplied at schools versus health centers or clinics.
- Define a snack food. Identify who controls its composition.

Selected readings

Andlaw, R.J. 1978. Oral hygiene and dental caries—a review. *Int Dent J* 28:6.

Bellini, H.P., Arneberg, P., and von der Fehr, F.R. 1981. Oral hygiene and caries, a review. *Acta Odontol Scand* 39:257–265.

Burt, B.A. (ed) 1978. *Relative Efficiency of Preventive Procedures in Dental Public Health.* Ann Arbor: University of Michigan School of Public Health.

Ericsson, Y. (ed) 1978. Twenty-five Years of Caries Prevention. *Caries Res* 12(Sp. Suppl).

Glickman, I. (ed) 1972. Symposium on Chairside Preventive Dentistry. *Dent Clin North Am* 16:607–813.

Horowitz, A.M. 1981. *Preventing Tooth Decay: A Guide for Implementing Self Applied Fluorides in School Settings.* NIH Publication No. 82-1196, Bethesda, Maryland.

Katz, S., McDonald, J.L., and Stookey, G.K. 1976. *Preventive Dentistry in Action.* 2nd ed. Upper Montclair, N.J.: Dental Control Products, Inc.

Stallard, R.E. (ed) 1982. *A Textbook of Preventive Dentistry.* 2nd ed. Philadelphia: W.B. Saunders.

References

1. Agerholm, D.M., and Sidi, A.D. 1988. Reasons given for extraction of permanent teeth by general practitioners in England and Wales. *Br Dent J* 164:345–348.
2. Ainamo, J., Sarkki, L., Kuhalampi, M.L., Palolampi, L., and Piirto, O. 1984. The frequency of periodontal extractions in Finland. *Community Dent Health* 1:165–172.

3. Alban, A.L. 1970. Putting prevention into practice. 21st National Dent. Health Conference. Chicago: American Dental Association, pp. 440–448.
4. Anderson, J.L. 1972. Integration of plaque control into the practice of dentistry. *Dent Clin North Am* 16:621–630.
5. Ashley, F.P., and Sainsbury, R.H. 1981. The effect of a school-based plaque control programme on caries and gingivitis. *Br Dent J* 150:41–45.
6. Axelsson, P., and Lindhe, J. 1974. The effect of a preventive programme on dental plaque, gingivitis and caries in schoolchildren. Results after one and two years. *J Clin Periodontol* 1:126–138.
7. Axelsson, P., and Lindhe, J. 1975. Effect of fluoride on gingivitis and dental caries in a preventive program based on plaque control. *Community Dent Oral Epidemiol* 3: 156–160.
8. Axelsson, P., Lindhe, J., and Wäseby, J. 1976. The effect of various plaque control measures on gingivitis and caries in schoolchildren. *Community Dent Oral Epidemiol* 4:232–239.
9. Badersten, A., Egelberg, J., and Koch, G. 1975. Effect of monthly prophylaxis on caries and gingivitis in schoolchildren. *Community Dent Oral Epidemiol* 3:1–4.
10. Barkley, R.F. 1972. How to make an effective plaque control program part of the practice of dentistry. *Dent Clin North Am* 16:631–646.
11. Barkley, R.F. 1973. Prevention—facts, fad or myth. *J Am Coll Dent* 40:209–213.
12. Barnard, P.D., Gillings, B.R.D., and Gillings, K.J.R. 1974. Assessment of a preventive dentistry programme in private practice. *N Z Dent J* 70:15–24.
13. Bibby, B.G. 1966. Do we tell the truth about preventing caries? *J Dent Child* 33: 269–279.
14. Bouma, J., Schaub, R.M.H., and VandePoel, A.C.M. 1985. Periodontal status and total tooth extraction in a medium-sized city in The Netherlands. *Community Dent Oral Epidemiol* 13:323–327.
15. Bradford, E.W., and Crabb, H.S.M. 1961. Carbohydrate restriction and caries incidence. A pilot study. *Br Dent J* 111:273–279.
16. Cahen, P.M., Frank, R.M., and Turlot, J.C. 1985. A survey of the reasons for dental extractions in France. *J Dent Res* 64:1087–1093.
17. Chauncey, H.H., Glass, R.L., Alman, J.E., and Feller, R.F. 1987. Dental caries: the primary cause of tooth extraction in a sample of U.S. male adults. *Caries Res* 21:161.
18. Clark, C.A., Fintz, J.B., and Taylor, R. 1974. Effects of the control of plaque on the progression of dental caries. Results after 19 months. *J Dent Res* 53:1468–1474.
19. Dahl, L.O., and Davis, B.B. 1954. Oral hygiene habits of young children. *J Periodontol* 25:209–213.
20. Dahl, L.O., and Muhler, J.C. 1955. Oral hygiene habits of young adults. *J Periodontol* 26:43–46.
21. De la Rosa, M.R., Guerra, J.C., Johnston, D.A., and Radike, A.W. 1979. Plaque growth and removal with daily toothbrushing. *J Periodontol* 50:661–664.
22. Driezen, S., and Brown, L.R. 1976. Xerostomia and dental caries. In *Microbial Aspects of Dental Caries*, H.M. Stiles, W.J. Loesche, and T.C. O'Brien (eds), Sp. Suppl. Microbiol. Abstr. 1:263–273.
23. Emling, R.C., Flickinger, K.C., Cohen, D.W., and Yankell, S.L. 1981. A comparison of estimated versus actual brushing time. *Pharmacol Therap Dent* 6:93–98.
24. Gibbons, R.J., and van Houte, J. 1975. Dental Caries. *Annu Rev Med* 26:121–136.
25. Granath, L.E., Martinsson, T., Mattsson, L., Nilsson, G., Schröder, U., and Soderholm, B. 1979. Intra-individual effect of daily supervised flossing on caries in schoolchildren. *Community Dent Oral Epidemiol* 7:147–150.
26. Hamp, S.E., Linke, J., Fornell, J., Johnsson, L.A., and Karlsson, R. 1978. Effect of a field program based on systematic plaque control on caries and gingivitis in schoolchildren after 3 years. *Community Dent Oral Epidemiol* 6:17–23.
27. Hawkins, B.F., Kohout, F.J., Lainson, P.A., and Heckert, A. 1986. Duration of toothbrushing for effective plaque control. *Quintessence Int* 17:361–365.
28. Heifetz, S.B., Bagramian, R.A., Suomi, J.D., and Segreto, V.A. 1973. Programs for the mass control of plaque. An appraisal. *J Public Health Dent* 33:91–95.
29. Honkala, E. 1984. Frequency, pattern and duration of habitual toothbrushing in children. *J Pedodont* 8:367–376.
30. Honkala, E., Nyyssonen, V., Knuuttila, M., and Markkanen, H. 1986. Effectiveness of children's habitual toothbrushing. *J Clin Periodontol* 13:81–85.
31. Horowitz, A.M., Suomi, J.D., Peterson, J.K., Mathews, B.L., Vogelsong, R.H., and Lyman, D.A. 1980. Effect of supervised daily dental plaque removal by children after 3 years. *Community Dent Oral Epidemiol* 8:171–176.

32. Horowitz, H.S., Heifetz, S.B., and Law, F.E. 1972. Effect of school water fluoridation on dental caries. Final results in Elk Lake, Pa., after 12 years. *J Am Dent Assoc* 84: 832–838.
33. Horowitz, H.S., Heifetz, S.B., Meyers, R.J., Driscoll, W., and Korts, D.C. 1977. Evaluation of a combination of self-administered procedures for the control of dental caries in a non-fluoride area. Findings after 2 years. *Caries Res* 11:178–185.
34. Kay, E.J., and Blinkhorn, A.S. 1986. The reasons underlying the extraction of teeth in Scotland. *Br Dent J* 160:287–290.
35. Kleber, C.J., Putt, M.S., and Muhler, J.C. 1981. Duration and pattern of toothbrushing in children using a gel or paste dentifrice. *J Am Dent Assoc* 103:723–726.
36. Koch, G., and Martinsson, T. 1971. Socio-odontological investigation of school children with high and low caries frequency. II. Parents' opinion of dietary habits of their children. *Odontol Revy* 22:55–64.
37. Krasse, B. 1976. Approaches to prevention. In *Microbial Aspects of Dental Caries,* H.M. Stiles, W.J. Loesche, and T.C. O'Brien (eds), Sp. Suppl. Microbiol. Abstr. 3:867–876.
38. Leske, G.S., Ripa, L.W., and Barenie, J.T. 1976. Comparisons of caries prevalence of children with different daily toothbrushing frequencies. *Community Dent Oral Epidemiol* 4:102–105.
39. Ludwig, T.G., Denby, G.C., and Struther, W.H. 1960. Dental health. I. Caries prevalence amongst dentists' children. *N Z Dent J* 56:174–177.
40. MacGregor, I.D.M., and Rugg-Gunn, A.J. 1979. Survey of toothbrushing duration in 85 uninstructed English schoolchildren. *Community Dent Oral Epidemiol* 7:297–298.
41. MacGregor, I.D.M., and Rugg-Gunn, A.J. 1985. Toothbrushing duration in 60 uninstructed young adults. *Community Dent Oral Epidemiol* 13:121–122.
42. MacGregor, I.D.M., Rugg-Gunn, A.J., and Gordon, P.H. 1986. Plaque levels in relation to the number of toothbrushing strokes in uninstructed English schoolchildren. *J Periodont Res* 21:577–582.
43. Mosteller, J.H. 1973. Preventive dentistry. Fads and facts. *J Am Coll Dent* 40:225–235.
44. Newbrun, E. 1977. The safety of water fluoridation. *J Am Dent Assoc* 94:301–304.
45. Newbrun, E. 1980. Achievements of the seventies: community and school fluoridation. *J Public Health Dent* 40:234–247.
46. Nizel, A.E. 1972. Personalized nutritional counseling. *J Dent Child* 39:353–360.
47. Nizel, A.E. 1976. Nutrition for the caries-susceptible patient. In *Clinical Dentistry,* J.W. Clark (ed), vol. 2, Hagerstown, Md.: Harper and Row, pp. 1–12.
48. O'Shea, R.M., and Gray, S.B. 1968. Dental patients' attitudes and behavior concerning prevention. *Public Health Rep* 83:405–410.
49. Ostrom, C.A. 1978. Effectiveness of a preventive dentistry delivery system. *J Am Dent Assoc* 97:29–36.
50. Pengelly, J.P.B., and Smyth, J.F.A. 1972. Incisor caries and primary school tuckshops. *Public Health* 86:183–188.
51. Plasschaert, A.J.M., and König, K.G. 1974. The effect of information and motivation towards dental health, and the fluoride tablets on caries in school children. I. Increment of the initial 2-year experimental period. *Int Dent J* 24:50–65.
52. Poulsen, S., Agerbaek, N., Melsen, B., Korts, D.C., Glavind, L., and Rölla, G. 1976. The effect of professional tooth cleansing on gingivitis and dental caries in children after 1 year. *Community Dent Oral Epidemiol* 4:195–199.
53. Ripa, L., Levinson, A., and Leske, G. 1980. Epidemiological survey of caries-related behavior of caries-free children. *NY State Dent J* 46:78–80.
54. Robinson, H.B. 1946. Toothbrushing habits of 405 persons. *J Am Dent Assoc* 33: 1112–1117.
55. Roder, D.M. 1973. The association between dental caries and the availability of sweets in South Australian school canteens. *Aust Dent J* 18:174–182.
56. Rugg-Gunn, A.J., MacGregor, I.D.M., Edgar, W.M., and Ferguson, M.W. 1979. Toothbrushing behavior in relation to plaque and gingivitis in adolescent schoolchildren. *J Periodont Res* 14:231–238.
57. Silverstein, S., Gold, S., Heilbron, D., Nelms, D., and Wycoff, S. 1977. Effect of supervised deplaquing on dental caries, gingivitis and plaque. *J Dent Res* 56(Sp. Issue A):A85.
58. Sutcliffe, P. 1973. A longitudinal clinical study of oral cleanliness and dental caries in schoolchildren. *Arch Oral Biol* 18:765–770.
59. Torell, P., and Ericsson, Y. 1965. 2-year clinical tests with different methods of local caries-preventive fluorine application in Swedish schoolchildren. *Acta Odontol Scand* 23:287–322.
60. U.S. Department of Health, Education and Welfare. Food and Drug Administration.

1980. Anticaries drug products for over-the-counter human use. Establishment of a monograph; notice of proposed rulemaking. *Federal Register* 45:20666–20691.

61. U.S. Department of Health and Human Services, National Institutes of Health. 1981. The prevalence of dental caries in United States children. 1979–80. NIH Publication No. 82-2245, Bethesda, Maryland.
62. U.S. Department of Health and Human Services, National Institutes of Health. 1983. Challenges for the eighties. N.I.D.R. Long-range research plan. U.S. Government Printing Office, p. 4.
63. Wright, G.Z., Banting, D.W., and Feasby, W.H. 1977. Effect of interdental flossing on the incidence of proximal caries in children. *J Dent Res* 56:574–578.
64. Wright, G.Z., Banting, D.W., and Feasby, W.H. 1979. The Dorchester dental flossing study. Final report. *Clin Prevent Dent* 1:23–26.

Index

A

Accretion 178
Acesulfame-K 139, 161
Acid etching 319
Acids,
  acetic 21
  and caries 16, 17, 18
  organic,
    dissociation constants 23, 24
    in plaque 20, 21, 22, 23
    production in plaque 20, 23, 24
  volatile 22
Actinomyces,
  acid accumulation by 21
  anaerobic 87
  cariogenicity 88
  characteristics 87
  facultative 87
  oral 87
  plaque and 88
Adhesion,
  dental materials 317, 318
  mechanisms 318
  principles 318
Aldoximes 165
Alexidine 224
American Dental Association, Council on Dental Therapeutics 39, 297, 305, 306, 307, 308, 322, 342, 344
Amine hydrofluoride, organic 306
2-Amino-4-nitrophenyl n-propyl ether. *See* 5-Nitro-2-propoxy-aniline.
2-Amino-4-nitrotoluene 139
Ammoniated glycyrrhizin 154
Animal model, caries etiology study 65
Animal, gnotobiotic. *See* Germ-free animal.
Animal studies,
  cariogenic diet 63, 112
  oral actinomyces 87
  pit and fissure caries 65
  Streptococcus mutans host factors 44, 46
p-Anisylurea 138
Antacids, sucrose content 36, 141
Anticholinergic drugs 31, 33, 37, 38
Anxiety 31
Arachnia 21
Arch form 52, 53
Asialia 31
Aspartame 153
L-Aspartyl L-phenyl-alanine methyl ester 139, 153

B

Bacitracin 223
Bacteria,
  aerobic, oral cavity 207
  anaerobic,
    action on plaque 24
    oral cavity 207
  carious lesion and 88
  interactions of 71–73, 74
  opsonization 44
  oral cavity types 206, 207
Bacteriocins 73, 74
Bacteroides melaninogenicus 24
Benzethonium chloride 226
Beverages. *See* Foods.
BIS-GMA 321
Bis-biguanides 224
1-Bromo-5-nitroaniline 139
Buffer, 40
  salivary 40
Buffer capacity test 278

C

Calcium 17, 18
Carbohydrates,
  and caries 103–104
  cariogenicity 115–121
  metabolism 119, 120
  plaque pH and 20
Caries,
  animal model system types 65
  arch form and 52, 53
  bacteria and 88
  carbohydrate and 103–104
  control 357–375
  defined 13
  dental pulp involvement 262
  desalivation effects on 30
  development,
    speed of 246
    time factors 246–248
  diet and, 99–134, 107, 362, 365, 369
    texture relation 101–102
  epidemiological studies 100, 248
  etiology, 29–61
    acids 15
    animal model 65
    bacterial interaction 73
    bacterial role 15, 63–64
    eating frequency 102, 124, 125, 126, 127
    food 14, 16
    lactobacilli 15, 86, 87
    occupational 106
    radiation therapy 246, 247
    Streptococcus mutans 73
    sucrose 15, 115
    theories,
      bacterial 15, 16
      chemical 15
      chemo-parasitic 15, 19, 20
      early 13
      history 13–19
      humors 14
      nutritional deficiency 19
      other 19
      parasitic 15
      phosphate sequestration 19
      proteolytic 16, 25
      proteolytic-chelation 17, 18, 25
      septic 15
      vital 14
      worms 13
  experimental,
    animal 112–115, 116–121
    snack foods in 113, 114
  fluoride relation 54
  formation speed 246, 247
  hereditary fructose intolerance and 104, 105, 106
  histology 249, 250, 251, 252
  histopathology 245–272
  host factors in 29
  host susceptibility 29, 52, 53
  iatrogenic 33
  immunity assessment 45
  immunization and, 51
    by antigens 44
    by *Streptococcus mutans* 44
  Immunoglobulin A and 48
  incidence, desalivation effects 30
  industrial 106
  interventional studies 102–104
  local immunization and 47
  microradiography of 245
  models,
    in vitro 108
    in vivo/in vitro 108
  noninterventional studies 107
  occlusal,
    extension for prevention 316
    impregnation 316
    prevention, historical efforts 315
    prophylactic odontotomy 316
    sealant development 317
    susceptibility 315
  oral flora localization 64
  pit and fissure,
    etiology 72
    microorganisms in 65
    susceptibility 52
  plaque relation to 245
  prediction of 283
  prehistoric times 13
  prevalence, 336, 358
    cumulative 101
    epidemiology 332, 333, 334, 335, 336, 337
    syrup medicine use 142
    water fluoride relation 332, 333, 334, 335, 336, 337
  prevention, 29, 39, 357–375
    combination fluoride therapy 369
    community programs 367–370, 371
    dietary 135, 359, 362, 365
    extension for prevention 316
    fluoridation 333, 334, 335
    fluoride,
      dentifrice 361
      supplements 361
      systemic 361

topical 361
historical efforts 315
host resistance 29, 359
immunization for 44, 51
impregnation 316
in dental office 362–367, 371
in home 359–362, 371
lipids and 122
microorganism decrease 29
nonadhesive materials 317
occlusal 315
of microbial agent 359
phosphate salts and 19
phosphates and 121
pit and fissure eradication 316
prophylactic odontotomy 316
sealants for 325
strategies for 359
substrate modification 29
time factors 29
trace elements and 123
probability curves 247
proximal 253
radiation induced 33, 246
rampant 31, 32, 36, 37, 141, 350
rate variation 100, 102, 103
recurrent, fluoride therapy 350
reduction by fluoridation 334, 335, 336, 337
root surface,
characteristics 67
dental management 68
described 67, 265
etiology,
bacterial interaction 72, 73
radiation therapy 68
microorganisms in 65, 68
prevalence,
age relation 69
ancient man 68
contemporary populations 68, 69
geriatric patients 68
primitive societies 68
progression 67
pulp involvement 68, 69
sequelae 68, 69
saliva composition and 39, 40
sealed in tooth 325
smooth surface, 254, 255
etiology, carbohydrates 116
microorganisms in 65
special populations and 101–102, 103–104, 104–107
Streptococcus interactions and 73
sucrose and 100, 101, 102
therapy, fumigation 14
tooth composition and 53, 54
vaccine against 50, 51
Caries activity tests, 273–293
cariogenic factor relation 285, 286
cariogenic substrate relation 287, 288
characteristics 285
host resistance relation 288
uses 275
value in disease control 289
Carious process, diagrammed 29
Cementum, caries 265, 266, 267
Cetylamine hydrofluoride 345, 347
Cetylpyridinium chloride 226
Chelate,
defined 17
structure 18
Chelating agent 17
Chewing gum 111, 113, 122, 125, 141, 149, 150, 162
Chewing sticks 219, 230
Chlorhexidine 224
Chloroform,
dentifrice 302
relative sweetness 138
Chlorogenic acid 158
6-Chlorosaccharin 139
Citrate 17, 18
Cloning, genes 51
Coating 178
Contour lines of Owen 261
Corn syrup, high-fructose,
relative sweetness 151
utilization, US 144, 151
Cuticle,
defined 178
primary enamel 178
Cyclamate, 147, 159, 162
carcinogenicity 164
consumption 162
dentifrice 302
metabolism 163
relative sweetness 162
toxicity 162
Cyclohexylsulfamate. *See* Cyclamate.
Cynarin 158

D

Def rate 103, 125
DFI rate, fluoridation relation 333, 334
DMF rate,

dietary control and 103
fluoridation relation 333, 334
sucrose relation 102, 103
DMFS score 105, 106
DMFT score 50, 103, 106, 126
Decalcification 18, 19, 53
Demineralization. *See* Decalcification.
Dental arch form 52
Dental calculus 185
Dental cavity preparation 316
Dental deposits, 177–243
in history 177
terminology 178
Dental disease, plaque relation 218
Dental floss 232
Dental materials, retention 317, 318
Dental pulp, caries effect on 262
Dental tape 232
Dental visits 362–363
Dentifrices, 295–313
abrasives in 296, 343, 345
abrasivity of 296, 297, 298, 343
ammonia 305
antibiotic 305
anticalculus claims 308
antiplaque claims 308
binders 299
chemotherapeutic 305
chlorophyll 305
claims for 306, 308, 309
coloring agents 302
composition 296–302, 296
contact sensitivity 304
cosmetic 295, 308
cost 309, 310
desensitizing 306–307
flavoring 162, 301
fluoride, 303, 306, 343, 345, 346, 347
concentration 226, 344
dose-response 344, 346
history 344
safety 344
fluoride-abrasive 345
functions 295
humectants 299
ingestion 303
irritation by 304
natural 308
organic 308
packaging, 302–303
pumps 303
shelf life 302
tubes 303
preservatives 302
shelf life 302
surface-active detergents 300, 301
sweetening agents 302
therapeutic 299, 304–305
titanium dioxide in 304
urea 305
xylitol 150
Dentin,
caries,
bacterial invasion 261
classification 263, 264
coronal 258–265
crystal deposition 264
deep dentinal 65, 66
filamentous organisms in 75
odontoblast process changes 264
recalcification 264
root, 265, 266, 267, 268, 269
advanced 268
microbiology 68
zones of 260
clefts 261, 262
dead tracts in 262, 263
lactobacilli of 86
macroscopic changes 258
microscopic changes 260, 261, 262, 263, 264
tubule,
caries 269
cleavage 261, 262
dilation 261
"liquifaction foci" 261
morphological changes 264
ultrastructural changes 265
Deposit 178
Depression 31, 33
Desalivation, effect on caries 30, 31
Dewar test 279
Dextranase 227, 228
Diabetes mellitus 31, 148
Diet,
abnormal habits 113
and caries 99–134, 135, 362, 365, 367, 369
carbohydrates and caries 103–104
changes in 126, 127, 362, 365, 367, 369
counselling 365
defined 99
diary 367
epidemiological studies 100, 102
evaluation chart 367
history, value of 99
plaque relation 190
texture effect on caries 101–102
Diethanol aminopropyl-N- 344, 347

ethanol octyldecylamine-
dihydrofluoride
Dihydrochalcones 156, 157
Disclosing agents 230
Domiphen bromide 226
Drugs, xerostomia-inducing 32, 33, 34, 37, 38
Dulcin 139, 159, 165
Dulcitol 138

E

Eating, frequency 102, 124, 125, 126, 127
Embden-Meyerhof pathway 104, 105, 120
Enamel,
acid attack on 15, 16
acid etching 319
acquired pellicle 180
caries, 248–258, 255, 256, 257, 258, 259
composition 53, 54
macroscopic changes 248
prevalence, ancient man 68
zones of 250, 253
chemical composition 16
composition 53
conditioning 319
cuticle 178
decalcification 18, 19, 54, 252
epithelium 179
fluoride uptake 340, 347
focal hole 252, 354
integument,
of embryonic origin 179
of posteruptive origin 179
terminology 179
macroscopic changes 248
microdefects 53, 54
microscopic changes 250–255
mottled 333, 334
perikymata 248, 249, 254
photodensity 252, 255
plaque relation 245
polishing 182, 183
posteruptive "maturation" 54
primary cuticle 178
prism structure 249, 252, 256
pretreatment for retention 319
retention 318
surface defects 53, 54, 184, 185
surface lesions 250, 251, 252, 253, 254
surface minerals 53
ultrastructural changes 255
white spot lesion 53, 54
Enzymes, proteolytic 16
Epithelium, enamel 179
Erythromycin 223
p-Ethoxyphenylurea. *See* Dulcin.
Ethylene glycol 138

F

Fermentation,
bacterial 20, 21, 22, 23, 24
heterolactic 20, 21
homolactic 20, 21
"First Law of Oral Biology" 200
Fissures. *See* Pits and fissures.
Flora,
cariogenic,
oral localization 64, 65, 71
specificity of 64, 65, 70
transmissibility 70, 71
types 65
oral,
localization 64
pit and fissure 66
pit and fissure lesions from 72
Flossing 232, 360
Fluoridation,
caries reduction 332, 333, 334, 335, 336, 337, 368
cost of 368
discontinuance 336
epidemiological surveys 368
opponents 337
safety of 337, 368
water supply, 332, 333, 334, 335, 336, 337, 368
school 337
Fluoride,
acidulated phosphate (APF) 226, 340, 347, 364
amine 344, 345, 347
anticaries mechanism 331, 332
application procedures 342, 343, 344
caries relation 54
cetylamine hydrofluoride 345, 347
concentration 331
conditions of use 331
dentifrices 226, 303, 343, 345, 346, 347, 361
diethanol aminopropyl-N-ethanol octadecylamine-dihydrofluoride 344

difluorosilane 341
effectiveness 331
enamel uptake 340, 342, 347
gel 340, 341, 342, 365
guide to agents 349
in human milk 339
ingestion, dentifrices 303
mechanism of action 331, 332
mouthwashes 226, 343, 347, 369
organic amine 227
patient needs 349
preventive dentistry and 331–355
prophylaxis paste 363
safety of 337, 341
sodium 306, 341, 343, 344, 345, 346, 349, 361, 364
sodium monofluorophosphate (MFP) 306,344, 345, 346, 361, 364
stannous 306, 340, 342, 343, 345, 347, 364
supplements, 338, 361
community programs 369
dosage 338, 339
prenatal 339
sample prescription 339
systemic 332–340, 350, 361
therapy, 39, 361, 364
immunization as adjuvant 52
multiple 336, 363
toxicology 348
uptake-time relation 342
water supplies, 332, 333, 334, 335, 336, 337
caries relation 333, 334, 335
discontinuance 336
optimal 333
school 337
survey 333
Fluoride, topical, 332, 340–347, 361, 364
acidulated phosphate fluoride 340, 347
amine fluoride 347
ammonium fluoride 347
caries reduction by 336, 337, 338, 346
concentration range 226
gel 341, 342
ingestion minimization 341, 342
professional application 340, 347, 350, 364
safety of 341, 342
self-applied 342, 350, 361
sodium fluoride 347
stannous fluoride 347
titanium tetrafluoride 347
varnish 341, 347
Fluorine, occurrence 331
Fluorosis 333, 334
Foods,
adhesiveness 102, 103, 109
advertising 135
algae 145
beverages,
carbonated 111
"diet" 159
biscuits (cookies) 111, 152, 370
bread 16, 102, 103, 105, 110, 127, 154, 157
cake 109, 154
candy 111, 149, 152
caramel 101, 109, 111, 127
cariogenic potential 107–112
cereal, breakfast 111, 114
cereals 103, 105, 109, 110, 111, 114, 150
chocolate 102, 109, 111, 127, 149, 152
clearance 109
coffee 110
cookies 111, 152, 370
corn chips 113
corn flakes 109
dairy products 103, 105, 109, 110, 111, 112, 113, 114, 126, 154
dates 109
debris 180
dessert 126
dietetic 150, 149
doughnuts 370
dried liver substance 112
dry products 162
eggs 110
fish 149
fructose content 112
fruit 103, 105, 109, 110, 111, 112, 126, 128, 135, 145, 148, 156, 157, 158
fruit drink 111
fruit juice 111
glucose content 112
honey 135
ice cream 111, 149
iced buns (pastries) 370
jam 152
jelly 152
junk 370
labeling 110
meat 16
meringue 111
milk 105, 109, 113
molasses 103

noodles 105
nuts 103, 110, 113, 148
oats 103, 105
potatoes 103
rice 103, 105
"safe for teeth" 110, 147
seaweed 145
semolina 105
serving changes 126
snack 113, 114, 126, 149, 370
soft drinks 126, 370
soya beans 103
spaghetti 105
sucrose content 109, 111, 112, 113, 114, 127
sugar 15, 16, 99–136, 110, 115
sugar beet 142
sugar cane 106
sugar-coated flakes 109
sugar-containing, "rich in energy" 135
sweets 105, 109, 111, 113, 122, 126, 145, 148, 149, 152, 154, 162, 370
toffee 101, 109, 127
treacle 103
vegetables 103, 105, 109, 111, 113, 148, 150, 154, 158
wheat germ 103
wine 157
Fosdick calcium dissolution test 278
Free energy of hydrolysis 118
Fructose, 20
food content 112
plaque pH and 150
relative sweetness 138, 151
Fructosyltransferase 116, 119
Fusobacterium nucleatum 24

G

GALT. *See* Peyer's patches.
Galactose,
plaque pH and 146
relative sweetness 138
Genetic bioengineering 51
Germ-free animal,
caries studies 25, 44, 46, 63, 70, 87
defined 64
Gingival index, syrup medicine use 142
D-Glucitol. *See* Sorbitol.
Glucose,
food content 112
metabolism 21, 22, 23
plaque pH and 20, 148
relative sweetness 138, 151
Glucosyl donors 118
Glucosylsucrose 152
Glucosyltransferase 44, 51, 116, 119
Glycerol 138
Glycine 138
Glycyrrhizin 138
Gnotobiotic animal. *See* Germ-free animal.

H

Heart muscle 50, 51
Hereditary fructose intolerance, 104–106
and caries 104, 105, 106
enzyme defect 105
oral hygiene in 106
plaque microbiota 106
Hexose sugars,
glycolytic bacterial fermentation 20, 22, 23
metabolism 20, 22, 23
n-Hexylchloromalonamide 139
Hexylresorcinol 226
High-fructose corn syrup (HFCS) 151
Hopewood House study 103–104, 107
Host factors, 29
animal studies 44
dental arch form 52
immune mechanisms 44
immunization 44–52
saliva, 30–44, 288
desalivation effects 30
terminology 30
tooth, 52–54, 288
composition 53
morphology 52
Hydroxyapatite 256, 259
3-Hydroxy-2-methyl-4-pyrone. *See* Maltol.

I

Immune system,
antigen study 45
cellular factors 44, 45
humoral factors 44, 45

Immunity,
  local 46, 47
  passive 50
Immunization,
  animal studies 44, 45, 46, 47
  as fluoride adjuvant 52
  host factors 44–52
  human studies 48
  immune mechanisms 44
  in perspective 51
  oral 46, 47
  salivary agglutinin titer effect 47
Immunoglobulins, in saliva 43, 44
Immunoglobulin A,
  agglutinating activity 43, 51
  and caries prevalence 48, 49
  deficiency 49
  in saliva 43
  secretory 45, 48
  stimulation 45, 46, 47
  structure 43
Immunoglobulin G,
  agglutinating activity 43
  in saliva 43
Immunoglobulins, salivary 43, 44, 48
Integument,
  defined 178
  enamel 179
Intraoral caries test (ICT) 108
Iodine permeability test (IPT) 108

J

Juvenile periodontitis 208

K

Kanamycin 223

L

Lactate 17, 18, 23
Lactobacilli,
  acid accumulation by 21
  bacterial interactions 72
  cariogenicity 86
  characteristics 86
  dentin 86
  described 86
  heterobacilli 86
  homofermentative 86
  oral 86–87
Lactobacillus colony count 274–275
Lactose 20, 118, 138
Ligand 17
Lipids 122
Lipoteichoic acid 50
Lycasin 147
Lysozyme 42

M

Maltol 154
Maltose 118, 138
Mannitol 138
Materia alba 180
Medicinals,
  saccharin in 160
  sugar-based 111, 141, 142, 149, 162
  xylitol in 150
5-Methylsaccharin 139
Metronidazole 227
Microflora, 63–97
  See also Flora, oral.
Microorganisms, oral,
  adsorption variations 85
  agglutination variations 85
  salivary factor regulation 42, 43
Microradiography 245
Mikulicz's disease 31
Miraculin 157
Monellin 139, 157
Mouth, microorganisms 44
Mouthrinses. *See* Mouthwashes.
Mouthwashes,
  community programs 369
  dextranase 227, 228
  flavoring 160, 162
  fluoride, 342, 347, 364
    concentration 226
Myocarditis 50

N

beta-Naphthol 226
Naringin dihydrochalcone 139, 156
Neisseria, 23
  acid accumulation by 21
Neohesperidin dihydrochalcone 139, 156
Niddamycin 223
5-Nitro-2-ethoxyaniline 139

5-Nitro-2-methoxyaniline 139
5-Nitro-2-propoxyaniline 139, 159, 166
p-Nitrosuccinanilide 139
Nutrition 99

O

Oligosialia 31
Oral cavity, bacteria in 206, 207
Oral hygiene, 359, 364, 366
  instruction 364
Oral prophylaxis,
  effectiveness 364

P

P-4000. *See* 5-Nitropropoxyaniline.
Palatinose 138
Parasympatholytic drugs 31, 33
Parkinson's disease 31, 32, 33
Pellicle,
  acquired, 180, 181–188, 211, 212
    bacterial colonization 189
    composition 185, 186, 187
    conversion to plaque 185, 192
    formation 181, 212
    functions 187
    histology 185, 186, 187, 188
    schematic diagram 212
  defined 178
Penicillin 223
Peptostreptococci, 24
  acid accumulation by 21
Perikymata 248, 249, 254
Perilla sugar. *See* Pellartine.
l-Perillaldehyde alpha-anti-aldoxime 139, 159
Pellartine 139, 165
Periodontal diseases,
  etiology 210
  microbiology 197, 203, 209, 210
Periodontitis 208
Periodontosis. *See* Juvenile periodontitis.
Peroxidase system, in saliva 42
Peyer's patches 46, 47
Pharmaceutical products, 111, 141,
  sugar-based 142, 149, 162
p-Phenetolcarbamide 4-ethoxyphenylurea. *See* Dulcin.
Phenol 226
Phyllodulcin 139
Pits and fissures,
  "artificial" 66
  caries susceptibility 52
  cross section diagram 67
  eradication 316
  flora 66
  morphology 248, 249, 250, 251, 254
  nonadhesive dental materials for 317
  plaque in 199, 203
  prophylactic odontotomy 316
  sealant development 317
Plaque,
  Actinomyces in 21, 88
  ammonia release from 24
  anaerobic bacterial action 24
  autogenic succession 212
  body of 192
  "bristle brush" 198
  carbohydrate pathways 117, 118, 119
  carbohydrates 215
  caries relation 245
  cellular factors in 44, 45
  characteristics 189
  composition,
    chemical 214–217
    inorganic 216
    microbial 32, 116, 206, 207, 215
    pathogenic 217, 218
  condensed microbial layer 192, 193, 195
  "corncob" 192, 193, 194, 198, 199
  defined 178, 180
  detection 230
  development 209–214
  diet relation 189
  enamel relation 245
  environmental relation 198
  enzymes 114, 115
  fissure 199, 203
  flora,
    distribution 209
    variations in 197, 198, 201
  formation, 209–214, 213
    from acquired pellicle 182, 211, 212
  fractionation 215
  general features 189
  glucans 114
  growth 74, 189, 191
  histology 190, 193, 195, 196, 197, 198
  humoral factors 44, 45

hypotheses 218
inorganic components 216
interface with tooth 192, 194, 195, 196, 197
levans 116
microbiology, 21, 83, 200–214, 200, 201, 202
culture preparation 204, 205, 206
culture problems 75
dispersion 203, 205
hereditary fructose intolerance 106
isolation procedures 204, 205, 206
sampling procedures 201
study methods 200, 201
microorganism,
identification 205
quantitation 205, 206
morphology 189–199
organic acids in 20, 21, 23, 24
oxidation-reduction potential 212, 213
pH, 19, 20, 21, 23, 24, 41, 42
diet relation 21, 108, 109, 110
measurement 109, 110
sweetening agent relation 146, 149
pathogenic potential, 217, 218
constituents 217
polysaccharides 116, 117, 118, 215
prevention, dietary 190
proteins 216
remodelling phase 212
sampling procedures 201
smooth surface, 191
bacterial progression 73
bacteriology 73–75
filamentous organisms 73, 75
subgingival 194, 208
supragingival, 189, 190, 208, 213
chemical composition 214
"corncob" 198
microbial composition 213
smooth surface 191
surface of 192
"test-tube brush" 198
Plaque control, 219–232
antibacterial 226
antibiotic, 221, 222, 223
bis-biguanide 224
antimicrobial 221, 222
bacterial attachment 227, 228, 229
chemotherapeutic agents 221
dextranase 227, 228
disclosing agents 230
drug therapy, 220
problems of 220
substantivity 220
glucan hydrolases 227, 238
mechanical, 229–232
cultural aspects 229
dental tape 232
floss 232
history 229
plaque detection 230
toothbrushing 231
methods 219–232
perspectives 219
problems 219–221
prospects 219
Plaque index, syrup medicine use 142
Polymyxin B 223
Polysaccharides,
free energy of hydrolysis 118, 119
plaque 116, 117, 119, 121
Preventive dentistry,
community programs 366–370
dental office programs 363
fluorides in 331–355, 368
in dental office 362–366
in home 359–362
Prophylaxis paste, fluoride 364
Propionibacteria, acid accumulation by 21
1-Propoxy-2-amino-4-nitrobenzene. *See* 5-Nitro-2-propoxyaniline.

R

Radiation effects 31, 32, 33, 68, 246, 304, 342
Raffinose 118, 138
Reductase test 277
Rhamnose 138

S

Saccharin, 159–161
cariogenicity 164
dental aspects 161
in dentifrices 302
metabolism 160
powdered forms 160
sodium 139

toxicity 160
Saliva,
and caries 39, 40
antibacterial factors 42
artificial 38, 39
buffers 40, 41
composition 38, 39
"critical pH" 41
defined 30
desalivation,
and caries 30, 31, 32
drug-inducing 32, 38, 39
host factors 30–44, 288
immunoglobulins 43, 49
lactobacilli-caries relation 86
lysozyme in 42
peroxidase system 42
proteins as buffer 41
Streptococcus mutans, 84
antigens 48
submandibular, bacterial binding by 85
Salivary agglutinin titer 47
Salivary gland,
abnormalities 31
infection 31
neoplasms 31, 32
removal effects 30
secretions, 40
antibacterial 42
immunoglobulins 43, 48
lysozyme 42
peroxidase-thiocyanate 42
Salivary peroxidase system 42
Sarcoidosis 31
Sealants, occlusal, 315–330, 364, 365
acceptance 327
adhesion principles 318
application technique 324
BIS-GMA 321, 322, 323
clinical effectiveness 324
clinical use factors 324, 326
cyanoacrylate 320
development 317–320
glass ionomer cement 323
indications for use 326
loss of 325
materials for 320–323
polyurethane 321
public health use 326
requirements for 317
retention-tooth relation 325
sodium fluoride varnish 323
tooth preparation 323
use techniques 323
"Serendipity berries" 157
Serum antibodies,
age dependence 49
caries relation 49, 50
stimulation 45, 46
titer-age relation 49
Sharpey's fibers 268
Sjogren's syndrome 31
Snyder test 276
Sodium cyclohexylsulfamate. *See* Cyclamate.
Sodium 3-methylcyclopentyl-sulfamate 138
Sorbitol, 20, 138, 145–148
bacterial adaptation 148
cariogenicity 147
dental aspects 146
fermentation 146
in dentifrices 299
plaque pH and 146, 150
relative sweetness 146
Sordes 180
Staphylococcus aureus 16
Staphylococcus pyogenes 17
Starch, 20
hydrolyzate 147, 150
Stevioside 139, 155
Stickland reaction 24
Stomatitis sicca 31
Streptococci,
acid accumulation by 21
antibody control of 44
described 75
glucose metabolism 21, 22, 23
group interactions 71–73
oral 75–86
Streptococcus faecalis 46
Streptococcus milleri 85
Streptococcus mitior 85
Streptococcus mitis 21
Streptococcus mutans,
acid accumulation by 21
adherence to tooth 83, 121
agglutination 121
antibody activity 48, 49
antibody levels 47, 49, 50
antigens 50, 82
bacterial interactions 72, 73
bacteriocin production 74
cariogenic strains 79
cariogenicity 21, 80
cell wall,
biochemical composition 81
diagram 83
characteristics 76, 83
colony morphology 76, 77
colony variants 77
culturing 76, 77

differences 78
ecology 82
glucose metabolism 21, 22, 23
immunization by 44
in subacute bacterial endocarditis 84
intragroup differences 78, 79, 81
opsonization 48
oral implantation of 70
pandemicity 83
phagocytosis 48
plaque level 83
properties 76, 77
saliva concentration 84
salivary antigens 48
serological classification 79–81
serum antibodies 49, 50
Streptococcus mutans 279–283
screening tests,
adherence 281
dip-slide 281
plaque/toothpick 279
saliva/tongue blade 280
replicate 282
Streptococcus "mutans-like" 79
Streptococcus oralis 85
Streptococcus s.b.e. See Streptococcus sanguis.
Streptococcus salivarius,
carcinogenicity 84
colony morphology 84
Streptococcus sanguis,
acid accumulation by 21
bacterial interactions 72
cariogenicity 75
chemical composition 214
colony morphology 75
serum antibodies 49
Stress, mental 31
Striae of Retzius 248, 251, 252
Subacute bacterial endocarditis 75, 84
Sucrol. *See* Dulcin.
Sucrose,
antacid content of 36
caries relation 115
cariogenicity 115–121
chemical structure 118
consumption, 162
and DMF rate 102
form 102, 127
rate 100, 102, 123, 126
timing 102
world 143–145
food content 111, 112, 113, 114
history 135, 140–142
manufacture 142
medicinals, content 111, 141, 142
plaque pH and 20
relative sweetness 138, 152, 153, 154, 155, 159, 161, 162, 165, 166
snack food-caries relation 113, 114
solutions of 102
sources 140, 142
Sugar, 135–175
and food adhesiveness 109
cane 106, 140, 141, 142
coupling 152
hexose 20, 22
invert 138
replacement possibilities 370
substitutes 135–175
See also specific material.
o-Sulfobenzimide. *See* Saccharin.
Suosan 139, 159
Sweetening agents,
aldoximes 165
consumer acceptance 166
noncaloric 135–175, 159–166
plaque pH and 20, 146
price comparisons 151
problems in use 167
relative sweetness 138, 139, 166
taste 136–140
utilization, US 143, 144
See also individual materials.
Sweetness, theories of, 136
bifunctional molecular 136, 137
complex formation 136, 137
hydrogen and hydrophobic bonding 136
sweet-sensitive protein 136, 137

T

Talin 139
Taste,
basic modalities 136
receptor response 137
sweetening agents and 136–140
theories,
bifunctional molecular 136, 137
complex formation 136, 137
hydrogen and hydrophobic bonding 136
Tetracycline 223
Thaumatin 139, 157
Tomes process 254

Tooth,
  caries susceptibility, 52, 53
    intraoral variation 52
  composition 53
  discoloration 32
  extraction, reasons for 358
  host factors 52–54, 288
  morphology 52
  preparation for sealant 323
  surface change and integument 229
  "surface membrane" 15
Tooth sponges 230
Toothbrushes, history 229, 230
Toothbrushing, 229, 231
  effectiveness 359, 360
  time 361
Toothpicks 219, 229, 230
Trace elements 121, 122
Tranquilizers 32
Treponema 24

U

Ultrasüss. *See* 5-Nitro-2-propoxy-aniline.

V

Vaccine, caries preventive 50, 51
Valzin. *See* Dulcin.
Vancomycin 223
Veillonella 21, 23
Vesiculoerosive disease 304
Vipeholm study 101–102, 104, 107, 123, 126, 127

W

World Health Organization Global Oral Epidemiology Bank 102

X

Xerostomia,
  caries prevention and 39, 342, 350
  DMF rate in 37, 39
  defined 31
  drugs-inducing 32
  etiology, 31
    medications 31, 32, 33, 34, 36
    radiation effects 31, 32, 33, 342
  management, 39
    physiological 39
Xylitol, 148–150
  cariogenicity 149
  plaque pH and 149, 150
  relative sweetness 138, 148
D-Xylose 138